Get ahead!
specialties
250 SBAs for Finals

Second edition

Get ahead!

specialties

250 SBAs for Finals

Second edition

Fiona Bach MBChB, MRCOG, BSc
Speciality Registrar in Obstetrics and Gynaecology, London, UK

Elizabeth Waddington BSc, MBChB, MSc, MRCP
Consultant Paediatrician, Mid Yorkshire Hospitals NHS Trust, UK

Peter Cartledge BSc MBChB MRCPCH PCME MSc
Leeds Children's Hospital, Leeds, UK

Mahesh Jayaram MB BS, DPM, MMedSci, MRCPsych, FRANZCP
Senior Lecturer, Department of Psychiatry,
University of Melbourne, Australia

Hannah Roberts MBBS, MRCGP, DFSRH
Salaried General Practitioner, North East Essex, UK

Series Editor

Saran Shantikumar BA, BSc, MBChB, MRCS
Academic Clinical Fellow in Public Health,
University of Warwick, UK

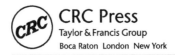

CRC Press
Taylor & Francis Group
Boca Raton London New York

CRC Press is an imprint of the
Taylor & Francis Group, an **informa** business

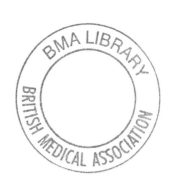

CRC Press
Taylor & Francis Group
6000 Broken Sound Parkway NW, Suite 300
Boca Raton, FL 33487-2742

© 2016 by Taylor & Francis Group, LLC
CRC Press is an imprint of Taylor & Francis Group, an Informa business

No claim to original U.S. Government works

Printed on acid-free paper
Version Date: 20150721
Printed by CPI Group (UK) Ltd, Croydon CR0 4YY

International Standard Book Number-13: 978-1-4822-5318-4 (Paperback)

Library of Congress Cataloging-in-Publication Data

Bach, Fiona, author.
    Specialties : 250 SBAs for finals / Fiona Bach, Elizabeth Waddington, Peter Cartledge, Mahesh Jayaram, Hannah Roberts. -- Second edition.
        p. ; cm. -- (Get ahead!)
    Includes bibliographical references and index.
    ISBN 978-1-4822-5318-4 (pbk. : alk. paper)
    I. Waddington, Elizabeth, author. II. Cartledge, Peter, author. III. Jayaram, Mahesh, author. IV. Roberts, Hannah, 1983- , author. V. Title. VI. Series: Get ahead! (CRC Press)
    [DNLM: 1. Pregnancy Complications--Great Britain--Examination Questions. 2. Genital Diseases, Female--Great Britain--Examination Questions. 3. Mental Disorders--Great Britain--Examination Questions. 4. Pediatrics--methods--Great Britain--Examination Questions. WQ 18.2]
    RG111
    618.076--dc23   2015027402

Visit the Taylor & Francis Web site at
http://www.taylorandfrancis.com

and the CRC Press Web site at
http://www.crcpress.com

Contents

Preface   vii
Introduction   ix

Practice Paper 1: Questions   1

Practice Paper 1: Answers   19

Practice Paper 2: Questions   67

Practice Paper 2: Answers   85

Practice Paper 3: Questions   121

Practice Paper 3: Answers   141

Practice Paper 4: Questions   185

Practice Paper 4: Answers   205

Practice Paper 5: Questions   247

Practice Paper 5: Answers   263

Preface

Welcome to *Get ahead! Specialties*. This book contains 250 Single Best Answer questions (SBAs) covering various topics within obstetrics, gynaecology, paediatrics and psychiatry. These are arranged as five practice papers, each containing 50 questions. Allow yourself 60 to 90 minutes for each paper. You can either work through the practice papers systematically or dip in and out of the book using the SBA index as a guide to where questions on a specific topic can be found. We have tried to include all the main conditions about which you can be expected to know, as well as some more detailed knowledge suitable for candidates aiming towards distinction. As in the real exam, these papers have no preset pass mark. Whether you pass or fail depends on the distribution of scores across the whole year group, but around 60% should be sufficient.

We hope this book fulfils its aim of being a useful, informative revision aid. If you have any feedback or suggestions, please let us know (RevisionForMedicalFinals@gmail.com).

Fiona Bach
Elizabeth Waddington
Peter Cartledge
Mahesh Jayaram
Hannah Roberts

Introduction

Single Best Answer questions (SBAs) are becoming more popular as a method of assessment in summative medical school examinations. Each clinical vignette is followed by a list of five possible answers, of which only one is correct. SBAs have the advantage of testing candidates' knowledge of clinical scenarios rather than their ability at detailed factual recall. However they do not always parallel real-life situations and are no comparison to clinical decision making. Either way the SBA is here to stay.

The *Get ahead!* series is aimed primarily at undergraduate finalists. Much like the real exam, we have endeavoured to include commonly asked questions as well as a generous proportion of harder stems, appropriate for the more ambitious student aiming for honours. The Medical Schools Council Assessment Alliance (MSCAA) is a partnership of UK medical schools aiming to improve undergraduate assessment. The MSCAA has been compiling a bank of SBAs and extended matching questions (EMQs) to be used in summative examinations. The questions in the *Get ahead!* series are written to follow the 'house style' of the MSCAA SBAs, and thus are of a similar format to what many of you can expect in your exams. All the questions in the *Get ahead!* series are accompanied by explanatory answers including a succinct summary of the key features of each condition. Even when you answer a question correctly, I strongly suggest you read these summaries. I guarantee you'll learn something. For added interest, we have included details of eponymous persons ('eponymous' from Greek *epi* = upon + *onyma* = name; 'giving name') and, as you have just seen, some derivations of words from the original Latin or Greek.

HOW TO PASS YOUR EXAMS

The clinical scenarios given in SBAs are intended to be based on 'house officer knowledge'. Sadly this is not always the case, and you shouldn't be surprised when you get a question concerning the underlying histology of testicular tumours (as I was). Start revising early and don't restrict yourself to the given syllabus if you can avoid doing so. If your exam is only two weeks away, then CRAM, CRAM, CRAM – you'll be surprised at how much you can learn in a fortnight.

During the exam ...

1. Try to answer the questions first, without looking at the responses – the questions are written such that this should be possible.
2. Take your time to read the questions fully. There are no bonus marks available for finishing the paper early.
3. If you get stuck on a question, then make sure you mark down your best guess before you move on. You may not have time to come back to it at the end.
4. Answer all the questions – there is no negative marking. If you are unsure, go with your instinct, it's probably going to be your best guess.
5. Never think that the examiner is trying to catch you out. Red herrings are not allowed so don't assume there is one. If a question looks easy, it probably is!

Although this may be obvious, there is no substitute for learning the material thoroughly and practicing as many questions as you can. With this book, you're off to a good start!

A final word ...

The *Get ahead!* series is written by doctors who have recently finished their finals and/or who have experience teaching and examining students. As such, I hope the books cover information that is valuable and relevant to you as undergraduates who are about to sit finals.

I wish you the best of luck in your exams!

Saran Shantikumar
Series Editor, *Get ahead!*

Practice Paper 1: Questions

1. BLEEDING IN PREGNANCY (1)

A 26-year-old multigravid woman is in spontaneous labour at 41 weeks. She has no antenatal risk factors with normal ultrasound scans. On examination, the head is two-fifths palpable per abdomen. She has a spontaneous rupture of membranes at 3 cm with heavily blood-stained liquor. The cardiotocograph (CTG) shows significant abnormalities. The midwife performs a vaginal examination and there is no cord protruding through the cervix, which is now 4 cm dilated. The mother feels no pain.

What is the most likely diagnosis?

A. Bloody show
B. Placental abruption
C. Placenta praevia
D. Uterine rupture
E. Vasa praevia

2. CAESAREAN SECTION (1)

Which of the following conditions is a medical indication for routine delivery by caesarean section?

A. Hepatitis C virus
B. Preterm labour
C. Previous lower segment caesarean section
D. Twin pregnancy with first twin breech and second twin cephalic
E. Twin pregnancy with first twin cephalic and second twin breech

3. VAGINAL DISCHARGE (1)

A 25-year-old woman attends the genitourinary medicine (GUM) clinic complaining of increased vaginal discharge that has an unpleasant odour. She says sexual intercourse with her partner is uncomfortable. A swab is taken and sent to the lab. On direct microscopy, a flagellated protozoan is seen.

Which is the most likely pathogen?

A. *Candida albicans*
B. *Chlamydia trachomatis*
C. *Gardnerella vaginalis*
D. *Neisseria gonorrhoeae*
E. *Trichomonas vaginalis*

4. MANAGEMENT OF INCONTINENCE (1)

A 57-year-old woman presents with a history of having to run to the toilet to pass urine and occasionally not getting there in time. She needs to wear pads every day and this is having a negative impact on her life. She also complains of waking up two or three times per night to pass urine. She has had two children by normal delivery and has never had any surgery on her bladder. She says she has been doing occasional pelvic floor exercises with little success.

Considering her diagnosis, what is the first-line treatment?

A. Bladder training
B. Botulinum toxin
C. Oxybutynin
D. Pelvic floor exercises with a trained physiotherapist
E. Tolteridone

5. CARDIOTOCOGRAPHY (1)

You are looking at a CTG of a woman of 39 weeks' gestation who has come to the antenatal day unit as she has had reduced fetal movements. There is a baseline rate of 170 with four accelerations in a 20-minute section. The variability is more than 10 beats. There are no decelerations.

What could explain the features of this trace?

A. Maternal pyrexia
B. Normal trace
C. Pre-terminal trace
D. Sleep pattern of fetus
E. Thumb sucking of fetus

6. FETAL POSITION (1)

You are examining a woman in established labour with the midwife, and she asks you to tell her how you would describe the examination. You explain that the cervix is fully dilated. Anteriorly, you feel a diamond-shaped fontanelle and, if you follow a line posteriorly, you then feel a Y-shaped depression in the skull bones.

How is the position best described?

A. Brow
B. Left occipitotransverse
C. Occipitoanterior
D. Occipitoposterior
E. Right occipitotransverse

7. GENITAL TRACT

In which anatomical location does fertilization normally occur?

A. Ampulla of fallopian tube
B. Cervix
C. Fimbriae of fallopian tube
D. Infundibulum of fallopian tube
E. Uterus

8. INDUCTION OF LABOUR (1)

A 21-year-old woman at 40 weeks + 12 days is being induced. She has received two doses of prostaglandins after examination revealed a low Bishop score. She is experiencing mild contractions with good fetal movements. Her CTG trace is normal. She is frustrated and tired and is becoming angry with the midwives as she thought she would have delivered sooner. On abdominal palpation, there is cephalic presentation with two-fifths palpable. On vaginal examination, 6 hours after the second dose of prostaglandin, she is 3 cm dilated with a partially effaced cervix.

What would be the next course of action?

A. Artificial rupture of membranes
B. Caesarean section
C. Further prostaglandin
D. Observation alone
E. Oxytocin

9. FETAL ULTRASOUND (1)

Which measurement is the most reliable indicator of gestational age in the first trimester?

A. Biophysical profile
B. Biparietal diameter
C. Crown–rump length
D. Femur length
E. Nuchal translucency

10. MANAGEMENT OF SMEAR RESULTS (1)

A 32-year-old woman has had a smear test, and the lab has found low-grade dyskaryosis with a negative HPV test. She has never previously had an abnormal smear.

What would be the next stage in her management?

A. Colposcopy
B. Recall in 6 months
C. Recall in 1 year
D. Recall in 3 years
E. Repeat the test today

11. OVARIAN CANCER (1)

Which one of the following factors increases one's risk of developing ovarian cancer?

A. Early menopause
B. Late menarche
C. Multiparity
D. Nulliparity
E. Oral contraceptive pill

12. INDUCTION OF LABOUR (2)

A 22-year-old woman attends the labour ward for induction of labour; she is 40 weeks + 12 days. She has had an uncomplicated pregnancy. She has no pain in her abdomen but says that although the baby is moving, the movements are fewer than has been normal. A CTG is performed and the baseline rate is 135, variability is more than 10, accelerations are present and there are no decelerations. You examine her and find a cephalic presentation and a Bishop score of 2.

What would be your next course of action?

A. Artificial rupture of membranes
B. Elective caesarean section
C. Emergency caesarean section
D. Oxytocin
E. Prostaglandin

13. INFECTION IN PREGNANCY (1)

A 27-year-old woman is at 19 weeks' gestation. She has a 3-day history of flu-like symptoms with a macular rash over her body. Her doctor performs serological testing. When he has the results, he tells her that her baby is at increased risk of sensorineural deafness, cataracts, congenital heart disease, learning difficulties, hepatosplenomegaly and microcephaly.

What is the underlying causative agent?

A. Chickenpox
B. Cytomegalovirus
C. Listeria
D. Parvovirus
E. Rubella

14. MECHANISMS OF LABOUR (1)

The midwife is delivering a term baby. The head has been delivered. Which movement should the midwife wait for before delivering the shoulders?

A. Descent
B. Extension
C. External rotation
D. Flexion
E. Internal rotation

15. MENSTRUAL HORMONES (1)

Which of the following hormones stimulate the growth of primary follicles?

A. Activin
B. Follicle-stimulating hormone
C. Inhibin
D. Oestrogen
E. Progesterone

16. METHODS OF DELIVERY (1)

The obstetric registrar is called to a 28-year-old primigravida who went into spontaneous labour at 39 + 5 weeks. She is now fully dilated after having an epidural and oxytocin (for failure to progress). She has been actively pushing for 2 hours, is exhausted and tells you she cannot push any longer. On examination, there is no head palpable abdominally and an occipitoanterior position is felt vaginally. The station is +2 with a small caput and no moulding.

How should the baby be delivered?

A. Elective caesarean section
B. Emergency caesarean section
C. Kielland's forceps
D. Manual rotation followed by Neville Barnes forceps
E. Neville Barnes forceps alone

17. OBSTETRIC EMERGENCIES (1)

A 31-year-old primigravid woman with a body mass index (BMI) of 31 had a positive glucose tolerance test at 28 weeks consistent with gestational diabetes mellitus. Although she was advised to change her diet, she did not do this and her glucose control has been suboptimal. An ultrasound scan demonstrated macrosomia.

Which emergency condition does this put her at a greater risk of?

A. Amniotic fluid embolization
B. Disseminated intravascular coagulation
C. Shoulder dystocia
D. Uterine inversion
E. Uterine rupture

18. CHRONIC PELVIC PAIN (1)

A 32-year-old woman complains of long-standing painful, heavy periods. She has had two normal vaginal deliveries after difficulty conceiving with both pregnancies. She suffers from significant pain on intercourse. Her past history includes an appendicectomy at age 10. Pelvic examination reveals a fixed retroverted uterus that is tender. Interestingly, the pain settled when she was pregnant.

What is the most likely explanation for her pain?

A. Adhesions from surgery
B. Chronic pelvic inflammatory disease
C. Endometriosis
D. Fibroid degeneration
E. Ovarian cyst

19. SCREENING (1)

A 41-year-old woman has conceived naturally for the first time despite two failed *in vitro* fertilization (IVF) attempts. She is very concerned about Down syndrome as she received a high-risk screening result. She would like a test performed as soon as possible that would give a firm diagnosis. She is currently at 12 weeks' gestation.

Which test would be most appropriate?

A. Amniocentesis
B. Chorionic villus sampling
C. Combined test
D. First trimester ultrasound scan
E. Nuchal translucency measurement

20. TWINS (1)

A 26-year-old woman with a twin pregnancy has developed twin-to-twin transfusion syndrome at 34 weeks' gestation.

What type of twins is she likely to have?

A. Dizygotic dichorionic diamniotic
B. Dizygotic dichorionic monoamniotic
C. Dizygotic monochorionic monoamniotic
D. Monozygotic dichorionic diamniotic
E. Monozygotic monochorionic diamniotic

21. OBSTETRIC EMERGENCIES (2)

A 32-year-old woman at 40 weeks + 6 days is having induction of labour for mild pre-eclampsia. She has had two doses of vaginal prostaglandins. On abdominal examination, the head is five-fifths palpable, and on vaginal examination, she is 3 cm dilated with intact membranes and a station of –3. She has mild contractions. She would like to proceed with artificial rupture of membranes.

Which emergency condition does this put her at a greater risk of?

A. Cervical shock
B. Cord prolapse
C. Shoulder dystocia
D. Uterine inversion
E. Uterine rupture

22. PERINEAL TEARS

You are asked to examine a woman's perineum after she has delivered vaginally. You see that the perineal skin and muscles are torn. On examination of the anus, the external anal sphincter is torn (but less than 50%) and the internal sphincter is intact.

What degree of perineal tear has this woman sustained?

A. First-degree tear
B. Second-degree tear
C. Third-degree tear, 3a
D. Third-degree tear, 3c
E. Fourth-degree tear

23. MENSTRUAL HORMONES (2)

Which hormone, produced by the corpus luteum, is low in the follicular phase and maximal in the luteal phase?

A. Follicle-stimulating hormone
B. Inhibin
C. Luteinizing hormone
D. Oestradiol
E. Progesterone

24. METHODS OF DELIVERY (2)

A 29-year-old woman is in spontaneous labour at 40 weeks. The CTG is normal. She has had one previous lower segment caesarean section. On abdominal examination, the head is zero-fifths palpable. On vaginal examination, she has been fully dilated for 20 minutes. There is an occipitoanterior presentation with a flexed head. The head is at station +1, and there is no caput and no moulding.

How should one plan for delivery?

A. Elective caesarean section
B. Emergency caesarean section
C. Kielland's forceps
D. Normal delivery
E. Neville Barnes forceps

25. RHESUS DISEASE (1)

A 31-year-old pregnant woman was involved in a minor road traffic collision where she banged her abdomen on the steering wheel. Serious injury has been excluded, but she is concerned about the baby. She has good fetal movements and has had no bleeding *per vaginam*. The fetal heart is heard and is regular. She is at 25 weeks' gestation and is RhD negative. She has had no previous children.

What action needs to be taken with regard to anti-D prophylaxis?

A. Give antenatal anti-D prophylaxis 250 IU and take Kleihauer test
B. Give antenatal anti-D prophylaxis 500 IU and take Kleihauer test
C. Give postnatal anti-D and take Kleihauer test
D. Give routine antenatal anti-D prophylaxis at 28 weeks and take Kleihauer test
E. No action needed at present

26. BISHOP SCORE

You examine a woman who has attended a labour ward for induction of labour at term + 12 days. She has a cephalic presentation that is three-fifths palpable. The cervix is not dilated at all, is 3 cm long, is of average consistency and is in a mid-position. The station is –2.

What is her Bishop score?

A. 0
B. 2
C. 4
D. 6
E. 8

27. PATHOGENESIS OF CERVICAL CANCER (1)

A 43-year-old woman has recently been diagnosed with cervical cancer.

Which of the following are risk factors for the development of cervical cancer?

A. Early menarche
B. Early menopause
C. Increased number of sexual partners
D. Nulliparity
E. Progesterone-only pill

28. BLEEDING IN PREGNANCY (2)

A 39-year-old primigravid woman attends a labour ward at 39 weeks' gestation. She has forgotten her notes. She complains of heavy, unprovoked, painless vaginal bleeding. On examination, she has a soft non-tender abdomen and the head is not engaged. She is passing clots *per vaginam*. She has a pulse rate of 112/min, and her blood pressure is 96/56 mmHg. The CTG is non-reassuring.

What is the most likely diagnosis?

A. Cervical ectropion
B. Placental abruption
C. Placenta praevia
D. Uterine rupture
E. Vasa praevia

29. MISCARRIAGE (1)

A 23-year-old woman with a positive pregnancy test complains of lower abdominal cramping with what she describes as a period-type bleed at home. On abdominal palpation, there is mild suprapubic discomfort. On speculum examination, a small amount of blood is seen in the vagina and the cervical os is closed. Urine dipstick is unremarkable.

What is the most likely diagnosis?

A. Complete miscarriage
B. Incomplete miscarriage
C. Inevitable miscarriage
D. Menstruation
E. Threatened miscarriage

30. PAIN IN PREGNANCY (1)

A 34-year-old woman who has had four previous normal deliveries attends the antenatal day unit at 40 weeks complaining of abdominal pain associated with fever and sweating. Initially, she thought she was in labour as she had spontaneous rupture of membranes 4 days ago, but she says the pain has become increasingly worse. On examination, her uterus is very tender and the cervix is long and closed with an associated yellow–green discharge. Her temperature is 39.7°C. She has a raised white cell count and C-reactive protein.

What is the likely diagnosis?

A. Abruption
B. Acute pyelonephritis
C. Chorioamnionitis
D. Uterine rupture
E. Urinary tract infection

31. ACUTE PELVIC PAIN (1)

A 33-year-old woman attends the emergency department complaining of an aching pain in her left iliac fossa. This has been present intermittently for a few months. She says the pain is significantly worse today but remains focused in the left iliac fossa. She has vomited four times. She denies being sexually active. On examination, she is tender in the left iliac fossa with some voluntary guarding. Speculum examination revealed no abnormalities. There is left adnexal tenderness on vaginal examination but no cervical excitation. Her observations show heart rate 112/min, blood pressure 98/62 mmHg and temperature 36.8°C. A urine result is awaited.

What is the most likely diagnosis?

A. Appendicitis
B. Mittelschmerz
C. Ovarian cyst torsion
D. Pelvic inflammatory disease
E. Renal colic

32. EARLY PREGNANCY (1)

A 31-year-old woman who has recently had a positive pregnancy test has an early pregnancy transvaginal scan that shows no intrauterine pregnancy. She subsequently has two βhCG samples taken, the first on the day of the scan and the second 48 hours later. The first result was 578 IU and the second result was 1126 IU.

What is the most likely diagnosis for this pregnancy of unknown location (PUL)?

A. Ectopic pregnancy
B. Early intrauterine pregnancy
C. Inevitable miscarriage
D. Missed miscarriage
E. Threatened miscarriage

33. MENSTRUAL DISORDERS

A 23-year-old woman complains of intense cramping pains that start on the second day of her period and last for 2 days. She has experienced these since menarche. She is otherwise fit and well.

What is the diagnosis?

A. Primary amenorrhoea
B. Primary dysmenorrhoea
C. Primary menorrhagia
D. Secondary dysmenorrhoea
E. Secondary menorrhagia

34. MECHANISMS OF LABOUR (2)

Which term describes the transition from a left occipitotransverse position to an occipitoanterior position as the fetal head passes through the pelvis?

A. Effacement
B. Extension
C. External rotation
D. Flexion
E. Internal rotation

35. ACUTE PELVIC PAIN (2)

A 25-year-old woman is brought into the resuscitation area having collapsed. She is maintaining her airway, is breathing with a non-rebreathe bag and has a weak pulse. The nurse informs you her observations are heart rate 125/min, blood pressure 86/48 mmHg, saturations 98% and temperature 37.2°C. After fluid resuscitation, the patient is responsive enough to tell you she had some right-sided lower abdominal pain earlier in the day but cannot remember anything else. She says she uses the copper coil for contraception. Her last menstrual period was 6 weeks ago and is normally regular every month. On examination, she is tender with guarding in the right iliac fossa. On speculum examination, there is brown discharge seen in the vagina. Threads from the coil are seen, and cervical excitation is present. A urine result is awaited.

What is the most likely diagnosis?

A. Appendicitis
B. Dislodged coil to a cervical location
C. Ectopic pregnancy
D. Ovarian cyst torsion
E. Pelvic inflammatory disease

36. PAIN IN PREGNANCY (2)

A 29-year-old primigravid woman of 38 weeks + 5 days' gestation attends the antenatal day unit after suddenly feeling unwell. She has vomited five times and complains of severe right upper quadrant pain. On examination, she is tender in the right upper quadrant only. Her blood results show mild anaemia, low platelets, deranged liver enzymes and a normal white cell count. Observations reveal temperature 36.7°C, blood pressure 168/96 mmHg and pulse rate 76/min. Her blood glucose level is 5 mmol/L.

What is the most likely diagnosis?

A. Acute fatty liver of pregnancy
B. Acute pyelonephritis
C. Cholecystitis
D. HELLP syndrome
E. Obstetric cholestasis

37. PARITY AND GRAVIDA

A 38-year-old woman is seen at 29 weeks' gestation. She has had one normal delivery at 41 weeks, one emergency caesarean section at 30 weeks, two miscarriages at 10 and 12 weeks and also a termination of pregnancy at 13 weeks with a different partner when she was 16 years old.

How would you describe her gravidity and parity?

A. G2 P6+3
B. G5 P2+3
C. G6 P2+3
D. P3 G5+2
E. P6 G2+3

38. EARLY PREGNANCY (2)

A 25-year-old woman has an early transvaginal ultrasound scan due to some vaginal brown spotting with a positive pregnancy test. The scan showed no intrauterine pregnancy. She had two βhCG serum tests taken: the first on the day of her scan showed a result of 653 IU and the second 48 hours later had a result of 623 IU.

What is the most likely diagnosis of this pregnancy of unknown location?

A. Early intrauterine pregnancy
B. Ectopic pregnancy
C. Inevitable miscarriage
D. Missed miscarriage
E. Threatened miscarriage

39. OVARIAN CANCER (2)

A 42-year-old woman was seen by the general practitioner after she complained of fatigue, weight loss and more recently a change in bowel habit. On examination, her abdomen was distended and the doctor elicited a positive fluid thrill test. She was urgently referred to the bowel surgeons; however, on CT scanning, bilateral ovarian cysts were seen. After referral to the gynaecology oncologists, she had an operation, and the histological findings were of psammoma bodies. Her diagnosis is the most common ovarian carcinoma.

Which type of ovarian cancer did she have?

A. Clear cell tumour
B. Endometrioid tumour
C. Mucinous tumour
D. Serous tumour
E. Urothelial-like tumour

40. POSTPARTUM HAEMORRHAGE (1)

A B-Lynch brace suture is used in management of this cause of postpartum haemorrhage.

A. Third-degree perineal tear
B. Fourth-degree perineal tear
C. Atonic uterus
D. Cervical tear
E. High vaginal tear

41. PROLAPSE

A 59-year-old woman who has had three previous vaginal deliveries complains of a feeling of 'something coming down' at the front of her vagina and increased urinary frequency. On examination, there is a bulge at the front of her vagina which is easily visible with a Sims' speculum. It is worse when she coughs.

What is the most likely diagnosis?

A. Cystocele
B. Enterocele
C. Procidentia
D. Rectocele
E. Vault prolapse

42. VAGINAL BLEEDING (1)

A 26-year-old female student is seen in the emergency department with postcoital bleeding which she has experienced for 2 weeks. She has no other abnormal discharge. She uses the oral contraceptive pill and has a long-term partner with whom she always uses barrier contraception. Her last smear was a year ago and was normal. On examination, you see an abnormal area of skin surrounding the os. It is flat with a florid appearance. There is contact bleeding when a swab is taken.

What is the most likely diagnosis?

A. Cervical cancer
B. Cervical ectropion
C. Cervical polyps
D. Endometrial carcinoma
E. Endometrial polyps

43. PRE-ECLAMPSIA (1)

A 30-year-old primigravid woman who is 34 weeks' pregnant attends the antenatal clinic. She has persistent hypertension of 164/112 mmHg and protein in her urine on dipstick testing. She has no visual disturbances, no epigastric pain and complains of mild headaches that are generally relieved with paracetamol. On examination, her abdomen is soft and non-tender; she has mild pedal oedema, normal reflexes and one beat of clonus. Her bloods are all normal. She has asthma, for which she uses a salbutamol inhaler when required.

Which antihypertensive should you use to manage her hypertension?

A. Furosemide
B. Labetalol
C. Magnesium sulphate
D. Nifedipine
E. Ramipril

44. CONTRACEPTION (1)

A 31-year-old nulliparous woman is requesting the combined oral contraceptive pill. On further questioning, she reveals she smokes 15 cigarettes per day, she occasionally suffers from migraines with typical focal aura and her mother had a pulmonary embolism at age 50 that was associated with abdominal surgery. She has a BMI of 26. There is no other relevant history.

Can you safely prescribe her the combined oral contraceptive pill and, if not, why not?

A. No – family history of thromboembolic disease
B. No – intends on having children in future
C. No – migraines with aura
D. No – smoker
E. Yes

45. PREMATURE LABOUR (1)

A 27-year-old para 1 + 0 woman attends the labour ward with regular painful contractions at 31 weeks' gestation. On abdominal examination, a cephalic presentation is felt with the head three-fifths palpable. The contractions are palpable and regular every 3 minutes, lasting 30 seconds.

What drug would you give to the mother now to reduce the risk of respiratory distress syndrome if the baby is born prematurely?

A. Amoxicillin
B. Betamethasone
C. $MgSO_4$
D. Salbutamol
E. Theophylline

46. FEMALE INFERTILITY

A 24-year-old woman who has been with her current partner for 5 years has been trying to conceive for 2 years. They are now being investigated for subfertility. She has previously had a chlamydia infection. Her BMI is 26. The woman is being investigated for tubal patency.

What should her first-line investigation be?

A. Laparoscopy and dye test
B. Hysterosalpingo-contrast sonography
C. Hysterosalpingogram
D. Hysteroscopy
E. Salpingoscopy

47. RHESUS DISEASE (2)

A 32-year-old pregnant woman attends the emergency department with a history of bleeding *per vaginam*. She says the bleeding is lighter than her normal period and has lasted for 2 days. She is at 9 weeks' gestation and this is her first pregnancy. She knows she is RhD negative as she gives blood regularly.

What needs to be done today with regard to anti-D prophylaxis?

A. Give antenatal anti-D prophylaxis 250 IU and take Kleihauer test
B. Give antenatal anti-D prophylaxis 500 IU and take Kleihauer test
C. Give postnatal anti-D and take Kleihauer test
D. Give routine antenatal anti-D prophylaxis at 28 weeks
E. No action is needed at present

48. OBSTETRIC EMERGENCIES (3)

A 29-year-old woman who is 38 weeks + 3 days attends the antenatal clinic after being referred by the midwife for measuring smaller than her dates. The presentation is cephalic. The baby is on the twenty-fifth centile for all measurements, and there is a normal liquor volume. The placental site is fundal.

Which emergency does this make her more at risk of when she is in labour?

A. Cord prolapse
B. Fetal distress
C. Stillbirth
D. Uterine inversion
E. Uterine rupture

49. POSTPARTUM HAEMORRHAGE (2)

Which of the following is the most common cause of primary postpartum haemorrhage?

A. Atonic uterus
B. Disseminated intravascular coagulation
C. Infection
D. Perineal trauma
E. Retained placental fragments

50. GAMETOGENESIS (1)

Which of the following is the by-product of female gametogenesis?

A. Mature oocyte
B. Oogonia
C. Polar body
D. Primary oocyte
E. Secondary oocyte

Practice Paper 1: Answers

1. BLEEDING IN PREGNANCY (1)

E – Vasa praevia

Vasa praevia is rare, occurring in only 1 in 3000 pregnancies. Normally the umbilical cord comes out of the centre of the placenta but, in vasa praevia, the umbilical cord vessels travel away from the placenta through the membranes and overlie the internal cervical os. The vessels can tear, leading to rapid exsanguination of the fetal circulation. The risk of vessels tearing is greatest when cervical dilation occurs and at rupture of membranes. A severely abnormal cardiotocograph (CTG) is seen with a small amount (<500 mL) of painless vaginal blood loss. Because it is fetal blood that is lost in vasa praevia, fetal mortality is very high (35%–95%), while there is little risk to the mother. Delivery must be expedited, normally with a caesarean section, and the neonate may need transfusion. There have been some studies into using ultrasound scans as a screening modality, but that is not commonly practiced due to limited evidence of benefit and rarity of the condition. Therefore, diagnosis is clinical and only confirmed when the placenta and membranes are examined after caesarean section.

Vasa, plural of Latin *vas* = vessel.

2. CAESAREAN SECTION (1)

D – Twin pregnancy with first twin breech and second twin cephalic

A caesarean section should be routinely offered to women with:

- HIV with high viral load or those not receiving anti-retroviral therapy
- Co-infection of HIV and hepatitis C
- Primary genital herpes in the third trimester (NB not a secondary attack)
- Placenta praevia major, i.e. grade 3 or 4
- Twin pregnancy where the first baby is breech
- Singleton breech at term but only after external cephalic version has been offered and failed, or is contraindicated

Women with the following should *not* routinely be offered a caesarean section:

- Twin pregnancy where the first twin is cephalic
- Preterm birth

- Small for gestational age baby
- HIV with low viral load on anti-retroviral medication
- Hepatitis B
- Hepatitis C virus without HIV
- Recurrent genital herpes at term

If a woman requests a caesarean section with no medical reason, the obstetric team (obstetrician, midwife, anaesthetist) must discuss in full why the woman wants to have a caesarean and her concerns about normal labour. She must also be informed about the risks and benefits of caesarean section compared with normal labour. Counselling can be offered if the woman has a fear of childbirth. The obstetrician may refuse to perform a section after a maternal request but is obligated to refer the woman to another clinician for a second opinion to determine if a caesarean section should be offered.

A previous caesarean section is not an indication for a repeat section. Women who have had one previous section should be informed about vaginal birth after caesarean (VBAC). The risks of VBAC compared with planned repeat caesarean section include a slight increased risk of uterine rupture with vaginal birth. Women who have had VBAC should be advised to have electronic fetal monitoring during labour and to deliver in a consultant-led unit. For more information, see the NICE 'caesarean section' clinical guideline.*

3. VAGINAL DISCHARGE (1)

E – *Trichomonas vaginalis*
Trichomoniasis is a sexually transmitted infection caused by the flagellated protozoan *Trichomonas vaginalis*, which invades superficial epithelial cells of the vagina, urethra, glans penis, prostate and seminal vesicles. Affected females present with an offensive frothy greeny-grey discharge, vulval soreness, dyspareunia, dysuria, vaginitis and vulvitis, although some are asymptomatic. On examination, the cervix may have a punctate erythematous (strawberry) appearance. Males are mostly asymptomatic. Diagnosis is by direct microscopy or culture of vaginal exudate. Treatment is with metronidazole.

Gonorrhoea is caused by the Gram-negative diplococcus *Neisseria gonorrhoeae* infecting the mucosal surfaces of the genitourinary tract, rectum and pharynx. The majority of females are asymptomatic (70%). Around 85% to 90% of cases involve the cervix, but only 10% of these cases have a significant increase in vaginal discharge. Seventy percent of cases involve the urethra and, again, it is generally asymptomatic although dysuria and urinary frequency may be seen. The vagina is not infected. Complications include Bartholin's abscess and gonococcal salpingitis

---

* National Institute for Health and Clinical Excellence. *Caesarean Section*. 2011.
  http://www.nice.org.uk/guidance/cg132/resources/guidance-caesarean-section-pdf

with irreversible tube damage. Infected males present with dysuria, frequency and/or a mucopurulent discharge after 3 to 5 days, coupled with urethritis and meatal oedema. Disseminated gonococcal infection occurs in <1% cases and causes pyrexia, a vasculitic rash and polyarthritis. Culture-sensitive antibiotics are used for treatment.

Chlamydia is caused by the oculogenital serovars D–K of *Chlamydia trachomatis.* Infection tends to be asymptomatic, although there can be increased vaginal discharge (30%), dysuria and urinary frequency. On examination, a 'cobblestone' appearance of the cervix may be noted. Ascending infection can cause salpingitis and, if it enters the abdominal cavity, perihepatitis (Fitz-Hugh–Curtis syndrome), which leads to right upper quadrant pain and tenderness. Chlamydia is a major cause for infertility and increases the possibility of ectopic pregnancy. In males, symptoms include mucopurulent discharge and dysuria (asymptomatic in 25%). Epididymo-orchitis is a complication. Diagnosis of chlamydia infection is by urine antigen detection or by vaginal swab culture. Treatment is with azithromycin or doxycycline.

Bacterial vaginosis (BV) is not a sexually transmitted infection. It is an infection caused by mixed anaerobic flora (commonly *Gardnerella vaginalis* and *Mycoplasma hominis*). It is often asymptomatic but can cause a creamy-grey discharge with a fishy odour. There is no itching. Diagnosis is by microscopy and treatment is with a single dose of metronidazole (2 g) in the non-pregnant population. It is currently not clear how the risk of preterm delivery and late miscarriage is related to BV, so only high-risk women should be screened for it. There is some evidence that oral clindamycin can reduce preterm delivery in this high-risk group.

Candidiasis (thrush) is caused by yeasts, particularly *Candida albicans* and *Candida glabrata*, and produces vulval *pruritis*, burning, swelling and dyspareunia. White discharge and plaques are seen in the vagina with redness of the vulva and labia minora. Candidiasis is seen more commonly with pregnancy, tissue maceration, diabetes mellitus, HIV infection and use of antimicrobial agents and immunosuppressive drugs. Diagnosis is confirmed by culture, and treatment is with antifungals, for example, topical imidazoles (Canesten) or oral fluconazole.

Chlamydia, from Greek *chlamys* = cloak (as chlamydia is often 'cloaked', i.e. asymptomatic).
Candida, from Latin *candidus* = clear and white.
Thomas Fitz-Hugh Jr, American physician (1894–1963).
Arthur Curtis, American gynecologist (1881–1955).

4. MANAGEMENT OF INCONTINENCE (1)

A – Bladder training
Urinary incontinence affects 10% to 20% of the adult female population. It is a social and hygienic problem. Incontinence occurs when the intravesical pressure exceeds the urethral closure pressure.

This woman is suffering from an overactive bladder (OAB), also known as unstable bladder or hyperactive bladder, which can be caused by detrusor instability. First-line treatment is bladder training for 6 weeks.

OAB is the second most common type of urinary incontinence in females (after stress incontinence). Other causes include retention with overflow, fistula and congenital abnormalities. OAB is where an involuntary detrusor contraction results in leakage of urine. It can occur in conjunction with stress incontinence. Women complain of frequency of micturition and urgency, which they describe as an overwhelming desire to pass urine with associated urge incontinence. This can also be associated with nocturnal frequency and nocturnal enuresis. It is important to establish how it affects the patient's life, dependent on severity, lifestyle and occupation, as this will impact on how aggressive the treatment strategies will be.

Investigations include examination of midstream urine (MSU), a frequency volume chart, filling urodynamic assessment and voiding urodynamic assessment. An MSU can indicate whether an acute or chronic urinary tract infection is present or, in the presence of red cells, a bladder tumour. A frequency volume chart (or urinary diary) shows the fluid intake and urinary volumes and times and how often the patient is wet. In OAB, passing frequent small volumes of urine is usual. Urodynamic assessments include filling and voiding studies. Filling studies involve filling the bladder with a catheter and assessing the detrusor pressure by measuring pressure inside the bladder and the abdomen. If leaking occurs with increase in detrusor pressure and total bladder pressure but without abdominal pressure increase, then this is detrusor overactivity. If leaking occurs on increased intra-abdominal pressure (e.g. a cough with no change in detrusor pressure), stress incontinence is demonstrated. Voiding studies measure total volume voided, peak flow of urine and detrusor activity required to create that flow. This can show high residual volumes and voiding difficulties if there is significant abdominal straining or reduced urinary flow rate. The normal flow rate is above 15 mL/sec.

Treatment of an OAB is initially conservative, then with the addition of medicine, although surgery can be done in some cases. First-line treatment is bladder training for 6 weeks. If this is not effective, an anticholinergic can be added (oxybutynin, tolterodine or darifenacin) as first-line drug treatment following counselling about the adverse antimuscarinic effects (i.e. dry mouth, blurred vision, constipation, urinary retention). If this class of medications does not work, then mirabegron (a β-3 adrenergic agonist that results in detrusor relaxation) should be used. If medical treatment is not effective, botulinum toxin A injections into the bladder wall should be offered provided the patient is willing and able to self-catheterize if needed. Rarely, sacral nerve stimulation and augmentation cystoplasty are required.

5. CARDIOTOCOGRAPHY (1)

A – Maternal pyrexia

Cardiotocography (CTG) measures the fetal heart rate with uterine activity. It can be used confidently after 32 weeks' gestation to monitor the condition of a fetus in correlation with the clinical situation. Prior to this gestation, the autonomic nervous system is not sufficiently developed to produce the predictable responses of the more mature fetus. A normal CTG is reassuring, but an abnormal CTG does not always mean the fetus is acidotic.

Indications for CTG monitoring can be maternal (previous caesarean section, pre-eclampsia, diabetes, antepartum haemorrhage), fetal (intrauterine growth restriction, prematurity, oligohydramnios, multiple pregnancy, breech) or intrapartum (oxytocin use, induction of labour). The CTG lead is placed on the mother's abdomen or attached vaginally to the fetal scalp. The use of CTG does not appear to improve long-term neonatal outcome.

A CTG tracing should be assessed as follows:

Baseline

The normal baseline fetal heart rate (FHR) is the mean FHR over 5 to 10 minutes. The normal range is from 100 to 160 beats/min. This represents a balance between sympathetic and parasympathetic systems. Sustained tachycardia may be due to prematurity with the rate slowing physiologically with advancing gestational age. It is also seen in hypoxia, fetal distress, maternal pyrexia (this case) and with the use of exogenous β-agonists (e.g. salbutamol). Baseline bradycardia may suggest severe fetal distress, possibly due to placental abruption or uterine rupture, but occurs more commonly with fetal hypoxia and acidaemia. A sustained baseline below 90 beats/min usually indicates impending fetal demise and should be acted on without delay.

Baseline variability

This describes the fluctuations in the FHR from one beat to the next. Variability is produced by the balance between the parasympathetic and sympathetic nervous systems. Minor fluctuations in the baseline FHR occur at three to five cycles per minute. Baseline variability is calculated by measuring the distance between the highest peak and the lowest trough in a one-minute segment of a CTG trace. Normal variability is between 5 and 25 beats/min and is a good indicator of fetal well-being. Reduced variability can be seen most commonly during phases of fetal sleep, which may safely last up to 40 minutes. It is also seen in early gestation (as the nervous system only develops later in pregnancy) and with certain drugs, particularly opiates or benzodiazepines. A prolonged reduced variability suggests fetal distress.

Accelerations and decelerations

Accelerations are defined as a rise in the FHR of at least 15 beats/min, for at least 15 seconds. Antenatally, you should expect at least two accelerations every 15 minutes. They are reassuring and often occur with fetal movements, although their absence in advanced labour is not uncommon. *Decelerations* are a fall in the FHR of at least 15 beats/min for more than 15 seconds. *Early decelerations* occur with contractions and return to normal by the end of the contraction. They are probably physiological and are thought to reflect increased vagal tone when fetal intracranial pressure increases during a contraction. They are uniform in depth, length and shape. *Late decelerations* occur during a contraction and only return to baseline after the contraction. They suggest fetal distress. Late decelerations are more worrying if they are shallow and late. *Variable decelerations* vary in timing and shape in relation to uterine contraction. They suggest cord compression, especially in oligohydramnios. 'Shouldering' is a sign that the fetus is coping well with the compression: this is when there is a small rise in FHR before and after the deceleration. These may resolve if the mother's position is changed.

A *sinusoidal trace* is a smooth undulating sine-wave-like baseline with no variability. The pattern lasts more than 10 minutes with an amplitude of 5 to 15 beats/min. A sinusoidal pattern may be physiological or can represent fetal anaemia/hypoxia but *must* be considered serious until proven otherwise. Sinusoidal patterns should be distinguished from *pseudosinusoidal traces,* which are a benign, uniform, long-term pattern. They are less regular in shape and amplitude when compared with sinusoidal traces.

Sinusoidal, from Latin *sinus* = curve or hollow space.

6. FETAL POSITION (1)

D – Occipitoposterior

Vaginal examination often involves a speculum examination and a digital examination but, in this case, there is no need for a speculum as it is already known that she is in established labour.

During labour, digital examinations are used to assess dilation of the cervix to ensure adequate progression. This is described in centimetres of dilation and in how effaced the cervix is. The fetal head is also examined to assess its position using fontanelles. Fontanelles are the soft spots on the baby's head in between the skull bones. They are covered with fibrous tissue and allow the bones to overlap to allow the head to pass more easily through the birth canal. The anterior fontanelle is a diamond-shaped structure formed at the junction of the two frontal bones, which cover the forehead, and the two parietal bones, which cover the side of the head. This fontanelle will become ossified by the child's second birthday. The posterior fontanelle is Y-shaped and is made from the junction between the two parietal bones and the occipital bone. This fontanelle will close during the first few months of life. The line felt in the question was the sagittal suture, which runs from the anterior to the posterior fontanelle between the two parietal bones.

The station of the head describes how far down the head is in relation to the ischial spines (in centimetres). If the head is at the spines, it is classed as 0; if it is above, then it is graded from −1 to −3; and if it is below, it is graded from +1 to +2. Moulding describes how much overlap of the fetal skull bones there is, and caput describes the localized swelling that is found on the baby's head due to pressure from the cervix or pelvic inlet.

The ideal position in which a baby's head should be is occipitoanterior (OA), so you would feel the posterior fontanelle towards the mother's symphysis pubis and the anterior fontanelle towards her back, meaning the baby would be born looking towards the mother's back. The baby in this case was 180° to this position (occipitoposterior), meaning the baby had the back of its head at the maternal posterior.

An occipitotransverse position describes when the occiput is at the side, either the left or right. A brow presentation is when the fetal head is more deflexed, meaning the anterior fontanelle would be in a central position and you might be able to feel the features of the face. A face presentation would mean that lips and nose would be easily felt and care must be taken not to injure the baby.

Another time when a digital examination is used is during induction, when the cervix is assessed using the Bishop score (see Question 26). A digital vaginal examination should be avoided if the membranes have ruptured but the woman is not in labour, as there is a risk of introducing infection, and in placenta praevia (risk of massive haemorrhage).

7. GENITAL TRACT

A – Ampulla of fallopian tube
Fertilization is defined as the union of the ovum and the spermatozoon. The ovum is normally released from the ovarian follicle every 28 days. The fimbrial end of the fallopian tube lies close to the release spot so the ovum is taken up into the fallopian tube. The lumen of the fallopian tube is lined by cilia, and it is the combination of the rhythmical movement of these cilia and the peristalsis created by the muscles of the fallopian tube that moves the ovum along towards the uterus. The ovum has a physiological pause when it reaches the ampulla of the fallopian tube. It is this physiological pause that means that fertilization normally happens in the ampulla. It also allows extra time for the sperm and ovum to be in the 'same place at the same time' as sexual intercourse happens at random in humans. The sperm can survive up to 7 days inside the female,

so, as long as ovulation occurs within 7 days of sexual intercourse, fertilization is feasible. After the pause, and possible fertilization, the rhythmic waves and peristalsis recommence and the ovum moves down into the uterus.

The lateral funnel-shaped end of the fallopian tube is called the infundibulum, which opens into the peritoneal cavity through the abdominal ostium. There are many finger-like projections known as fimbriae at the end of the infundibulum, which spread over the medial surface of the ovary to waft the released ovum into the fallopian tube. The ampulla is medial to the infundibulum and is the longest and widest part; this is where fertilization occurs. The isthmus enters the uterine horn and is thick-walled. The uterine portion travels through the uterine wall to terminate in the uterine cavity at the uterine ostium.

8. INDUCTION OF LABOUR (1)

A – Artificial rupture of membranes

Induction of labour is offered if pregnancy continues past 40 weeks; each unit will define the specific gestation at which they induce women. The process involves vaginal prostaglandins with artificial rupture of membranes (ARM) and the use of oxytocin.

This woman has received two doses of vaginal prostaglandins (PGE_2) to initiate contractions and to encourage cervical ripening. Prostaglandins are given 6 to 8 hourly or in slow release form on a small tampon. In this case, they have clearly worked as she has progressed from a low Bishop score (see Question 26) to a cervical dilation of 3 cm. If the patient is progressing well with strong contractions, no other action is needed; however, if there is slow progress with minimal contractions (as in this case), an ARM can be performed. An oxytocin infusion is used to maintain the contractions after membrane rupture. Further prostaglandins are contraindicated due to the risk of hyperstimulation as she already feels some uterine activity.

An amnihook is used to pierce the membranes surrounding the baby. The colour of the amniotic fluid should be recorded; any meconium or blood should be noted and appropriate action should be taken if required. The fetal heart should always be checked after an ARM. If there is a high head, an ARM may be performed in theatre due to the higher risk of a cord prolapse, in which case an immediate caesarean section may be needed.

Complications of induction and augmentation of labour include:

- Failure of induction – requiring operative delivery
- Uterine hyperstimulation (>7 contractions/15 min) – this can cause maternal and fetal distress. An oxytocin infusion must be stopped and continuous monitoring is needed. Tocolysis (suppression of contractions) can be used but, if there is suspicion of fetal compromise, delivery is needed as soon as possible.

- Nausea, vomiting, diarrhoea – systemic side effects of prostaglandins
- Uterine rupture

Toco-, from Greek *tokos* = childbirth.

9. FETAL ULTRASOUND (1)

C – Crown–rump length

Ultrasound scanning is a means of monitoring pregnancy and, to date, is without proven maternal or fetal risk. Scans can be performed abdominally or transvaginally.

The scan at 10 to 14 weeks is used to date the fetus by measuring crown–rump length (CRL). The estimated delivery date (EDD) is calculated roughly from the last menstrual period (LMP), but the ultrasound scan (USS) can give a more accurate date. As the fetus grows, it becomes more flexed in shape, which makes the CRL unreliable. If CRL measures more than 84 mm, which correlates to 14 weeks, the head circumference (HC) becomes a more reliable indicator of gestational age.

An EDD can be calculated from the LMP; however, LMP may not be accurately recalled, there may be an irregular cycle, and bleeding early in the pregnancy may be mistaken for a period. The EDD is 40 weeks after the first day of the LMP and not from the date of conception, although this is only true if the cycle is 28 days and regular. If the cycle is known to be shorter or longer, then days can be added or subtracted accordingly. The first date of a positive pregnancy test can be useful as it will generally become positive on the day the next period would have been due; therefore, when a positive pregnancy test is seen, the gestation must be at least 4 weeks.

Every woman should be offered an ultrasound scan early in pregnancy (between 10 and 14 weeks). There are a number of reasons for this:

- To establish viability and ensure that either a molar pregnancy or missed miscarriage has not occurred
- To detect multiple pregnancies and to determine chorionicity and amnionicity (most reliably done in the first trimester)
- The nuchal translucency test is done between 11 and 14 weeks to assess risk for Down syndrome.
- Gross anatomical anomalies can be detected in the first trimester scan, such as major anterior abdominal wall defects, cystic hygroma, anencephaly and bladder outflow obstruction.

10. MANAGEMENT OF SMEAR RESULTS (1)

D – Recall in 3 years

The aim of the cervical screening programme is to detect early changes in the cervix that may progress to cancer if not treated. Liquid based cytology (LBC) is the method used to take a sample of cells from the cervix, which is then sent to the lab to be tested. HPV infection can also be tested on the sample if required. The previous method, known as a smear test, used a spatula to scrape cells from the cervix, which were then 'smeared' onto a slide and examined under a microscope. The spatula has been replaced by a brush, which collects the cells from the cervix. The sample is then spun to separate the cells, and they are examined under a microscope. The cells could be normal or could show features of borderline abnormalities, low-grade dyskaryosis or high-grade dyskaryosis. Cytologically, the dyskaryotic cell is characterized by anaplasia, increased nuclear:cytoplasmic ratio and hyperchromatism with changes in the nuclear chromatin, multinucleation and abnormalities in differentiation.

If the cells are normal, there is no need for an HPV test and the woman can return to normal recall. In this patient, the cells have shown mild dyskaryosis, which means HPV should be tested as the result of this will change the management. If HPV is negative, the woman returns to normal recall, which would be 3 years in this patient as she is under 50 years old. If the HPV had been positive, she would require a colposcopy referral as she is at much higher risk of having a histological abnormality. 'Normal recall' is 3 years in women between 25 and 49 years; this extends to 5 years in women from 50 to 65 years, when the programme usually ends. The frequency of recall varies with age to ensure a targeted and effective screening programme; it is done via the general practice on a computer recall system. A woman may be recalled if there are inadequate cells for the study – this should be in 3 months.

Colposcopy is where the cervix is examined in greater detail using a binocular microscope known as a colposcope. The patient is placed in the lithotomy position (supine with knees and hips flexed and spread apart with stirrups) and the squamocolumnar junction (SCJ) of the cervix is visualized. Initially the cervix is inspected using a high-power microscope to study the general appearance and vasculature of the cervix. Subsequently, two different stains can be applied to the cervix in colposcopy: acetic acid and Lugol's iodine. Acetic acid stains abnormal areas white ('acetowhite'). Lugol's iodine stains glycogen. As pre-malignant and malignant cervical tissue lacks glycogen, it does not retain the iodine. These unstained areas can be biopsied or excised, a histological diagnosis can be made of cervical intraepithelial neoplasia (CIN) 1/2/3 and a management plan can be formulated.

It is important to remember that the smear gives a cytological (cells) result, but colposcopy biopsies give a histological (tissue) diagnosis.

CIN is a pre-malignant phase of cervical cancer. It is seen where cells from the endocervix are exposed to the environment of the vagina in the area known as the transformation zone. Under the influence of oestrogen, the endocervix (canal of the cervix) everts and exposes the columnar epithelium cells it is lined with to the chemical environment of the upper vagina. The change in the pH and other factors cause metaplasia of these columnar epithelium cells to squamous epithelium, with which the ecto-cervix (vaginal part of the cervix) is lined. CIN can then develop in this area of metaplasia at the transformation zone.

Lithotomy, from Greek *lith* = stone. This position was originally used to remove bladder stones via a perineal incision.

11. OVARIAN CANCER (1)

D – Nulliparity

Ovarian cancer is the fifth most common cancer in females in the UK. It is seen mainly in the fifth, sixth and seventh decade. It has a 5-year survival rate of 43%. There is currently no screening test as it has not been proven to be of benefit.

Like all cancers, there are numerous risk factors for its development. It may be related to ovulation, due to the repair of the ovarian epithelium required following each ovulation. This means the more you ovulate the more you increase your risk of developing cancer of the ovary. Hence nulliparity, infertility, late menopause and early menarche all increase your risk, whereas risk is lowered by the contraceptive pill, breastfeeding and pregnancy. Pelvic surgery decreases the risk (including hysterectomy without oophorectomy, unilateral oophorectomy and sterilization) for reasons that are not fully understood.

The risk of ovarian cancer is increased with a positive family history, and this is much more significant if there was early onset and more than one primary relative affected. Around 5% to 10% of ovarian cancers have a direct genetic link with the most significant being *BRCA1* and *BRCA2*. Affected women have a lifetime risk of up to 50% of developing ovarian cancer; hence, close monitoring is needed using CA125 and pelvic ultra-sounds. Furthermore, a prophylactic bilateral oophorectomy may be considered by some once the family is complete. Other cancers that are linked are breast, endometrial and colonic.

12. INDUCTION OF LABOUR (2)

E – Prostaglandin

Induction of labour (IOL) is used as there is an increased risk of still-birth with increasing gestation over 37 weeks. The current data suggest the stillbirth rate is 1 per 3000 at 37 weeks, 3 per 3000 at 42 weeks and 6 per 3000 at 43 weeks. About 20% of women need IOL. If a woman declines IOL at 42 weeks, they should be offered twice-weekly cardioto-cograph (CTG) and ultrasound scans to measure maximum amniotic pool depth.

A stretch and sweep should be done prior to formal IOL. A finger is inserted into the cervix and the membranes are stripped from the uterine wall with the aim of inducing labour more naturally.

Prior to IOL, the woman's cervix should be assessed using the Bishop score (see Question 26). If the Bishop score is very low, such as in this case, IOL involves vaginal prostaglandins (PGE_2) as either tablets or gels or slow release from a small tampon to initiate contractions and to encourage cervical ripening. The tablets are given 6 to 8 hourly, and the tampon is left by the cervix for 24 hours. The CTG has to be reassuring for prostaglandins to be given, and there should be no evidence of contractions; otherwise, the risk of uterine hyperstimulation is increased.

If women are progressing well, they can be left to labour; however, if there is slow progress, an artificial rupture of membranes can be performed along with an oxytocin infusion to maintain the contractions. If there has been pre-labour rupture of membranes, the oxytocin can be started regardless of the state of the cervix.

A CTG should be performed prior to IOL and following insertion of prostaglandin, and continuous monitoring should be used once on oxytocin. If there is uterine hyperstimulation, the oxytocin should be stopped or decreased; tocolytics can be used if the hyperstimulation is not resolving and is causing a suboptimal CTG.

Indications for IOL include:

- Post-term pregnancy
- Women with pre-labour rupture of membranes (PROM) at term should be offered a choice of immediate induction or expectant management but this should not exceed 24 hours after membrane rupture
- Diabetes in pregnancy
- Fetal indications (e.g. intrauterine growth restriction)

13. INFECTION IN PREGNANCY (1)

E – Rubella

Rubella (German measles) is a viral infection spread by person-to-person contact. It has an incubation period of 14 to 21 days. Rubella is rare nowadays thanks to immunization (MMR vaccine) and UK immunity is 97%. Women develop a non-specific flu-like illness with a macular rash covering their trunk (20%–50% of infections are asymptomatic). Diagnosis is confirmed by serological antibody testing. Rubella antibodies are checked at booking and postnatal vaccination is offered to those with low titres. There is an 80% risk of infection to the fetus if rubella develops in the first trimester, dropping to 25% at the end of the second trimester. Teratogenic effects are worse at earlier gestations, with a 50% risk of abnormalities if the fetus is under 4 weeks, 25% at 5 to 8 weeks, 10% at 9 to 12 weeks and 1% over 13 weeks. The characteristic abnormalities from maternal rubella infection are sensorineural deafness, cataracts, congenital heart disease, learning difficulties, hepatosplenomegaly, jaundice, microcephaly and spontaneous miscarriage.

Rubella is also known as German measles as the first three reported cases were described by German physicians in the mid-eighteenth century, who all thought the condition was a variant of measles.

Listeria is a rare bacterial infection. The Gram-positive coccus, *Listeria monocytogenes,* is found in soil, animal faeces, pâté and unpasteurized dairy products such as soft cheese. Pasteurized milk carries no risk. The incubation period is 3 to 70 days. The incidence and severity of infection is increased in pregnancy. Symptoms include fever, headache, malaise, backache, abdominal pain, pharyngitis or conjunctivitis. Diagnosis is by blood cultures or placental/neonatal swabs. Treatment is with high-dose penicillin. Listeria infection during pregnancy can lead to miscarriage, stillbirth, preterm delivery and neonatal listeriosis, which carries 50% mortality.

Parvovirus B19 infection is spread by respiratory droplets with an incubation period of 18 days. It is often seen in outbreaks at schools and manifests in children as erythema infectiosum – a 'slapped cheek' appearance. Erythema infectiosum is also known as the fifth disease – so-called because it is the fifth of the classical childhood skin rashes (the others being measles, chickenpox, rubella, scarlet fever and roseola infantum). In adults, parvovirus infection presents with fever, malaise and arthralgia. In women with parvovirus infection, fetal death is seen in 9% of cases. The second trimester holds the highest risk of fetal infection. The fetal sequelae are non-immune hydrops due to chronic haemolytic anaemia and myocarditis. *In utero* blood transfusion of hydropic fetuses may prevent demise. There are no long-term sequelae among survivors.

Parvovirus B19 is so called because it was first discovered in well B19 (row B, column 19) of a large series of microtitre plates. It was noted by chance in 1975 by Australian virologist Yvonne Cossart (1934–2014).

14. MECHANISMS OF LABOUR (1)

C – External rotation

Labour describes the expulsion of the fetus and the placenta by the uterus. There are regular, painful uterine contractions associated with dilation and effacement of the cervix. A normal spontaneous labour is divided into three stages.

The *first stage* is divided into a latent and active phase. In the latent phase, there are contractions and cervical effacement and dilation to 4 cm. The active phase is when there are regular painful contractions and the cervix dilates from 4 to 10 cm. The latent phase is a slow process and may take hours to days; however, the active phase is faster and women should progress by at least 2 cm every 4 hours. The *second stage* is from full dilation to delivery of the fetus. The passive phase of the second stage is from full dilation until the woman feels an urge to push as the head reaches the pelvic floor. The active phase of the second stage is where the pressure on the pelvic floor generates an irresistible desire to push or where the woman is directed to push.

The *third stage* is from delivery of the fetus to delivery of the placenta. The placenta is sheared from the uterine wall due to the contraction of the uterus constricting the supplying blood vessels. This is often indicated by lengthening of the cord associated with a rush of dark blood.

The 'three Ps' make up the mechanical aspect of labour. The *power* is the uterine contractions that force the fetus out along the birth canal. In labour, contractions should last 40 to 60 seconds and occur every 2 to 3 minutes. This is associated with shortening and dilation of the cervix. The pacemakers for the contractions are in the cornuae of the uterus. Irregular contractions are often seen in primigravid women. The *passage* is the bony pelvis and its associated soft tissues. The important dimensions of this passage are the pelvic inlet (transverse diameter 13 cm, anteroposterior [AP] diameter 11 cm) and the pelvic outlet (transverse diameter 11 cm, AP diameter 13 cm). These dimensions are important in the descent and rotation of the baby. The soft tissues are the pelvic floor muscles that help the head rotate down the pelvis through the vagina to crown in the occipitoanterior (OA) position at the introitus. The *passenger* is the fetus. Factors that determine the ease of transfer of the passenger through the passage include degree of flexion of the head, position of the head and size of the head. The smallest diameter of the head is at full flexion (chin on chest, average 9.5 cm). Any degree of deflexion will increase the diameter. The position of the head can be described by feeling the fontanelles and sutures. The head will enter the pelvis in a right or left occiput transverse position (i.e. baby looking sideways) and then rotate by 90° as it passes though the pelvis to give an OA position (i.e. baby looking at mother's back). Some, however, do not rotate or rotate the wrong way resulting in more difficult vaginal births. Moulding is where fetal head bones overlap, and this can be felt on vaginal examination.

Passage of the head through the pelvis can be summarized as follows:

- Descent – descent of the head into the pelvis, which usually occurs in the last few weeks of pregnancy in a nulliparous woman but much later in multiparous women.
- Engagement – when the maximum transverse diameter of the head has passed below the pelvic inlet. Engagement is when less than two-fifths of the head can be palpated above the pelvic brim abdominally.
- Flexion – as the head descends through the pelvis, it flexes to give the smallest diameter for easy passage through the pelvis. The posterior fontanelle should be palpable vaginally with maximum flexion.
- Internal rotation – this is the rotation of the head that occurs in the mid-pelvis; from the occiput transverse position, it enters the pelvic inlet to the OA position required for easy delivery.
- Extension – the head only extends as it reaches the perineum and 'crowns' as delivery is imminent.

- External rotation (restitution) – on delivery, the fetal head reverts back to its earlier transverse position.
- Lateral flexion – this is the movement needed for the shoulders and trunk to be delivered.

15. MENSTRUAL HORMONES (1)

B – Follicle-stimulating hormone

Menstruation is controlled by the hypothalamic–pituitary–ovarian axis. There are two phases: the follicular phase (days 1–14) and the luteal phase (days 15–28). During these phases, there are changes in hormone levels, in endometrial thickness and in cervical mucus.

Follicle-stimulating hormone (FSH) is a glycoprotein produced by the anterior pituitary gland in response to gonadotrophin-releasing hormone (GnRH) from the hypothalamus. The concentrations of FSH and luteinizing hormone (LH) are allowed to rise during early follicular phase due to the low levels of oestrogen and progesterone at the end of the previous cycle. The action of FSH along with LH is to stimulate the growth of 6 to 12 primary follicles each month during the follicular phase of the cycle (days 1–14). As the follicles mature, there is a rise in oestrogen due to increased production from the granulosa cells of the developing follicles; this increase in oestrogen inhibits the release of FSH and LH (by negative feedback). This mechanism avoids hyperstimulation of the ovary and the resultant maturation of multiple follicles. Thus, only one of these follicles will reach full maturation at the mid-follicular phase with the others undergoing atresia.

As the oestrogen levels continue to rise throughout the follicular phase, there is a mild surge in FSH mid-cycle due to the *very* high levels of oestrogen (positive feedback). More importantly, there is a concurrent surge in LH which initiates ovulation. The gonadotrophins LH and FSH are low in the luteal phase and do not rise again until degeneration of the corpus luteum; there is a subsequent decrease in steroid hormones (oestrogen and progesterone) at days 26 to 28 to repeat the cycle.

FSH is low during childhood, increases with puberty to become cyclical throughout a woman's reproductive lifetime and is very high after menopause as there are no follicles left to be released so there is no negative feedback mechanism from oestrogen and progesterone.

16. METHODS OF DELIVERY (1)

E – Neville Barnes forceps alone

Delay in the second stage of labour (if birth is not imminent after 2 hours in nulliparous women, or 1 hour in parous women) should be managed by a trained obstetrician. Forceps are made of two interlocking blades, which fit around the baby's head and are used to guide it out. When correctly applied, they should lock together easily and not be forced. Neville Barnes forceps have both a cephalic curve to fit the baby's head and a pelvic curve, which follows the contours of the sacral hollow. These are used to aid delivery when rotation is not required, such as in this case.

With all instrumental deliveries, a maximum of three contractions associated with traction should be used to deliver the baby. If more than this is required, then a caesarean section should be performed. The patient should have adequate analgesia, which is ideally a spinal or epidural but, if this is not possible, a pudendal block or local infiltration of the perineum can be used for non-rotational forceps in an emergency situation. Risks of all forceps include failure to deliver requiring caesarean section, vaginal tears and fetal trauma including facial bruising or abrasions.

Kielland's forceps are rotational forceps and therefore do not have a pelvic curve as this would damage soft tissue during rotation. Rotation can be used to turn the baby to the occipitoanterior position and then traction can be applied to deliver the baby. These deliveries are usually done in theatre, so a caesarean section could be undertaken if the head does not rotate. Rotation of a baby can also be achieved manually or by using a ventouse. A *ventouse* is a suction cap which is attached to the baby's head at a specific point before traction is applied. A combination of traction and maternal effort can rotate the baby to an occipitoanterior position (if not in this position initially). There is an element of operator choice when determining whether forceps or ventouse is used.

Prerequisites for all instrumental deliveries include patient consent, valid indication for instrumental delivery, fully dilated cervix with ruptured membranes, no head palpable per abdomen, head at or below the level of the ischial spines, maternal bladder empty and adequate analgesia. Position of the head must be determined, and there must be no excessive moulding.

Christian Kielland, Norwegian obstetrician (1871–1941).

17. OBSTETRIC EMERGENCIES (1)

C – Shoulder dystocia

Shoulder dystocia describes impaction of the fetus's anterior shoulder behind the symphysis pubis after delivery of the head, impeding delivery of the rest of the body.

This woman has gestational diabetes mellitus and is more likely to develop macrosomia. Macrosomia – an abnormally large fetus – occurs in maternal diabetes due to excessive production of fetal insulin and an increased deposition of glycogen in the fetus. Macrosomia increases the risk of shoulder dystocia due to the size of the shoulders. Other risk factors for shoulder dystocia include a past history of dystocia, maternal obesity, prolonged first stage of labour, secondary arrest >8 cm cervical dilation, mid-cavity arrest and forceps/ventouse delivery. Consider shoulder dystocia if the head delivers slowly or with difficulty and the neck does not appear, or if the chin retracts against the perineum (the turtle sign).

Fetal morbidity and mortality occur due to compression of the umbilical cord between the fetal trunk and the maternal pelvis, which rapidly leads to fetal hypoxia and death. Nerve injury can also occur due to downward traction on the head during attempts to deliver the baby (Erb's palsy or Klumpke's palsy). Fracture of the fetal humerus or clavicle may also occur but may be necessary for delivery. Maternal complications include birth canal injuries, femoral nerve injury from excessive hip flexion and an increase in maternal blood loss.

Emergency management

Excessive traction should not be put on the baby's head as this can lead to further impaction of the shoulder and nerve damage. An *aide memoire* to management is 'HELPERR'.

H Call for *help* including obstetricians, anaesthetists and paediatricians. It is very important to have a 'scribe' who can write down the timings to ensure good standards of care are achieved in emergency situations.

E *Evaluate* for an *episiotomy* – not to help directly with delivery, but it allows more room for manoeuvres and reduces genital trauma to the mother.

L The mother's *legs* should be put into the McRoberts' position (flexion and abduction). This allows delivery of the baby in 40% to 60% of cases as it straightens the sacrum relative to the lumbar vertebrae.

P Suprapubic *pressure* (Mazzanti technique) is applied abdominally on the posterior aspect of the fetus's anterior shoulder in an attempt to disimpact the shoulder and rotate it from an anteroposterior direction to an oblique line in the pelvis. This is attempted first with continuous pressure and then with a rocking motion.

E *Enter* the pelvis and perform various manoeuvres. The Rubin manoeuvre involves placing your fingers directly on the posterior aspect of the anterior shoulder *per vagina* and applying pressure with the contraction to move the baby's shoulders into a more favourable oblique position in the pelvis to allow the anterior shoulder to deliver. The Woods' screw manoeuvre involves attempting to rotate the baby by 180° using pressure on the posterior aspect of the anterior shoulder and pressure on the anterior aspect of the posterior shoulder to move the anterior shoulder to a posterior position. This should allow the anterior shoulder to be delivered under the pubic arch. This can then be attempted in reverse.

R *Remove* the posterior arm in an attempt to deliver the posterior shoulder first, thereby leaving more room in the pelvis. Find the fetal elbow and flex the forearm and deliver it by sweeping it over the chest and face.

This should allow the anterior shoulder to deliver by normal traction on the head, but if it does not then rotate the baby and deliver the initial anterior shoulder in a similar way.

R *Roll* the mother over and attempt all manoeuvres again.

Each manoeuvre should be attempted for 20 to 30 seconds.

If all these methods fail, more invasive and 'last resort' procedures must be performed including symphysiotomy (where a scalpel is used to split the symphyseal joint), deliberate fracture of the anterior clavicle to reduce bisacromial distance, or the Zavanelli manoeuvre, which involves pushing the fetus's head back with flexion and rotation and performing a caesarean section.

18. CHRONIC PELVIC PAIN (1)

C – Endometriosis

Endometriosis is the most likely diagnosis, with the typical symptoms of abdominal pain, dyspareunia, secondary dysmenorrhoea and subfertility. Bimanual palpation in this case has revealed a tender fixed uterus, but there can also be uterosacral nodules, endometriomas, uterine or ovarian enlargement or adnexal tenderness.

Endometriosis is where functioning endometrial tissue is seen outside the cavity of the uterus. This tissue responds to the cyclical hormonal changes and bleeds at the time of menstruation forming abdominal deposits. The ovaries, uterosacral ligaments or ovarian fossae are common sites of this endometrial tissue. If there is deposition near the bowels, rectal bleeding can be seen. It is most common in 25- to 35-year olds. The aetiology is unclear and likely to be multifactorial.

An ultrasound is useful to exclude other pathology but is not diagnostic of endometriosis. It may pick up an endometrioma (a blood-filled ovarian cyst often seen in endometriosis). Endometriomas are also known as chocolate cysts due to their dark, reddish brown appearance. Diagnosis can only be made by clinical appearances on laparoscopy. Treatment choices depend on the patient's age, fertility wishes and location and severity of disease. Medical treatment includes analgesia, the combined oral contraceptive pill, progestogens and gonadotrophin-releasing hormone analogues. Although useful for symptomatic relief, many of these options are not appropriate if the woman is trying to conceive. Surgical treatment is used where fertility is required. Infertility is common even without visible tube blockage. *In vitro* fertilization may be required.

Chronic pelvic inflammatory disease describes episodes of recurrent acute pelvic infection that result in chronic inflammation of the pelvic organs with multiple adhesions causing abdominal pain, dyspareunia and subfertility. Chronic pelvic pain can be caused by adhesions from previous surgery; however, the significant menstrual symptoms again point one away from this diagnosis. Treatment options for this include adhesiolysis; this is more likely to be effective if there are large adhesions and if it is done laparoscopically. There is still a significant risk of visceral damage and a chance of further adhesions developing.

The pain from an ovarian cyst can be due to torsion, cyst rupture or bleeding into a cyst. This would be unlikely to give menstrual and fertility problems. Other causes of chronic pelvic pain can be functional pain, constipation or irritable bowel syndrome.

19. SCREENING (1)

B – Chorionic villus sampling

Chorionic villus sampling is a diagnostic test, which means a definite diagnosis can be given rather than a 'risk' of a condition being present. A biopsy of the chorionic villus is taken either transabdominally or transcervically under ultrasound guidance. Obtained cells are analyzed and a result is ready in 48 hours. The risk of miscarriage is around 1%; therefore couples must be counselled appropriately before undertaking this test. It is performed at 11 to 14 weeks, which means this woman could proceed with this test after appropriate counselling. The early gestation means a decision regarding termination of pregnancy can be made as early as possible before a pregnancy becomes easily visible under clothes. Chorionic villus sampling is not performed before 9 to 11 weeks as fetal limb abnormalities can occur. There are cases where inconclusive results can occur due to placental mosaicism; this would mean that amniocentesis would have to be performed later. There can be maternal contamination, which would lead to false-negative results. Rhesus D negative women must receive anti-D immunoglobulin. Amniocentesis is where amniotic fluid is collected transabdominally. This is performed at a later gestation as prior to 14 weeks there is a higher chance of talipes.

The screening test that she has had would have been the *combined test,* which is the combination of nuchal translucency and two serum markers from a maternal blood test (βhCG and PAPP-A) to indicate the risk of the fetus having Down syndrome. It is performed between 11+0 and 13+6 weeks' gestation.

Nuchal translucency is the measurement of the thickness of the skin over the back of the fetal neck. If thickened, it is a marker of fetal abnormalities, and the patient should be referred to a fetal medicine specialist. A *first trimester ultrasound scan* is used to establish fetal number, viability and gestation during the first trimester. It detects defects in gross anatomy and determines the chorionicity and amnionicity of multiple pregnancies.

Non-invasive prenatal testing (NIPT) is not currently widely available, but it is important that you have knowledge of it, as it is likely to significantly change the way fetal chromosomal abnormalities are detected. Fetal DNA is found in maternal plasma; therefore, by taking a blood sample from the mother it is possible to gain information about fetal conditions. It can be used to test for aneuploidy, especially Down syndrome, for assessing a fetus at risk of haemolytic disease of the newborn and for determining sex in cases where high-risk, sex-linked conditions may be present. It is much more accurate than existing screening strategies, but it is not yet regarded as a diagnostic assay. At present, a diagnostic test such as CVS or amniocentesis would still be used to confirm the diagnosis.

20. TWINS (1)

E – Monozygotic monochorionic diamniotic

The incidence of twins is 1 in 100, and triplets 1 in 1000. Predisposing factors are increasing maternal age and parity, personal or family history, race and assisted conception. Multiple pregnancies need closer monitoring as fetal and maternal mortality and morbidity are greater. The mother has a greater risk of hyperemesis, miscarriage, hypertension and pre-eclampsia, gestational diabetes, polyhydramnios (especially with monozygotics), anaemia, antepartum and postpartum haemorrhages and placenta praevia. The fetal risks include increased perinatal mortality, increased congenital abnormality, preterm labour, placental insufficiency or intrauterine growth restriction (especially in monozygotics), malpresentation, twin-to-twin transfusion and vanishing twin syndrome.

Twin-to-twin transfusion is where, due to anastomosis of vessels in the single placental mass of a monochorionic twin pregnancy, one twin gains at the other's expense. It does not happen in dichorionic twin pregnancies. One twin becomes anaemic, hypovolaemic, oligohydramniotic and growth-restricted while the other one develops polycythaemia, hypervolaemia, polyuria and polyhydramnios. It occurs in varying degrees in up to 35% of monochorionic twins and accounts for 15% of perinatal mortality. Ultrasound scan is used to look at fetal well-being and to identify any abnormalities such as liquor volume that may suggest twin-to-twin transfusion. Therapeutic amniocentesis may be used to reduce the amniotic fluid pressure. Laser ablation of placental vessels can be useful although there is a risk of fetal demise.

Vanishing twin syndrome is where a fetus in a multiple-gestation pregnancy dies *in utero* and is subsequently reabsorbed by the mother (either partially or completely).

The delivery of twins requires special management. If the first twin is cephalic, a trial of labour is normally attempted regardless of the presentation of the second twin, but there is no definitive evidence comparing vaginal delivery to caesarean section. If the first twin is breech or transverse lie, a caesarean section is offered. Problems with delivery include cord prolapse, entanglement or knotting, locking, postpartum haemorrhage, thrombosis, fetal distress (especially in the second twin) and inefficient uterine activity after the first twin is delivered.

Monozygotic twins result from the mitotic division of a single fertilized ovum (zygote) into identical twins. They may or may not share the same chorion and amnion depending on when the mitotic division occurs. Monozygotic monochorionic monoamniotic twins occur rarely when the mitotic division occurs after 8 days. If this occurs prior to the formation of the primitive streak, there will be a single amniotic cavity and chorion. If the division occurs after primitive streak formation, conjoined (Siamese) twins develop.

Monozygotic monochorionic diamniotic twins result if division occurs between 4 and 7 days (during formation of the inner cell mass). There is a single placenta but, if the amnion has not developed, each fetus will have its own amniotic membrane. This is the most common type of monozygotic twin (66%) compared with monozygotic dichorionic diamniotic (30%), monozygotic monochorionic monoamniotic (3%) and conjoined (1%).

Monozygotic dichorionic dizygotic twins result if the division occurs at less than 3 days after fertilization (at the 'eight-cell' stage). The two embryos implant at separate sites and have a separate chorion, amnion and placenta. They will have the same structural appearance *in utero* as dizygotic twins do but will be identical.

Dizygotics are the most common type of twins (60%). They develop due to fertilization of two different ova, from the same or opposite ovaries, by two different sperm, and are therefore not identical. They can be of different sexes and are no more genetically similar than siblings would be. They are *always* dichorionic and diamniotic, which means each fetus has its own chorion, amnion and placenta. Options B (dizygotic dichorionic monoamniotic) and C (dizygotic monochorionic monoamniotic) are nonsense!

The term *Siamese twins* originated with Chang and Eng Bunker, a famous pair of conjoined twins who travelled the world with a circus in the nineteenth century. They were born in Siam (now Thailand).

21. OBSTETRIC EMERGENCIES (2)

B – Cord prolapse

Cord prolapse is when the cord passes through the cervix before the baby has been delivered. Cord presentation is where the cord lies below the presenting part with intact membranes, meaning it is more likely to prolapse when the waters break. Cord prolapse is life-threatening for the baby as the supply of blood can be greatly reduced due to either mechanical compression of the umbilical cord by the presenting part or to spasm of the umbilical vessels due to cooling, drying, pH change and handling. The cardiotocograph (CTG) will reflect the effect of these changes by indicating fetal distress, showing deep decelerations or a prolonged bradycardia.

There is an increased risk of cord prolapse in ARM due to the sudden rush of fluid, particularly with a high presenting part. Therefore, it is important to perform a vaginal examination following an ARM to ensure there is no cord prolapse. In this case, it may be prudent to perform the ARM in theatre, so an emergency caesarean section could be performed immediately if the cord did prolapse.

As seen in this case, cord prolapse is more likely in cases where there is not a close fit between the presenting part and the pelvic inlet such as a high head, malpresentation such as transverse or oblique lie, breech presentation particularly footling breech, prematurity, polyhydramnios and fetal growth restriction. It is also seen where there is a long umbilical cord or in a second twin. Of course it can occur without risk factors, and a vaginal examination should be done to rule out a cord prolapse if there are CTG abnormalities after spontaneous rupture of membranes.

Management, as with all emergencies, is to call for help including senior obstetricians and anaesthetists, and to alert theatre staff as it is important to deliver the baby as soon as possible. If the woman is fully dilated, forceps or ventouse delivery should be attempted and, if she is not fully dilated, an emergency caesarean section (category 1) should be performed. On the way to theatre, pressure must be taken off the cord, so a 'head down, bottom up' position is adopted on the bed with the woman placed on all fours with her buttocks uppermost. A hand can be placed in the vagina to lift the presenting part off the cord to prevent compression. In a community setting, the maternal bladder can be filled with saline, via a catheter, which keeps the presenting part off the cord.

22. PERINEAL TEARS

C – Third-degree tear, 3a

Tears of the perineum can occur in normal deliveries but are often more severe in operative delivery, particularly if an episiotomy is not performed.

Tears are graded as follows:

- *First degree* – injury to perineal skin only. There is no need for routine suturing unless haemostasis is a problem.
- *Second degree* – injury to perineum involving perineal muscles without involvement of the anal sphincter. These should be sutured to ensure correct apposition of the perineal muscles and skin and to secure haemostasis. Many midwives will suture second-degree tears. These can be repaired using local anaesthetic.
- *Third degree* – injury to perineum involving the anal sphincter complex. These must be sutured in theatre with adequate analgesia, spinal or epidural top-up, by a trained surgeon, normally the obstetric registrar or consultant. The anal sphincter must be repaired to avoid incontinence.
  - 3a – less than 50% external anal sphincter (EAS) thickness torn
  - 3b – more than 50% EAS thickness torn
  - 3c – both EAS and internal anal sphincter (IAS) torn

- *Fourth degree* – injury to perineum involving the anal sphincter complex and anal/rectal epithelium. These must be repaired in theatre with adequate analgesia by a trained obstetrician with the assistance of a general surgeon, if required.

Third- and fourth-degree tears can lead to faecal incontinence if unrecognized. Obstetric anal injury is seen in 1% of vaginal deliveries with increased risk seen with high birthweight babies (>4 kg), persistent occipitoposterior position, nulliparity, induction of labour, epidural, prolonged second stage (>1 hour), shoulder dystocia, midline episiotomy and forceps delivery.

Post-repair advice should be given to all women, which includes performing regular pelvic floor muscle exercises, avoiding constipation, good hygiene measures and antibiotics. Follow-up should be offered, which may include endo-anal ultrasound if symptomatic.

An episiotomy is a mediolateral cut through the perineum from the posterior end of the vaginal opening generally at a 45° angle towards the woman's right side. It is important to perform this under local anaesthetic in the absence of any regional block.

23. MENSTRUAL HORMONES (2)

E – Progesterone

Progesterone is a steroid hormone produced by the corpus luteum. The corpus luteum is the remnant of the Graafian (ovarian) follicle after the oocyte and cumulus oophorus have been expelled. After ovulation, the remnants are penetrated by capillaries and fibroblasts while the granulosa cells undergo luteinization to collectively form the corpus luteum (yellow body).

There are very low levels of progesterone during the follicular phase. There is an immediate rise in progesterone following ovulation due to the formation of the corpus luteum; progesterone concentration is maximal in the luteal phase of the menstrual cycle (days 15–28). If conception does not occur, the corpus luteum will degenerate after 14 days, production of both steroid sex hormones declines and the next cycle begins. If conception and implantation occur, the corpus luteum is maintained by gonadotrophin released by the trophoblast.

The luteal phase of the menstrual cycle correlates to the secretory phase of the endometrium. The high level of progesterone means secretory vacuoles develop in the glandular epithelium below the nuclei, which then release secretions into the lumen of the glands, which become tortuous. After ovulation, the rise in progesterone opposes the action of oestrogen and stimulates production of thick cervical mucus – which is less penetrable by sperm – and contraction of the cervical os.

Luteum, from Latin *luteum* = yellow.
Regnier de Graaf, Dutch physician and anatomist (1641–1673).

24. METHODS OF DELIVERY (2)

D – Normal delivery

This case describes very good conditions for a normal delivery. Most importantly, the cardiotocograph is normal, so labour can continue without intervention.

The head is low in the pelvis, as shown by there being no head palpable per abdomen and a station of +1, which increases the chances of a normal delivery. Abdominal examination of the fetal head is described by 'fifths' of the head palpable. The head is five-fifths palpable when all the head can be felt *per abdomen* and, if it is free, it can be balloted between the examiner's hands. The head is described as engaged if there is less than two-fifths palpable. In this case, the head cannot be palpated abdominally so it is described as zero-fifths palpable. Station describes the position of the presenting part in relation to the ischial spines. A station of 0 is where the presenting part is level with the ischial spines. A station above the ischial spines is described as –1 to –3, and below the ischial spines (closer to the introitus) is described as +1 to +2. A vaginal delivery is more likely with a more positive station.

She has reached full dilation, and a flexed head in the occipitoanterior position is the optimal position of the fetal head to achieve a normal delivery. There is no caput or moulding, which indicates there is adequate room in the pelvis for the head to descend as there has been minimal compression on the fetal head.

Vaginal delivery is not contraindicated following one caesarean section and is known as vaginal birth after caesarean (VBAC). In these cases, there is increased monitoring and more cautious use of induction and augmentation agents due to the risk of scar rupture.

25. RHESUS DISEASE (1)

B – Give antenatal anti-D prophylaxis 500 IU and take Kleihauer test

At booking, all women are offered blood tests to screen for infection and to establish maternal blood group. Fifteen percent of women are rhesus D negative (RhD –ve), which means their red blood cells lack the rhesus D antigen (compared to RhD +ve women who do carry the D antigen). The rhesus status of a woman must be clearly documented on her antenatal notes as, if there is any passage of fetal blood into the maternal circulation, there can be serious consequences for subsequent pregnancies.

The lack of rhesus D antigen in RhD –ve women means they are at risk of developing anti-D antibodies to an RhD +ve fetus. If any fetal blood cells from an RhD +ve fetus cross into the circulation of an RhD –ve woman, she will react to the 'foreign' anti-D antigens on the fetus's red blood cells and produce antibodies. This is known as a sensitizing event. This is of no consequence in the current pregnancy but, in future pregnancies, the maternal anti-D antibodies can cross the placenta and destroy the blood cells of a subsequent RhD +ve fetus resulting in haemolytic disease of the newborn (varies from subclinical disease to severe disability or death). Anti-D prophylaxis prevents production of anti-D antibodies by providing anti-D immunoglobulins either routinely or after a sensitizing event. The frequency of haemolytic disease of the newborn was 1% of all births before immunoprophylaxis. Now it is reduced to 1 in 21,000 births.

The RCOG guidelines describe when anti-D prophylaxis must be given. All women who are RhD −ve are offered routine antenatal anti-D prophylaxis 500 IU at 28 and 34 weeks (or in some units a larger single dose at 28 weeks) regardless of sensitizing events or previous administration of anti-D. RhD −ve women are offered antenatal anti-D prophylaxis at the time of any possible sensitizing event (as described above) where fetal blood could enter the maternal circulation, such as antepartum haemorrhage, abdominal injury, external cephalic version of the fetus, invasive prenatal diagnosis (amniocentesis, chorionic villus sampling, fetal blood sampling), other intrauterine procedures (insertion of shunts, embryo reduction) or intrauterine death. The dose is 250 IU before 20 weeks and 500 IU after 20 weeks' gestation. Postnatally, if an RhD −ve woman has given birth to an RhD +ve baby, 500 IU anti-D prophylaxis should be offered. The anti-D Ig is given intramuscularly as soon after the sensitizing event as possible and ideally within 72 hours; however, there is evidence that it still provides some protection if given within 10 days. Women only require anti-D prophylaxis if they have not previously been sensitized (as this would mean antibodies to the D antigen would already be present in the blood). This is detected by a blood test at the start of the pregnancy.

After all sensitizing events and delivery, a Kleihauer blood test should be taken to ensure a higher dose of anti-D is not required if there has been particularly large fetomaternal haemorrhage (FMH). The test measures the amount of fetal haemoglobin in the maternal blood.

The rhesus system is named after the rhesus macaques (rhesus monkeys), who were first shown to possess the antigens. The five main rhesus antigens are C, c, D, E and e.

26. BISHOP SCORE

C – 4

The Bishop score is a classification system used to describe the 'favourability' of the cervix. A higher score is associated with an easier, shorter labour that is less likely to fail. Although it is a universal system, it is subject to examiner variation. Therefore, the same person should examine the woman to assess progress.

The modified Bishop scoring system is as follows:

Cervical feature	0	1	2	3
Dilation (cm)	<1	1–2	2–4	>4
Consistency	Firm	Average	Soft	–
Length of cervix (cm)	>4	2–4	1–2	<1
Position	Posterior	Mid/anterior	–	–
Station of presenting part (related to ischial spines)	−3	−2	−1 or 0	Below spines

This woman scores 0 for dilation, 1 for length of cervix, 1 for station, 1 for consistency and 1 for position, giving a score of 4.

Labour is unlikely to be imminent if the score is less than 6, so induction with vaginal prostaglandins would be indicated. If the score is above 9, labour is likely to progress without medical assistance although a stretch and sweep may speed up the process or, if possible, an artificial rupture of membranes could be performed. At a score between 6 and 9, management will depend on the indication for induction.

The original Bishop score included effacement of the cervix instead of length of cervix.

27. PATHOGENESIS OF CERVICAL CANCER (1)

C – Increased number of sexual partners

Cervical cancer is largely a disease of sexually active women. Women with the disease have generally had more sexual partners, are likely to have started having intercourse earlier and are less likely to have used barrier protection. (Always remember that the sexual behaviour of their partners is also important.) The reason for this correlation is that cervical cancer has a strong association with the human papillomavirus (HPV), a sexually transmitted DNA virus. There is a link between HPV serotypes 16, 18 and 33 with pre-invasive disease and invasive cancer.

There is some evidence to suggest that prolonged use of the oral contraceptive pill produces a moderately increased risk of cervical cancer of both the squamous cell and the rarer adenocarcinoma type. There is also an associated increase in mortality. It has been suggested that this effect may be due to differences in sexual behaviour in women who use the oral contraceptive pill compared with those who do not; however, there is no evidence demonstrating that the progesterone-only pill increases cervical cancer risk. Such studies cannot be corrected for all variables as it is difficult to establish the exact sexual activities of both the women and their partners.

Smokers are at increased risk of cervical cancer. This may be due to chemical carcinogenesis or to alterations in immune function in the cervical epithelium as smoking is known to reduce the number of Langerhans' cells that are involved in local immune surveillance. Immunocompromised women are more likely to contract cervical cancer.

Unlike endometrial carcinoma, there is no link to the onset or arrest of menstruation in cervical cancer. Parous women are more likely to suffer from cervical carcinoma.

Cervix, from Latin *cervix* = neck.

28. BLEEDING IN PREGNANCY (2)

C – Placenta praevia

Antepartum haemorrhage is defined as bleeding after 24 weeks' gestation. Between 2% and 4% of women have antepartum haemorrhage. Bleeding can be maternal, fetal or placental. Sometimes no cause can be found.

Placenta praevia is where the placenta lies close to, or covers, the internal os. It occurs in 1% of pregnancies. It is more common in older women, previous caesarean section, increasing parity, previous placenta praevia, smoking and multiple gestations. Placenta praevia is graded from I to IV, or classified as major or minor, as follows:

Minor	I	Encroaches on lower segment
	II	Reaches internal os (marginal)
Major	III	Covers part of os (partial)
	IV	Completely covers the os (complete)

A placenta praevia may be found at the 20-week scan and, if seen, a repeat scan at 34 to 36 weeks is performed. Ninety percent of placenta praevia seen at the 20-week scan will no longer be praevia later on as the placenta moves away from the os due to uterine growth.

Clinically, there is sudden-onset painless unprovoked or postcoital fresh red blood *per vagina* in the second or third trimester. On abdominal examination, there is a soft non-tender uterus with a high head or mal-presentation as the placenta blocks the passage of the presenting part into the pelvis. The clinical condition of the mother correlates with the visible blood loss (unlike uterine abruption). Maternal blood is lost, so there is little risk to the fetus unless the mother becomes hypovolaemic.

Management depends on multiple factors including gestation and condition of the fetus and clinical condition of the mother. There could be sudden major haemorrhage at any time. For this reason, some women who have had heavy bleeds or who live far from the hospital are advised to be admitted from 30 to 32 weeks until delivery (which is generally planned for 38–39 weeks but may be earlier if indicated). If there is major haemorrhage that is threatening maternal or fetal life, a caesarean section should be performed. Risks include haemorrhagic shock, complications of caesarean section, transfusion-related complications and, if there is a concurrent placenta accreta, massive haemorrhage (which may need hysterectomy).

Placenta, from Greek *plakous* = flat cake.
Praevia, from Latin *prae* = ahead of + *via* = road (i.e. 'in the way').

29. MISCARRIAGE (1)

E – Threatened miscarriage

Miscarriage is defined (in the UK) as the loss of pregnancy before 24 weeks. It is the most common complication of pregnancy and occurs in 25% of all pregnancies. The risk of miscarriage is highest early in pregnancy and decreases as gestation increases. Most are unexplained, but underlying causes of miscarriage include fetal abnormality, infection (ToRCH – toxoplasmosis, other infections, rubella virus, cytomegalovirus and herpes simplex virus), increasing maternal age, maternal illness (diabetes, renal disease), abnormal uterine cavity (intrauterine device, congenital septum), antiphospholipid syndrome and intervention (amniocentesis and chorionic villus sampling). It is important to inform women that exercise, intercourse and emotional trauma *do not* cause miscarriage. Investigation into the cause of miscarriage is generally only performed if three miscarriages have occurred. Although miscarriages are very common, they are distressing to parents, so it is important to act with care and sensitivity.

Clinical presentation of miscarriage is varied with some women experiencing very little pain and bleeding and passing the fetus with no complications while other women have life-threatening vaginal bleeding and severe pain.

This scenario describes a threatened miscarriage. There can be cramping, lower abdominal pain with vaginal bleeding. On examination, the cervical os is closed. Only 25% of threatened miscarriages eventually miscarry. A scan should be arranged to investigate the bleeding and to confirm the viability of the pregnancy. This can be done in an early pregnancy assessment unit (EPAU).

An inevitable miscarriage generally presents with cramping abdominal pain and vaginal bleeding, but on examination the cervical os is open in contrast to a threatened miscarriage. The fetus may still be alive, but miscarriage *will* occur due to dilation of the cervical os. An incomplete miscarriage is where some fetal material has been passed but some products of conception are retained in the uterus (these are visible on ultrasound scanning). The cervical os remains open until all the products have passed (whether that be spontaneous or with medical or surgical assistance). This can be associated with a significant amount of bleeding. A complete miscarriage describes passage of all fetal tissue with closure of the cervical os. Hospital follow-up is generally not required, but a pregnancy test should be performed after 3 weeks to ensure it has returned to negative. Finally, a missed miscarriage (previously known as a delayed or silent miscarriage) is when the fetus dies *in utero* and the cervix stays closed. This is only discovered on an ultrasound scan. There may or may not be bleeding in this case. The management for this can be conservative, medical or surgical.

30. PAIN IN PREGNANCY (1)

C – Chorioamnionitis

Chorioamnionitis is infection of the amniotic cavity and the chorioamniotic membranes. Causative pathogens include *Escherichia coli*, *Streptococcus* and *Enterococcus faecalis*. Both mother and fetus can develop potentially life-threatening septicaemia. It is normally seen after rupture of membranes, particularly if this has been over a prolonged period of time, although it can occur with intact membranes. Other risk factors include prolonged labour, preterm labour, internal fetal monitoring, cervical examinations or urinary tract or vaginal infection.

A woman with chorioamnionitis can present with abdominal pain, uterine tenderness, fever and meconium or foul-smelling liquor. On examination and investigation, there may be maternal pyrexia and tachycardia, raised C-reactive protein and raised white cell count. There could be fetal tachycardia or a non-reassuring cardiotocograph. If there is chorioamnionitis, the baby must be delivered. Antibiotics are needed for the mother and baby, and the paediatricians should be present at the delivery. Often the baby will be admitted for antibiotics and observations, as infection can be serious in newborns.

If a woman attends with suspected pre-labour spontaneous rupture of membranes (SROM), a digital examination *must not* be performed as this increases the risk of introducing infection. Either a sample of liquor is obtained or a sterile speculum examination performed. The cervix should be visualized and the woman asked to cough to identify liquor coming from the cervix. If at term, they should be offered immediate induction of labour or expectant management, as they will often go into labour naturally: 70% by 24 hours. Expectant management should not exceed 24 hours.

Pregnant women are predisposed to urinary tract infections (UTIs) due to a short female urethra and gravid uterus. Increased urinary frequency, dysuria, offensive smelling urine, suprapubic pain, fever and tachycardia are seen. There can be uterine tightenings and a speculum examination must be done. A dipstick and midstream urine (MSU) culture are performed with the most likely organism being *E. coli*. Treatment is usually with cephradine or amoxicillin, which are both safe and effective in pregnancy, unless the organisms are resistant. Recurrent UTIs need further investigations.

The chance of ascending renal infection is increased in pregnancy due to higher levels of progesterone ($\rightarrow$ dilation of the urinary system) and the physical presence of the baby ($\rightarrow$ obstructive uropathy and urinary stasis). Presentation is of an unwell patient with fever and rigors, nausea and vomiting, typically loin to groin pain and urinary frequency with dysuria. A urine dip should be taken and MSU sent for culture. A renal ultrasound scan may show hydronephrosis. The patient may report uterine tightenings, which can occur due to general inflammation; for this reason, there is a risk of preterm labour with severe UTI and bacteraemia. A speculum must be performed as silent cervical dilation can occur. Treatment includes analgesia, fluids and intravenous antibiotics.

31. ACUTE PELVIC PAIN (1)

C – Ovarian cyst torsion

This case describes an intermittent ovarian cyst torsion, which has become an acute problem. Torsion of an ovarian cyst results in a sudden-onset severe, unilateral, colicky or twisting pain with intermittent pain if torsion is incomplete. Vomiting is common and tachycardia, hypotension and low-grade pyrexia can be found on examination. This must not be missed as delay can lead to irreversible ischaemia of the ovary. An urgent laparoscopy is needed where the pedicle is untwisted and ideally blood supply returns, but signs of irreversible ischaemia or necrosis warrant oophorectomy.

The management of untorted ovarian cysts varies depending on symptoms and investigation findings. For a cyst to be low risk, the patient would have a normal serum CA-125 and ultrasound would show a small, simple, unilateral, unilocular cyst. These can be managed conservatively if the patient is asymptomatic, as 50% resolve spontaneously, but must be followed up with an ultrasound scan in 3 to 4 months. If cysts are symptomatic, then surgical removal is considered. A cyst associated with an elevated CA-125, with ultrasound appearances of a complex, bilateral or multinodular cyst, or that is larger than 5 cm is considered to be at higher risk of cancer. The patient should be referred to the MDT where the images and biochemistry can be discussed if there is concern of cancer. Surgical removal may be needed in a specialist centre. A histological diagnosis is essential for appropriate follow-up.

Pelvic inflammatory disease (ascending infection through the genital tract via sexual contact) is unlikely in this case. The patient denies recent sexual contact, is apyrexial and has no abnormal discharge. Appendicitis tends to present with central abdominal pain, which later localizes to the right iliac fossa and is associated with anorexia, malaise and nausea. Renal colic presents with loin pain radiating to the groin.

Mittelschmerz is the name given to the lower abdominal pain that occurs during the middle of the menstrual cycle. It corresponds with ovulation. Mittelschmerz pains are benign and experienced by at least 20% of women, most commonly by teenagers and older women. Treatment is with simple analgesia or by use of the oral contraceptive pill (to suppress ovulation).

Mittelschmerz, from German *mittel* = middle + *schmerz* = pain (pain that occurs mid-cycle).

32. EARLY PREGNANCY (1)

B – Early intrauterine pregnancy

The fact that the βhCG was below 1000 IU on the day of the transvaginal scan explains the reason why an intrauterine pregnancy was not seen. Generally, a level of 1000 IU or more is associated with being able to visualize the gestational sac on transvaginal scan. The βhCG was therefore repeated 48 hours later and doubled, suggesting a healthy intrauterine pregnancy. An ultrasound scan can be repeated in a week to confirm viability of the pregnancy.

If the repeat βhCG is static or only slowly reducing, an ectopic pregnancy must be considered and further investigation or management should be initiated. If the βhCG level rapidly reduces, it is likely that it is a failing pregnancy and the patient can be treated conservatively with regular βhCG measurements to ensure resolution.

An empty uterus with a positive pregnancy test (i.e., a pregnancy of unknown location [PUL]) can mean three things: a complete miscarriage, a very early intrauterine pregnancy that is too small to visualize or an ectopic pregnancy. As seen in this question, βhCG can be used to aid diagnosis. If βhCG is >1000 IU, a gestational sac should be seen on a transvaginal scan; therefore, an empty uterus with this result could indicate an ectopic pregnancy. If βhCG is <1000 IU, it may be too early to visualize a gestational sac. In both cases, serial βhCGs must be used. Serum βhCG should double in 48 hours in viable intrauterine pregnancies. A plateau of βhCG suggests ectopic pregnancy, and a significant fall in βhCG suggests a miscarriage; however, this is not always true. An ultrasound can be repeated in 1 week if the βhCG doubles and the patient remains well. A diagnostic laparoscopy is considered if the βhCG levels are not rising satisfactorily or if there is pain.

33. MENSTRUAL DISORDERS

B – Primary dysmenorrhoea

Dysmenorrhoea describes cyclical cramping pains occurring before or during menstruation, which may be associated with malaise and gastrointestinal symptoms. Fifty percent of women have some pain during periods, with 10% describing it as severe. Primary dysmenorrhoea occurs from menarche, and there is often no cause found. Secondary dysmenorrhoea has an onset after menarche; it is often associated with pathology such as endometriosis, pelvic inflammatory disease, fibroids or iatrogenic causes including copper intrauterine devices or cervical stenosis after large loop excision of the transformation zone (LLETZ).

Treatment for primary and secondary dysmenorrhoea includes using a hot water bottle, transcutaneous electrical nerve stimulation, acupuncture and non-steroidal anti-inflammatory drugs (NSAIDs), especially mefanamic acid. (The latter reduce the uterine production of prostaglandins and can also reduce heavy blood loss.) Hormonal treatments include combined oral contraceptives, depot progestogens and the Mirena coil (levonorgestrel intrauterine device).

Amenorrhoea is the absence of menstruation. This would be a normal occurrence before puberty, during pregnancy and breastfeeding and after menopause. Primary amenorrhoea means the menstrual cycle never begins due to anatomical abnormalities, genetic disorders or hormonal imbalances or any of the secondary causes. Secondary amenorrhoea means menstruation stops, having previously been present, and can be due to disorders of the hypothalamic–pituitary axis, deficiency of ovarian or thyroid hormones, anorexia nervosa or significant change in surroundings or circumstances.

34. MECHANISMS OF LABOUR (2)

E – Internal rotation

35. ACUTE PELVIC PAIN (2)

C – Ectopic pregnancy

This is most likely to be an ectopic pregnancy that may have ruptured leading to bleeding into the abdominal cavity, causing the woman to collapse and become clinically shocked. Appendicitis, cyst torsion and pelvic inflammatory disease are possible, but with the history of 6 weeks of amenorrhoea and the severity of the presentation, ectopic pregnancy is the condition that must urgently be treated or ruled out as she is already compromised.

Ectopic pregnancy describes implantation of the embryo outside the uterine cavity, most commonly in the fallopian tube, but also in the cornu of uterus, cervix, ovary or abdominal cavity. Presentation is variable and ectopic pregnancy must always be considered in a woman of childbearing age with amenorrhoea, lower abdominal pain, abnormal vaginal bleeding associated with dizziness, fainting, shoulder pain or collapse. On examination there is abdominal tenderness with cervical excitation, tender adnexae or an adnexal mass in a shocked patient.

If the patient is shocked, resuscitation using ABC is required followed by urgent laparoscopy or laparotomy to remove the ectopic and stop the bleeding. In a stable patient, a transvaginal ultrasound scan should be performed. Depending on the scan result, management can be medical (methotrexate) with serial βhCG measurements, or surgical. Rhesus D negative women should be given anti-D immunoglobulin.

Ectopic pregnancies are becoming increasingly common in the UK. The incidence is 1:200–400 pregnancies. Risk factors include pelvic inflammatory disease, previous tubal surgery, previous ectopic pregnancy, assisted reproductive techniques, endometriosis, intrauterine contraceptive devices and the progesterone-only pill, although 50% occur in people with no predisposing risk factors.

Intrauterine coils can dislodge, resulting in discoloured vaginal discharge and lower abdominal pain. Speculum examination would indicate the position of the coil by seeing the threads through the cervix. If the threads are not present, an ultrasound scan or X-ray can be done to locate the coil. If the threads are present, the coil is likely to be in the correct place or it could be lodged in the cervix causing pain and discharge. It is unlikely to cause shock and collapse.

Ectopic, from Greek *ek* = away from + *topos* = place (i.e. in the wrong place).

36. PAIN IN PREGNANCY (2)

D – HELLP syndrome

HELLP syndrome is the hepatic manifestation of pregnancy-induced hypertension, characterized by hepatic and haematological dysfunctions. The name is an acronym of the biochemical findings: haemolysis, elevated liver enzymes and low platelets. The patient presents with nausea, vomiting and epigastric/right upper quadrant pain due to haemorrhage or distension of the liver capsule. There is often a sudden onset and, despite the normal association with pre-eclampsia, 10% to 20% of women with HELLP have no high blood pressure and therefore no warning that they will develop the condition. HELLP has high mortality and morbidity with progression to acute renal failure and disseminated intravascular coagulation, and there is increased risk of abruption. Treatment includes correction of coagulopathy, anti-seizure prophylaxis and antihypertensives. The fetus must be assessed with ultrasound and monitored by cardiotocograph. Delivery is the only cure, but deterioration can occur 48 hours after delivery. The woman must be counselled that the recurrence rate in subsequent pregnancies is 20%.

Acute fatty liver of pregnancy is rare but serious with a maternal mortality of up to 20%. Presentation is similar to cholecystitis with sudden-onset epigastric pain, anorexia, malaise, nausea, vomiting and diarrhoea. However, in acute fatty liver there is jaundice, mild hypertension or proteinuria, and it can progress to fulminant liver failure. Biochemically, there is raised bilirubin with abnormal liver enzymes, leukocytosis, thrombocytopenia, hypoglycaemia and coagulation defects. This is biochemically distinguishable from HELLP syndrome due to hypoglycaemia. Diagnosis is generally clinical with CT or MRI, but a liver biopsy can be taken if needed. Management is with strict fluid balance, correction of coagulopathy and electrolyte disturbances and hasty delivery. Depending on the severity of the condition, admission to a specialist liver unit or ICU may be needed.

The presenting feature of obstetric cholestasis is severe itching affecting the limbs and the trunk (classically, the palms of the hands and the soles of the feet). It can be quite debilitating for the mother. There is no abdominal pain. Obstetric cholestasis occurs due to impaired bile acid secretion. An increased serum total bile acid concentration confirms the diagnosis, although it can also be diagnosed with other elevated liver function tests (LFTs) provided other causes have been excluded. It generally occurs in the third trimester and is more common with a positive family history. There is an increased risk of iatrogenic preterm delivery, fetal intracranial haemorrhage, fetal distress and intrauterine fetal death; therefore, the fetus should be monitored closely. Delivery at 37 to 38 weeks reduces risk of intrauterine death while not increasing risks associated with prematurity, but the evidence of the optimal time for delivery is unclear. Women should be offered induction of labour after 37 weeks but informed of the additional risks of operative delivery with earlier induction. There are no long-term maternal risks. Chlorphenamine is used for simple relief of itching, but ursodeoxycholic acid can be used to reduce serum bile acids in more severe cases. No medication alters the outcome for the fetus. Other causes of itching and abnormal liver function should be investigated if there are other symptoms. Generalized itching in pregnancy can be caused by scabies, urticaria or eczema. LFTs should be measured postnatally to ensure a return to normal levels.

37. PARITY AND GRAVIDA

C – G6 P2+3

An obstetric history must include the number of pregnancies a woman has had and the outcomes, including gestation at delivery, listed in chronological order. If gestation was more than 24 weeks, a number of other details must be ascertained including mode of delivery, and if not a normal delivery, then why; any complications during pregnancy/delivery to mother/baby; the sex and weight of the baby; and the condition of the baby at birth. Some women have unfortunate obstetric histories, which can include multiple miscarriages or stillbirths, so be prepared to be sympathetic.

Gravida is the number of times a woman has been pregnant regardless of the gestation at delivery. In this case, the woman has been pregnant six times, which includes one normal delivery, one caesarean section, two miscarriages, one termination and the current pregnancy. This is indicated as G6.

Parity describes the number of potentially viable babies a woman has delivered; this includes all live births (even before 24 weeks) and stillbirths delivered after 24 weeks. The woman in the question would be a para 2 (P2) as she has had two deliveries of more than 24 weeks' gestation. The third number preceded by a '+' indicates all pregnancies up to 24 weeks that did not result in a live birth, so this includes miscarriages and terminations. A full description of parity would be para 2 + 3, indicating two miscarriages before 24 weeks and one termination.

Nulliparity describes a woman who has never delivered a potentially live baby (i.e. gestation more than 24 weeks), but she may have had miscarriages or terminations before 24 weeks' gestation. Multiparity describes a woman who has delivered at least one potentially live baby (i.e. gestation over 24 weeks). It is not relevant that there was a different partner, and the modes of delivery are not included in this nomenclature.

This nomenclature can be difficult to understand, and the following is an example of a particularly complex case. A pregnant woman who has had any of the following would be described as G9 P4+4:

- A live birth at 23 weeks
- A stillbirth at 38 weeks
- An emergency section at 37 weeks
- A normal delivery at 31 weeks
- An ectopic pregnancy removed by laparoscopy in the first trimester
- A miscarriage at 12 weeks
- A surgical termination of pregnancy at 11 weeks
- A miscarriage at 22 weeks

This case highlights the need for further information on the outcomes of each pregnancy, and this woman is likely to be particularly anxious around weeks 22–23 and 31 due to previous premature deliveries.

38. EARLY PREGNANCY (2)

B – Ectopic pregnancy

An ectopic pregnancy means the fertilized ovum has implanted outside the uterine cavity. The most common place is the fallopian tube, but they are seen on the ovary, in the cornua of the uterus and in the abdomen. Investigations for pregnancies of unknown origin depend on the clinical condition of the patient. If the patient is well and has no pain or cervical excitation on vaginal examination, outpatient investigations are considered. This includes serial βhCG measurements 48 hours apart and the next available ultrasound scan appointment. In the early stages of a normal pregnancy, the βhCG level should double every 48 hours. If the βhCG plateaus, an ectopic pregnancy must be ruled out. If the βhCG is falling, it is likely to represent a miscarriage. A gestational sac should generally be seen on transvaginal scan if the βhCG level is above 1000 IU (or >3500 IU for transabdominal scans).

Ectopic pregnancy is the most likely diagnosis in this case. Initially the scan is not worrying as a gestational sac should not be expected to be visualized with a βhCG level of 653 IU. The patient was quite rightly discharged and asked to return 48 hours later for a further βhCG test. She would have been advised to return sooner if she had any pain or was concerned by bleeding or feeling unwell. The second βhCG result has not doubled, which would lead us to the diagnosis of ectopic, and further investigation should be considered. If the βhCG had doubled, a repeat scan in one week could be arranged to ensure viability of the pregnancy. If the βhCG had rapidly fallen, a diagnosis of complete miscarriage could have been made and the patient would have been followed up using βhCG. In this case, where she has no pain, a further βhCG could be done to assess the trend and, if still static, methotrexate or laparoscopy could be considered as a treatment.

39. OVARIAN CANCER (2)

D – Serous tumour

The presentation of ovarian cancer is non-specific and varied, and most present late. Most patients present with vague lower abdominal discomfort and abdominal swelling. Women also present with pain, which can be caused by bleeding or ovarian torsion. Other symptoms include anorexia, nausea and vomiting, change in bowel habit, weight loss, abnormal vaginal bleeding, urinary symptoms, malaise, deep vein thrombosis and, rarely, hormonal effects such as virilization and precocious puberty. Signs include an abdominal/pelvic mass, ascites, pleural effusion, cervical lymphadenopathy and hepatomegaly.

Spread through the peritoneal cavity leads to intraperitoneal disease, which gives rise to intestinal obstruction and cachexia. More distant spread includes liver metastases and malignant pleural effusions. Investigations for ovarian cancer include blood tests for routine measurements and tumour markers, pelvic and abdominal ultrasound scan, CT/MRI and chest X-ray. Management must include a multidisciplinary team meeting where diagnosis and management are discussed with gynae-oncologists, pathologists, radiologists and nurse specialists.

Epithelial tumours are the most common of the ovarian tumours and are divided into serous, mucinous, endometrioid, clear cell and urothelial-like (Brenner) tumours. Serous tumours comprise approximately half of all ovarian cancers and are the most common ovarian neoplasm. They occur mainly in women of reproductive age. The benign form – serous cystadenomas – consists of unilocular cysts of variable sizes filled with straw-coloured fluid; 20% are bilateral. The malignant type – serous cystadenocarcinomas – consist of mixed solid areas with unilocular cysts. Histological findings are psammoma bodies that are concentric, laminated calcified concretions. They are bilateral in 30% to 50% of cases. Other types include sex cord/stromal tumours including granulosa cell, thecoma/fibroma tumours and Sertoli/Leydig cell tumours. Germ cell tumours include dysgerminomas, endodermal sinus or yolk sac tumours, choriocarcinomas and teratomas (dermoid cyst).

Treatment for suspected ovarian cancer should be undertaken in a specialist gynaecological cancer unit. Benign tumours are dealt with by simple excision or drainage under laparoscopic control. The problem is in not being sure clinically that the cyst is benign. Statistically, the younger the woman, the more likely it is to be benign. In general, benign cysts are unilateral, unilocular and have smooth internal and external surfaces with no solid elements. Six percent of all ovarian cysts are malignant.

Epithelial cancers can require radical surgical debulking, which involves hysterectomy and bilateral oophorectomy, infracolic omentectomy and inspection of liver and peritoneal surfaces with peritoneal washings or ascites sent for cytology. This may be accompanied by bowel resection and defunctioning colostomy, followed by chemotherapy. If the disease is confined to one ovary and the woman wishes to preserve her fertility, conservative surgery can be considered by doing a unilateral oophorectomy and partial omental biopsy. Often surgery is palliative as the disease presents at such a late stage.

40. POSTPARTUM HAEMORRHAGE (1)

C – Atonic uterus

Vaginal blood loss during a normal delivery is expected to be between 200 and 300 mL. A postpartum haemorrhage (PPH) describes blood loss of more than 500 mL or less than 500 mL if associated with haemodynamic changes in the mother. Around 5% of deliveries are reported to have been associated with PPH, but this number is probably higher as blood loss is often underestimated. Life-threatening PPH occurs in 1 in 1000 deliveries. Primary PPH occurs within the first 24 hours, and secondary PPH ranges from 24 hours to 6 weeks postpartum.

An atonic uterus causes 90% of primary PPH. This occurs when the uterus does not contract down enough, leading to inadequate compression of the intramyometrial blood vessels by the uterine muscles and continued bleeding. It is more common if there is a retained placenta or placental tissue as the physical presence of this prevents contraction of the uterus.

If medical options are not controlling the bleeding, surgical options must be used. A laparotomy is performed for better access to the uterus.

The uterus is massaged directly to attempt to initiate contraction of the uterine muscles. A B-Lynch suture can be used, which is a uterine compression stitch that opposes the anterior and posterior walls to apply continuing compression. The stitch starts on the front wall and goes all the way over the top of the uterus. A stitch is then taken into the posterior wall and is brought back over the top again to the front of the uterus to 'squash' or compress the uterus as much as possible; it looks a little bit like braces when the stitch is completed. Other surgical approaches include over-sewing the placental bed, creating a tamponade using a Rusch balloon, uterine artery or internal iliac artery ligation or hysterectomy as a last resort.

A third- and fourth-degree tear (see Question 22) should be repaired in theatre. A cervical tear could occur if delivery happens prior to full dilatation. A high vaginal tear can occur with a normal delivery but would be more likely if forceps are used.

Christopher B-Lynch, British obstetrician (contemporary).

41. PROLAPSE

A – Cystocele

Prolapse can be asymptomatic, but if symptoms are present they are often non-specific: general discomfort, dragging, a feeling of a lump or swelling that worsens as the day progresses and, rarely, coital problems.

Uterovaginal prolapse is descent of the pelvic organs into the vagina. Descent of a single organ rarely occurs due to the close proximity of the urethra, bladder, uterus, small bowel and rectum. The main predisposing factor allowing descent is weakening of the pelvic tissues by the trauma of childbirth, which is compounded by menopausal oestrogen deficiency and loss of connective tissue strength. Other contributing factors to prolapse formation are congenital causes, previous suprapubic surgery for urinary incontinence and genetic factors. These tend not to occur in isolation; rather, it is a combination of these factors, which are also aggravated by mechanisms that increase intra-abdominal pressure including obesity, cough, constipation, heavy lifting, ascites or a large pelvic mass.

Cystocele describes descent of the bladder through the anterior vaginal wall. This can occur in conjunction with an urethrocele (descent of the first 3–4 cm of the vaginal wall that overlies the urethra). Urinary symptoms occur due to alteration of the urethrovesical angle, which can lead to stress incontinence, urinary frequency or urgency and difficulties in emptying the bladder, which can lead to overflow incontinence. Patients with large cystoceles are predisposed to urinary tract infections due to incomplete emptying of the bladder.

A procidentia can develop where the cervix, uterus and vaginal wall prolapse outside the introitus, which can lead to ulceration and thickening of the vaginal wall. Total vault prolapse occurs after hysterectomy where the top of the vagina everts and protrudes outside the introitus.

A rectocele involves protrusion of the rectum into the lower vaginal wall, which can lead to feeling of incomplete evacuation of bowel. Some women will need to physically push the rectocele back to pass stool. An enterocele is a herniation of small bowel or omentum contained within a sac made of the peritoneal lining of the Pouch of Douglas. This can lead to general lower abdominal discomfort.

If a prolapse is an incidental finding, there is no need for further management. Conservative management such as pelvic floor exercises (PFEs) can be used initially and if the patient is either not suitable for surgery or awaiting surgery. PFEs can help with the associated urinary incontinence but will rarely improve the prolapse once it is established. Vaginal pessaries are very useful for women who want to avoid surgery or who are waiting for surgery. They are inserted into the vagina and push the excess mucosa back inside. Surgical options depend on the fitness of the patient, the type of prolapse and whether the woman wants to remain sexually active. They include anterior or posterior repair and vaginal hysterectomy.

Procidentia, from Latin *procidere* = to fall.
James Marion Sims, American gynecologist (1813–1883).

42. VAGINAL BLEEDING (1)

B – Cervical ectropion

Cervical ectropion is an entirely benign change in the area of mucosa surrounding the lower cervical canal. A florid appearance is described (signifying secretory glandular mucosa). It is often asymptomatic but may cause postcoital bleeding or persistent vaginal discharge. There may be no obvious cause, but it is associated with hormonal changes during puberty, pregnancy or the oral contraceptive pill. Sexually transmitted infections must be ruled out, and a normal smear test must be confirmed. If there is no reason to suspect anything more sinister, then it can be treated with diathermy or cryocautery.

It would be very rare for a woman this young to present with endometrial carcinoma. It is generally a disease of older women who present with postmenopausal bleeding. Prompt investigations must be initiated if there is any suspicion of endometrial cancer including hysteroscopy with endometrial sampling and ultrasound or MRI. Spread is seen directly through the endometrial cavity and cervix and along the fallopian tubes to the ovaries and peritoneal cavity.

Endometrial polyps are common adenomatous lesions, which present with menstrual irregularities. They can cause dysmenorrhoea or postcoital bleeding if they protrude through the cervix; however, they are usually found in the body of the uterus. If found, they should be excised and the tissue histologically analyzed. Cervical polyps usually arise from the endocervical mucosa and are pedunculated. They are seen as bright red growths up to a few centimetres in diameter protruding through the external cervical os. They can cause chronic discharge, postcoital or intermenstrual bleeding or may be asymptomatic and only discovered on routine smear tests. They can be avulsed and the base cauterized with diathermy. Cervical polyps are usually benign, and there is a very low risk of malignancy (1:6000) but any tissue removed should be sent for histology.

Ectropion, from Greek *ek* = out + *trope* = a turning ('an out-turning').

43. PRE-ECLAMPSIA (1)

D – Nifedipine

Pre-eclampsia and eclampsia are pregnancy-specific conditions. There is a spectrum of pathology that includes gestational hypertension/pregnancy-induced hypertension (hypertension alone), pre-eclampsia (hypertension and proteinuria, with or without oedema and involvement of other organs), eclampsia (generalized convulsions in the presence of pre-eclampsia) and HELLP syndrome (haemolysis, elevated liver enzymes and low platelets). Affected women can progress quickly from mild symptoms to convulsions, although some women look unwell but have no serious problems. The only cure is delivery of the baby and placenta. Screening tests of blood pressure and urine dip are done every time the woman sees her midwife or is seen in antenatal clinic.

Symptoms of pre-eclampsia include headache, blurred vision, epigastric pain and vomiting (although most cases are asymptomatic). Clinical signs are high blood pressure, hyperreflexia, proteinuria, hepatic tenderness, oliguria and spontaneous bleeding. Classification of pre-eclampsia is the presence of proteinuria with mild (140/90–149/99 mmHg), moderate (150/100–159/109 mmHg) or severe (>160/110 mmHg) elevations in blood pressure. Indicators of severe disease are cerebral or visual disturbances, abdominal pain, fetal growth restriction, oliguria (urine output <500 mL in 24 hours), impaired liver function tests and thrombocytopenia.

Pre-eclampsia has no definite pathophysiology, but it appears to be caused by a placental factor that leads to endothelial dysfunction. Maternal risk factors for pre-eclampsia include previous hypertensive disorders, chronic renal disease, autoimmune diseases (systemic lupus erythematosus, antiphospholipid disease), diabetes, first pregnancy, age over 40 years, BMI >35, family history of pre-eclampsia and multiple pregnancy.

Blood pressure control

All women with pre-eclampsia should be admitted, and when the blood pressure reaches the threshold of systolic >150 or diastolic >100 mmHg, antihypertensives should be started. Antihypertensives do not 'cure' the disease, but their use may avoid extreme prematurity by limiting the risk of vascular damage due to uncontrolled hypertension. Antihypertensive medication may need to be continued for 3 months postpartum.

Nifedipine is given orally. It is a calcium channel blocker and vasodilator. Side effects include flushing, headache and ankle swelling. This is the most suitable drug in this case.

Labetalol can be given orally but can also be used intravenously. It is an α- and a β-blocker. The side effects are tiredness and headaches. Although labetalol is the drug of choice in pre-eclampsia, it is not suitable in this case due to the history of asthma. Atenolol should be avoided as it is associated with fetal growth restriction. Hydralazine can be given orally, intravenously or intramuscularly and is a direct-acting vasodilator. An unfortunate side effect is that it may mimic impending eclampsia.

Methyldopa can be given orally and acts centrally to decrease the sympathetic outflow from the brain. The main side effect is initial drowsiness. Methyldopa is not used in the acute setting as it is slow to act and may take several days to decrease BP; however, it is a good first-line medication for essential hypertension in pregnancy or as an adjunct. Ramipril is an angiotensin-converting enzyme (ACE) inhibitor that is contraindicated due to adverse fetal effects. Furosemide is a diuretic and should only be used if pulmonary oedema is seen and not for hypertension alone. Magnesium sulphate is used for the prevention and treatment of fits, not hypertension.

44. CONTRACEPTION (1)

C – No – migraines

Migraines with typical focal aura are a contraindication to the combined oral contraceptive pill (COCP).

COCPs are widely used as first-line contraception and are more than 99% effective if taken appropriately. They prevent ovulation, thicken cervical mucus to prevent sperm reaching an egg and thin the lining of the womb to prevent ovum implantation by the action of two hormones: oestrogen and progesterone. Non-contraceptive advantages include a reduction in period pain, menstrual bleeding and premenstrual symptoms. They protect against cancer of the ovary, uterus and colon, as well as some pelvic infections. Fertility quickly returns to normal when the medication is discontinued, so a future desire for children would not be a reason not to prescribe the COCP for this woman. The disadvantages include temporary minor side effects such as headaches, mood changes and breast tenderness, and there is a slightly increased risk of venous thrombosis, breast cancer and cervical cancer. COCPs are less effective with some drugs, vomiting or severe long-lasting diarrhoea, or if pills are missed. In such instances, additional contraception needs to be used.

The UK Medical Eligibility Criteria (UKMEC) guidelines give four categories for use of reversible methods of contraception. '1' means there are no restrictions, '2' means the advantages outweigh the risks (so could be prescribed by a GP but with greater follow-up), '3' means that the risks outweigh the advantages (so would *only* be prescribed by a contraception specialist) and '4' represents an unacceptable risk.

The following are common category 3 or 4 conditions for COCP use and therefore should not be prescribed in a regular GP surgery – see the guideline for full information.

- Pregnancy related: breastfeeding up to 6 months, anyone within 21 days of birth
- Smoking: any smoker over the age of 35 years
- Obesity: BMI >35 kg/m^2
- Hypertension
- Venous thromboembolism (VTE): previous or current VTE, family history of VTE <45 years, immobility
- Known thrombogenic mutations
- Cardiac: current or previous IHD, complicated valvular disease
- Stroke
- Migraine with aura: current or previous history
- Breast disease: current or previous breast cancer, carriers of breast cancer-associated gene mutations
- Diabetes: with complications including nephropathy, retinopathy, neuropathy, vascular disease

45. PREMATURE LABOUR (1)

B – Betamethasone

Premature labour is defined as labour before 37 weeks. It occurs in 5% to 10% pregnancies and incidence is rising, but many women that have threatened preterm labour actually go on to deliver at term. Survival rates are improving with advances in neonatal medicine, but many believe that the limit of viability is reached at 24 weeks' gestation. Certainly the sequelae of extreme prematurity are potentially severe. Onset of labour is suggested by the presence of painful regular contractions associated with cervical change, although there may only be some lower abdominal pain or silent dilation of the cervix.

The causes of preterm labour are not fully understood, but there are a number of risk factors, the greatest of which is previous preterm labour. Maternal factors include extremes of maternal age, smoking, infection (including urinary tract infection, genital tract infection or chorioamnionitis) and low socioeconomic status. Pregnancy-related factors include uterine distension such as polyhydramnios or multiple pregnancies, pre-eclampsia, antepartum haemorrhage, placental abruption, uterine abnormalities (such as cervical incompetence or bicornuate uterus) and previous cervical surgery. Fetal factors include pre-labour rupture of membranes, intrauterine growth restriction and congenital abnormalities.

Examination includes abdominal examination, speculum examination with swabs, urine dip, maternal bloods, cardiotocograph and ultrasound to confirm presentation. The special care baby unit must be informed and the patient moved to a different hospital if there are no facilities to care for a premature baby. The woman should be counselled by the paediatrician about the problems prematurity can bring for babies.

Corticosteroids reduce the incidence of neonatal respiratory distress, intraventricular haemorrhage, necrotizing enterocolitis and neonatal death. There have been no adverse neurological or cognitive effects following steroid treatment after 12-year follow-up. Steroids cross the placenta to increase production and release of pulmonary surfactant by a complex mechanism involving receptor-mediated gene transcriptase. They are contraindicated if the mother has active septicaemia. They should also be used with caution in insulin-dependent diabetics as they can lead to ketoacidosis; a sliding scale may be required.

Tocolytics inhibit smooth muscle contraction in the uterus to delay, rather than stop, labour to allow time for steroids to take effect and to allow transfer of the mother to a hospital that has adequate facilities for neonatal resuscitation if needed.

Choice of mode of delivery of a preterm fetus is vaginal provided the fetus is not compromised. Instrumental delivery would be used in the same situations as in full-term delivery, but ventouse is not used before 34 weeks due to the immature fetal head and a risk of intracranial haemorrhage. Close monitoring is needed as complications such as abnormal lie, cord prolapse, placental abruption and intrauterine infection are more common.

An infusion of magnesium sulphate ($MgSO_4$) given to the mother prior to delivery of a preterm infant has been found to reduce the risk of cerebral palsy and to protect gross motor function in the baby. It should be given just prior to delivery and is thought to have greater benefit at the most preterm gestations.

46. FEMALE INFERTILITY

A – Laparoscopy and dye test

Diagnostic laparoscopy and dye is the best option for this patient as she has a risk factor for tubal damage: pelvic inflammatory disease (PID). Other reasons for a 'lap and dye' test are previous ectopic pregnancy or endometriosis as other pelvic pathology can be assessed at the same time and treatment performed simultaneously. A laparoscopy is performed, under general anaesthetic, to give a direct view of pelvic organs to assess abnormalities, damage or significant adhesions. During the operation, methylene blue dye is inserted into the uterus using a syringe via the cervix. If blue dye is seen coming from the fimbrial ends of the fallopian tubes, they are deemed patent.

A hysterosalpingogram involves passing radio-opaque fluid into the uterine cavity via the cervix to ascertain (via X-ray) if it leaks from the ends of both fallopian tubes. If it is normal, the result can be trusted 97% of the time. If it is abnormal, it is only correct in 34% of cases, and a lap and dye test would be needed to confirm the test. The advantages of this overlap and dye are that this avoids the risk of surgery and anaesthetic, and it can be done as an outpatient procedure. It is generally done in women with no risk factors for pelvic disease or those with high anaesthetic risk. Hysterosalpingo-contrast sonography involves inserting a galactose-containing ultrasound contrast medium into the uterine cavity. A standard ultrasound probe is then used to outline abnormalities such as submucosal fibroids, endometrial polyps and the patency of the fallopian tubes. It has a similar accuracy to the hysterosalpingogram.

Salpingoscopy involves inserting a fine telescope (salpingoscope) into the ampullary portion of the fallopian tube at laparoscopy to investigate the presence of fine intratubal adhesions. Falloposcopy involves insertion of a fibreoptic instrument (falloposcope) into the fallopian tube via the uterine cavity as an outpatient procedure. This is a new technique and is generally only used as a research tool as it is expensive and delicate.

47. RHESUS DISEASE (2)

E – No action is needed at present

It sounds as though this woman has a threatened miscarriage. The guidelines state that only those women with vaginal bleeding *after* 12 weeks require anti-D. As long as the bleeding is not heavy, this woman could be sent home after arranging a pelvic scan to assess the bleeding and viability of the pregnancy.

The RCOG guidelines provide advice on who should be given anti-D prophylaxis in the early stages of pregnancy. Threatened miscarriage: anti-D prophylaxis should be given to all RhD –ve women after 12 weeks in the event of a threatened miscarriage but not given before 12 weeks, as is seen in this case. Spontaneous miscarriage: a similar distinction is given for spontaneous miscarriage with those over 12 weeks requiring anti-D prophylaxis but not for those under 12 weeks' gestation unless uterine evacuation is required. Therapeutic termination of pregnancy: anti-D prophylaxis is needed in all non-sensitized RhD –ve women having medical or surgical termination of pregnancy regardless of gestational age. Ectopic pregnancy: anti-D prophylaxis should be given to all non-sensitized RhD –ve women who have ectopic pregnancy.

48. OBSTETRIC EMERGENCIES (3)

D – Uterine inversion

Uterine inversion is rare and describes the passage of the uterine fundus through the cervix into the vagina. The resultant stretch on the round ligament can cause profound shock due to vagal stimulation. The shock seen is out of proportion to the blood loss, and this increases suspicion of uterine inversion rather than haemorrhage.

A fundal placenta means there is an increased risk of uterine inversion, so it is particularly important not to attempt to remove the placenta before signs of placental separation have been seen (cord lengthening and a gush of dark blood). It is also important to only use controlled cord traction with counter-pressure on the uterus over the suprapubic region. Other risk factors for inversion are uterine atony and previous uterine inversion.

Presentation includes shock (primarily vasovagal), which is out of proportion to the amount of bleeding and pain. The uterine fundus will not be palpable abdominally – rather it will be seen or felt as a bluish-grey mass in the vagina. The placenta remains attached in 50% of cases and can be morbidly adherent, so further attempts to remove it should not be attempted.

As with all emergencies, call for help and start resuscitation of the mother. If the placenta is still attached to the uterus DO NOT attempt to separate it, instead attempt to replace the uterus and placenta inside as this will relieve the vasovagal shock. Tocolytic therapy may help. Johnson's method involves manual transvaginal fundal pressure. O'Sullivan's method of hydrostatic reduction can be used (2L of warmed fluid is passed into the vagina to encourage vaginal distension and allow the uterus to return to its normal position). The Huntington procedure involves traction on the round ligaments at laparotomy with vaginal pressure simultaneously. Haultain's procedure involves incising the uterine fundus and cervical ring to allow manual re-inversion. Hysterectomy is used as a last resort. Once the uterus is re-sited, prophylactic antibiotics and oxytocin are needed.

49. POSTPARTUM HAEMORRHAGE (2)

A – Atonic uterus

Ninety percent of primary postpartum haemorrhages (PPHs) are caused by an atonic uterus. Other causes include trauma (cervical tear, high vaginal tear, perineal tears, uterine rupture), retained placenta or placental fragments and clotting disorders. Risk factors include antepartum haemorrhage, previous history of PPH, over-enlarged uterus due to multiple pregnancy, polyhydramnios or macrosomic fetus, uterine fibroids, placenta praevia, prolonged labour, grand multiparity, chorioamnionitis and bleeding diathesis.

It is easy to remember the causes of PPH as the four Ts:

- Tone
- Tissue
- Trauma
- Thrombosis (i.e. clotting disorders)

Uterine atony occurs due to inadequate compression of the intramyometrial blood vessels by the uterine muscles leading to continued bleeding. It is more common if there is a retained placenta or placental tissue as the physical presence of this prevents contraction of the uterus occurring.

Initial management of an atonic uterus includes emptying the bladder and 'rubbing up uterine contractions' while administering oxytocics to contract the uterus. To 'rub up a contraction', the uterus is massaged through the abdominal wall. A bolus of intravenous ergometrine is given followed by infusion of oxytocin. If bleeding persists, bimanual compression can be employed, which involves inserting a fist into the vagina and using the other hand abdominally to compress the uterus between the two hands. For further persistent bleeding, carboprost (15-methylprostaglandin/Hemabate) can be given intramuscularly into the thigh or gluteal muscle. If the bleeding is not controlled, surgical options must be considered.

50. GAMETOGENESIS (1)

C – Polar body

Oogenesis begins in females during intrauterine life and is a protracted process with many stages of division being arrested for long periods of time. It is more complicated than the male pathway, although the same principles are followed. Primordial germ cells are present in the wall of the yolk sac at the end of the third week of embryological development. They migrate to the developing gonads by amoeboid movement, where they arrive by the beginning of the fifth week. They then divide by mitosis and differentiate into oogonia. Oogonia differentiate into primary oocytes and become surrounded by follicular (epithelial) cells. These are collectively named primordial follicles. Primary oocytes contain 46 double-structured chromosomes and enter prophase of meiosis I. Division is arrested at the dictyotene phase of meiosis I, and the first meiotic division is completed only with the pre-ovulatory luteinizing hormone/follicle-stimulating hormone (LH/FSH) surge to give a secondary oocyte and a polar body. The polar body is merely a useless by-product, which subsequently degenerates.

Secondary oocyte and polar bodies both contain 23 double-structured chromosomes. Meiosis I of the secondary oocyte is completed with the pre-ovulatory LH/FSH surge, but further division of the secondary oocyte only occurs if fertilization occurs. With fertilization, the secondary oocyte divides by meiosis II to give a mature oocyte and a further polar body. The mature oocytes and its polar body both contain 23 single chromosomes. The initial polar body also undergoes meiosis II to give a further two polar bodies, both containing 23 single chromosomes.

Primary oocytes therefore eventually give rise to four daughter cells, all of which contain 22 + X chromosomes. However, only one of these is a mature oocyte, the remaining three daughter cells being polar bodies.

Practice Paper 2: Questions

1. FETAL POSITION (2)

You examine the abdomen of a woman who has attended for induction of labour at 40 weeks + 12 days. The abdomen is soft and non-tender. It is difficult to feel any definite presenting part in the pelvis. The baby is longitudinal lie, you can feel a smooth part on the patient's left side and the right side feels more irregular. The fundus has a ballottable object. You find the fetal heart above the umbilicus.

How is the position best described?

A. Breech
B. Occipitoposterior
C. Occipitotransverse
D. Occipitoposterior fully engaged
E. Transverse lie

2. BLEEDING IN PREGNANCY (3)

A 21-year-old primigravida at 41 weeks' gestation rings the labour ward complaining of gradual-onset abdominal cramping pains approximately every 15 to 20 minutes. She is concerned as she has had a mucous-like pink loss vaginally. She has good fetal movements.

What is the most likely explanation for this?

A. Bloody show
B. Cervical ectropion
C. Cervical polyp
D. Placenta praevia
E. Vasa praevia

3. ACUTE PELVIC PAIN (3)

An 18-year-old female attends the emergency department with generalized lower abdominal pains, which have been present for a couple of days. She also complains of a purulent vaginal discharge. She recently had an intrauterine device inserted as emergency contraception after a condom she was using failed 5 days ago. Her periods are normally regular. Currently, she feels hot and sweaty. Observations show a heart rate 96/min, blood pressure 110/70 mmHg and temperature 38.8°C. Her abdomen is soft with moderate tenderness in the lower abdomen. There is no guarding or rebound tenderness. Speculum examination reveals a purulent discharge. Cervical excitation was detected on vaginal examination. A urine result is awaited. Prior to this she had never been sexually active.

What is the most likely diagnosis?

A. Ectopic pregnancy
B. Mittelschmerz
C. Ovarian cyst torsion
D. Pelvic inflammatory disease
E. Urinary tract infection

4. CARDIOTOCOGRAPHY (2)

A woman at term is in early labour. The cardiotocography (CTG) has been reactive with a baseline rate of 140, multiple accelerations, no decelerations and variability of 15 to 20. The trace 30 minutes later shows a baseline rate of 135, with no accelerations or decelerations and a variability of 5 to 7 beats.

What could explain the features of this trace?

A. Maternal pyrexia
B. Suspicious trace
C. Pre-terminal trace
D. Sleep pattern of fetus
E. Thumb sucking of fetus

5. CHRONIC PELVIC PAIN (2)

A 44-year-old woman is a regular attendee at the gynaecological clinic. At her current appointment, she complains of abdominal pain that has been present for over 10 years. She says the pain is low in her abdomen, aching in character with no radiation, associated with nausea but with no correlation to her periods. It is worse at night, and she finds it hard to sleep as she is concerned about the pain. She takes no painkillers as she does not want to 'put chemicals into her body'. She complains of dyspareunia and is concerned that she may have a sexually transmitted infection contracted from her husband despite his assurance to her that he has not been unfaithful. She has previously had two negative diagnostic laparoscopies, three negative hysteroscopies, a reassuring smear and negative swab tests. She is also seeing a neurologist for chronic headaches.

What is the most likely diagnosis?

A. Adhesions from surgery
B. Chronic pelvic inflammatory disease
C. Endometriosis
D. Functional pain
E. Ovarian cysts

6. MECHANISMS OF LABOUR (3)

Which of the following movements occurs during crowning of the head during labour of an occipitoanterior cephalic normal vaginal delivery?

A. Effacement
B. Extension
C. External rotation
D. Flexion
E. Internal rotation

7. CONTRACEPTION (2)

A 21-year-old woman is asking about contraception, specifically condoms.

How effective are condoms if used correctly?

A. 80% effective
B. 85% effective
C. 95% effective
D. 98% effective
E. 100% effective

8. SCREENING (2)

A 37-year-old woman at 17 weeks' gestation attends clinic after having had a high-risk screening test result for Down syndrome. After counselling, she and her partner decide they need to know definitely whether the pregnancy is affected by Down syndrome.

Which test would be most appropriate?

A. Amniocentesis
B. Chorionic villus sampling
C. Fetal tissue sampling
D. Nuchal translucency test
E. Routine anomaly scan

9. ENDOMETRIAL CANCER

Which of these increases your risk of developing endometrial carcinoma?

A. Combined oral contraceptive pill
B. Early menopause
C. Late menarche
D. Multiparity
E. Obesity

10. CAESAREAN SECTION (2)

You consent a woman for a caesarean section. Which out of the following would you say was a frequently occurring risk?

A. Bladder injury
B. Hysterectomy
C. Persistent wound and abdominal discomfort in the months after surgery
D. Risk of placenta praevia or placenta accreta in subsequent pregnancies
E. Ureteric injury

11. MENSTRUAL HORMONES (3)

A surge in which hormone occurs 18 hours before ovulation?

A. Activin
B. Follicle-stimulating hormone
C. Luteinizing hormone
D. Oestradiol
E. Progesterone

12. INDUCTION OF LABOUR (3)

A 28-year-old woman attends labour ward as her waters have broken at term + 12. She has good fetal movements. She has some contraction pains, but these are mild and she is not troubled by them. She has had an uncomplicated pregnancy and had two previous normal deliveries, both of which needed inducing due to post-maturity. The CTG is normal. A scan is done, which shows a transverse lie of the fetus. The cervix is long on speculum examination.

What would be the next course of action?

A. Artificial rupture of membranes
B. Caesarean section
C. Oxytocin
D. Prostaglandin
E. Stretch and sweep

13. GAMETOGENESIS (2)

How long does it take for a single sperm to be created from start to finish?

A. 12 hours
B. 64 hours
C. 12 days
D. 64 days
E. Varies from 12 hours to 12 days

14. CARDIOTOCOGRAPHY (3)

Which of these terms describes a dip in the fetal heart rate of 20 beats per minute that starts with the contraction and has recovered to normal by the end of the contraction?

A. Early decelerations
B. Late decelerations
C. Acceleration
D. Sinusoidal pattern
E. Variable decelerations

15. GENITAL ULCERATION

A 31-year-old woman attends the GUM clinic saying she had unprotected sexual intercourse with a new partner 3 weeks ago. She reports seeing a dull red spot on her labia, which has now turned into a single, painless, well-demarcated ulcer. She is otherwise well.

What is the most likely diagnosis?

A. Chancroid
B. Granuloma inguinale
C. Herpes simplex
D. Lymphogranuloma venereum
E. Syphilis

16. MALE INFERTILITY

A couple who are experiencing difficulties in conceiving are undergoing investigation. The semen analysis of the male partner reveals asthenospermia.

What does this mean?

A. Complete absence of sperm
B. Localized infection
C. Morphologically defective sperm
D. Poorly motile sperm
E. Reduced sperm count

17. INFECTION IN PREGNANCY (2)

A 29-year-old primigravida has just given birth to a baby who is unwell and has had to be taken to the special care baby unit. On examination of the baby, the paediatricians find dermatomal skin scarring, neurological defects, limb hypoplasia and eye defects. The woman states that during the pregnancy she had two episodes of vaginal bleeding at weeks 7 and 9. She also states she felt unwell at 14 weeks with a fever and general malaise followed by an itchy vesicular rash all over her body.

From the description of mother and baby, choose the most likely infection affecting this pregnancy.

A. Chickenpox
B. Cytomegalovirus
C. Parvovirus
D. Rubella
E. Salmonella

18. VAGINAL BLEEDING (2)

A 35-year-old woman presents with a long history of very heavy periods. She has visited you now as she cannot cope with the bleeding, and she has a swelling in her abdomen. On examination, you feel a uterus equivalent to pregnancy of 18 weeks; however, she says that she has not been sexually active for 3 years.

What is the most likely diagnosis?

A. Cervical cancer
B. Cervical ectropion
C. Endometrial carcinoma
D. Large endometrial polyps
E. Uterine fibroids

19. OBSTETRIC EMERGENCIES (4)

A 23-year-old woman has had two children, one by normal delivery and the other by caesarean section for fetal distress. She is now in labour. She is currently 7 cm dilated with membranes intact. The head is low in the pelvis.

Of which emergency is she at increased risk?

A. Cord prolapse
B. Fetal distress
C. Shoulder dystocia
D. Uterine inversion
E. Uterine rupture

20. FETAL ULTRASOUND (2)

Which measurement is the most reliable indicator of gestational age after 14 weeks?

A. Abdominal circumference
B. Amniotic fluid level
C. Crown–rump length
D. Femur length
E. Head circumference

21. POSTPARTUM HAEMORRHAGE (3)

Which of the following is the most common cause of secondary post-partum haemorrhage?

A. Atonic uterus
B. Disseminated intravascular coagulation
C. Infection
D. Perineal trauma
E. Retained placental fragments

22. PAIN IN PREGNANCY (3)

A 34-year-old woman who is 40 weeks + 4 days' gestation attends the antenatal day unit with constant pain in the suprapubic area that radiates to her upper thighs and perineum. It is worse on walking. She has not taken any analgesia. On examination, her abdomen is soft and non-tender with tenderness only elicited by compressing her pelvis. There is a cephalic presentation with the head two-fifths palpable and a right occipitotransverse position. Her urine dipstick showed only a trace of protein.

What is this most likely cause of her pain?

A. Braxton Hicks contractions
B. Labour
C. Round ligament stretching
D. Symphysis pubis dysfunction
E. Urinary tract infection

23. MANAGEMENT OF INCONTINENCE (2)

A 56-year-old woman has a history of leaking urine when lifting her grandchild. She can no longer participate in her aerobics class as she is afraid of the consequences of jumping up and down. She is distressed and wants something to be done about this. She is tearful during the consultation.

Considering the diagnosis, what is the first-line treatment?

A. Bladder training
B. Botulinum toxin A
C. Oxybutynin
D. Pelvic floor exercises with a trained physiotherapist
E. Surgery following urodynamics

24. MENOPAUSE

A 52-year-old woman attends the general practitioner saying that she last had a period many months ago. She is not sure if she has undergone the menopause as she has no symptoms.

A serum test of which of the following could aid a clinical diagnosis of menopause?

A. Follicle-stimulating hormone
B. Human chorionic gonadotrophin
C. Luteinizing hormone
D. Oestrogen
E. Progesterone

25. PHYSIOLOGICAL CHANGES IN PREGNANCY

You are asked to review some blood results taken in the emergency department of a woman at 34 weeks' gestation, who has been admitted following a minor road traffic collision. She is generally well and has no obvious trauma. On further questioning, she reveals an increased urinary frequency but no dysuria and the urine dip is clear. She also tells you she previously had a diagnosis of gallstones but has not been bothered by these for years.

Her blood results are as follows:

Ranges for non-pregnant women			
Haemoglobin	11.7 g/dL	Low	11.5–16.0 g/dL
White cell count	12.5 × 10⁹/L	High	4.0–11.0 × 10⁹/L
Platelets	142 × 10⁹/L	Low	150–400 × 10⁹/L
Alkaline phosphatase	367 IU/L	High	30–300 IU/L
Albumin	31 g/L	Low	35–50 g/L
Na	139 mmol/L	Normal	135–145 mmol/L
K	3.9 mmol/L	Normal	3.5–5.0 mmol/L
Ur	2.1 mmol/L	Low	2.5–6.7 mmol/L
Cr	64 µmol/L	Low	70–150 µmol/L

What would you tell the emergency department doctors about these results?

A. All normal physiological results for pregnancy
B. All normal physiological results apart from alkaline phosphatase
C. All normal physiological results apart from haemoglobin
D. All normal physiological results apart from urea
E. All normal physiological results apart from white cell count

26. PLACENTAL ABNORMALITIES

You are in the pathology department studying a uterus and placenta that were removed during an emergency hysterectomy. The pathologist shows how the placenta has invaded through the uterine wall and through the outer serosal layer, invading the bladder.

What is this known as?

A. Placental abruption
B. Placenta accreta
C. Placenta increta
D. Placenta percreta
E. Placenta praevia

27. MENORRHAGIA (1)

A 42-year-old woman has a 12-month history of heavy periods. She is a smoker. An ultrasound scan reveals nothing abnormal, and a recent outpatient hysteroscopy was normal. She would like a long-term treatment for menorrhagia and a form of contraception. She is unsure whether she would like more children.

Which treatment would you offer her?

A. Antifibrinolytics
B. Combined oral contraceptive pill
C. Endometrial ablation
D. Intrauterine or systemic progestogens
E. Prostaglandin inhibitors

28. MANAGEMENT OF SMEAR RESULTS (2)

A 55-year-old woman has had a smear test and the lab has found a high-grade dyskaryosis.

What is the next most appropriate step in her management?

A. Colposcopy
B. HPV test
C. Recall in 6 months
D. Recall in 3 years
E. Recall in 5 years

29. RHESUS DISEASE (3)

A 27-year-old attends the antenatal day unit to receive her routine antenatal anti-D prophylaxis at 28 weeks' gestation. This is her first child, and she is rhesus D negative. She has already received an anti-D injection after a bleed early on in pregnancy at 14 weeks.

What action needs to be taken with regard to anti-D prophylaxis?

A. Give routine antenatal anti-D prophylaxis 250 IU at 28 weeks
B. Give routine antenatal anti-D prophylaxis 500 IU at 28 weeks
C. Give routine antenatal anti-D prophylaxis 250 IU at 34 weeks
D. Give routine antenatal anti-D prophylaxis 500 IU at 34 weeks
E. No action needed at present

30. SCREENING (3)

A 22-year-old primigravid woman attends the general practice at 16 weeks' gestation. She explains that she would consider termination if she found out she was carrying a fetus affected by Down syndrome. After counselling, you agree to use an initial non-invasive screening test for Down syndrome.

Which of the following tests would you suggest?

A. Amniocentesis
B. Chorionic villus sampling
C. Fetal echocardiography
D. Nuchal translucency test
E. Serum quadruple test

31. TWINS (2)

A 25-year-old primigravid woman with a twin pregnancy has a 20-week ultrasound scan. She is excited to discover that she is carrying one girl and one boy.

How are these twins described?

A. Dizygotic dichorionic diamniotic
B. Dizygotic dichorionic monoamniotic
C. Dizygotic monochorionic monoamniotic
D. Monozygotic dichorionic diamniotic
E. Monozygotic monochorionic diamniotic

32. MENORRHAGIA (2)

A 29-year-old woman who has not completed her family has a diagnosis of large subserous fibroids and troublesome heavy periods. She feels medical treatments have made no difference to the bleeding.

Which treatment option should be offered?

A. Endometrial ablation
B. Hysterectomy
C. Hysteroscopic resection of fibroids
D. Myomectomy
E. Uterine artery embolization

33. PREMATURE LABOUR (2)

A 29-year-old woman at 33 weeks' gestation describes a sudden gush of water from her vagina. She has no abdominal pain and has felt good fetal movements. Abdominal examination reveals a cephalic presentation. Speculum examination shows a clear fluid draining from the cervix. The CTG shows a baseline rate of 140, with four accelerations in a 20-minute period, a variability of 5 to 15 beats and no decelerations. The tocograph shows a flat line.

What medication would you give her for prophylaxis against infection?

A. Atosiban
B. Betamethasone
C. Co-amoxiclav
D. Erythromycin
E. Gentamicin

34. CONTRACEPTION (3)

A 38-year-old woman is asking about the combined oral contraceptive pill (COCP). She used to be on it prior to having her family and is hoping to return to using it for contraception. She suffers from hypertension, for which she takes Ramipril. This adequately controls her blood pressure. Her body mass index is 28, and she is currently trying to lose weight.

Can you safely prescribe her the COCP and, if not, why not?

A. No – hypertension
B. No – weight loss
C. No – high body mass index
D. No – age
E. Yes

35. GAMETOGENESIS (3)

Which of the following is the male cell that contains 23 single chromosomes prior to spermiogenesis?

A. Primary spermatocyte
B. Secondary spermatocyte
C. Spermatid
D. Spermatogonia
E. Spermatozoon

36. INFECTION IN PREGNANCY (3)

A 31-year-old woman is admitted to labour ward in early labour. The midwife notices that she has had a positive vaginal swab taken that requires antibiotic treatment only when she is in established labour.

What organism was found on the swab?

A. Bacterial vaginosis
B. Cytomegalovirus
C. Group B streptococcus
D. Herpes
E. Toxoplasmosis

37. MENORRHAGIA (3)

A 45-year-old woman has been struggling with increasing heaviness of her regular menstrual periods over the past year. She now finds them unmanageable, with regular flooding. She has completed her family. She has a BMI of 23. She had a normal hysteroscopy, pelvic scan and Pipelle biopsy 4 months ago. She has had two large loop excision of the transformation zone (LLETZ) procedures in the last 5 years for cervical abnormalities and struggles with these examinations; she has further high-grade abnormalities on a recent colposcopy examination. Despite numerous medical options from her general practitioner, she still feels the condition is worsening and that she is at the end of her tether. She is requesting a hysterectomy.

What treatment would you suggest?

A. Endometrial ablation
B. Endometrial biopsy
C. Subtotal hysterectomy
D. Total hysterectomy
E. Uterine artery embolization

38. OBSTETRIC EMERGENCIES (5)

A 26-year-old primigravid woman with moderate pre-eclampsia has been induced at 38 weeks with vaginal prostaglandin and artificial rupture of membranes. She is not on an oxytocin infusion. There are no other antenatal complications. On vaginal examination, her cervix is 5 cm dilated and fully effaced, with the presenting part at station −1. She has an epidural in situ so she does not feel the contractions. Suddenly, she develops abdominal pain, and there are deep decelerations on the CTG. On examination, her uterus feels hard. She feels faint and her blood pressure is low with a maternal tachycardia.

What event has just occurred?

A. Amniotic fluid embolism
B. Epidural failure
C. Placental abruption
D. Uterine hyperstimulation
E. Uterine rupture

39. MENORRHAGIA (4)

A 16-year-old female attends her general practitioner with complaints of heavy and painful periods. She is normally fit and well and has never been sexually active. Her mother is with her at the consultation and would prefer her not to have hormone treatment.

What is the most appropriate treatment option?

A. Tranexamic acid and mefanamic acid
B. Combined oral contraceptive pill
C. Gonadotrophin-releasing hormone analogues
D. Intrauterine or systemic progestogens
E. Progesterone-only pill

40. PRE-ECLAMPSIA (2)

A 34-year-old primigravid woman at 37 weeks' gestation has been admitted to the labour ward with pre-eclampsia. Her blood pressure will not decrease below 166/114 mmHg despite being on maximum oral antihypertensive treatment, and it is decided she requires induction of labour, intravenous antihypertensive medication and medication for prevention of convulsions.

What infusion is used to prevent convulsions?

A. Carbamazepine
B. Diazepam
C. Gabapentin
D. Magnesium sulphate
E. Phenytoin

41. PREMATURE LABOUR (3)

A 24-year-old primigravid woman at 32 weeks' gestation attends the antenatal day unit with intermittent abdominal pains. Abdominal examination reveals a cephalic presentation and palpable contractions every 3 minutes lasting for 20 seconds. Speculum examination shows a long and closed cervix. The CTG has a baseline rate of 150 and variability above 5. There are two accelerations in 30 minutes. The tocograph shows regular uterine activity every 3 minutes.

Which oxytocin receptor antagonist would you use to attempt to delay labour?

A. Atosiban
B. Indometacin
C. Nifedipine
D. Ritodrine
E. Salbutamol

42. MENSTRUAL HORMONES (4)

Which hormone promotes proliferative endometrium growth in the follicular phase of the menstrual cycle?

A. Activin
B. Follicle-stimulating hormone
C. Luteinizing hormone
D. Oestradiol
E. Progesterone

43. RHESUS DISEASE (4)

A 34-year-old primigravid woman who is rhesus D negative has received routine antenatal anti-D prophylaxis at 28 and 34 weeks and a further dose of antenatal anti-D prophylaxis during her pregnancy. She has now delivered a rhesus D positive infant.

What action needs to be taken with regard to anti-D prophylaxis?

A. Give antenatal anti-D prophylaxis 250 IU and take Kleihauer test
B. Give antenatal anti-D prophylaxis 500 IU and take Kleihauer test
C. Give blood transfusion and take Kleihauer test
D. Give postnatal anti-D and take Kleihauer test
E. No action needed at present

44. MISCARRIAGE (2)

A 39-year-old woman with a positive pregnancy test complains of a 3-day history of lower, cramping abdominal pain. She complains of bleeding that started lightly and has become gradually heavier over the 3 days. On examination, she is tender suprapubically. Speculum examination reveals bright red blood in the vagina and an open cervical os. She has had two previous miscarriages.

What is the most likely diagnosis?

A. Complete miscarriage
B. Incomplete miscarriage
C. Inevitable miscarriage
D. Menstruation
E. Threatened miscarriage

45. OVARIAN CYSTS

A 22-year-old woman who has never been sexually active complains of sudden-onset sharp, left-sided abdominal pain that was localized to the left iliac fossa and is associated with vomiting. An ultrasound scan demonstrated a mass on the left ovary. Following the operation to remove the cyst, she was told that they had found hair and teeth inside.

Which tumour did this woman have removed?

A. Dysgerminoma
B. Fibroma
C. Granulosa cell tumour
D. Teratoma
E. Yolk sac tumour

46. TWINS (3)

A 33-year-old woman delivers genetically identical twins at 40 weeks. The midwife examines the placenta and finds a separate chorion, amnion and placenta. The registrar explains to the medical student that mitotic division to form twins must have occurred before day 3 of embryonic development.

How are these twins described?

A. Dizygotic dichorionic diamniotic
B. Dizygotic dichorionic monoamniotic
C. Dizygotic monochorionic monoamniotic
D. Monozygotic dichorionic diamniotic
E. Monozygotic monochorionic diamniotic

47. OVARIAN CANCER (3)

A 59-year-old woman presented with vague symptoms of abdominal distension and some weight loss associated with fatigue. On examination, a large pelvic mass was detected. An ultrasound scan showed a large multiloculated cyst on her right ovary and some uncertain areas in her abdomen. Her CA-125 was increased. She had a staging laparotomy and pseudomyxoma peritonei was seen.

Which ovarian tumour is she likely to have?

A. Brenner tumour
B. Clear cell tumour
C. Endometroid tumour
D. Mucinous tumour
E. Serous tumour

48. PATHOGENESIS OF CERVICAL CANCER (2)

A 37-year-old woman has recently been diagnosed with cervical cancer.

Which of these is related to cervical cancer?

A. Hepatitis B virus
B. Hepatitis C virus
C. Herpes simplex virus
D. Human papillomavirus 6b and 11
E. Human papillomavirus 16 and 18

49. EARLY PREGNANCY (3)

A 27-year-old woman has an early pregnancy transvaginal scan, which shows an empty uterus with a βhCG result of 2365 IU. She has no pain and is otherwise fit and well.

What is the most likely diagnosis?

A. Early intrauterine pregnancy
B. Ectopic pregnancy
C. Inevitable miscarriage
D. Missed miscarriage
E. Threatened miscarriage

50. VAGINAL DISCHARGE (2)

A 59-year-old woman attends clinic with one episode of watery, bloody vaginal discharge. She has never had any children, and she had menopause at age 55. On examination, she is obese, but her abdomen is unremarkable. On speculum examination you see some purulent bloody discharge and you take triple swabs.

Considering the likely diagnosis, what would be your next course of action?

A. Await results of triple swabs and follow-up in clinic in one month
B. Dilation and curettage
C. Ultrasound scan ± hysteroscopy and endometrial biopsy
D. Pipelle biopsy and follow-up in clinic in 1 month
E. Vabra biopsy and follow-up in clinic in 1 month

Practice Paper 2: Answers

1. FETAL POSITION (2)

A – Breech

This is a breech presentation for a number of reasons. First, no definite presenting is felt in the pelvis as the bottom is softer than the head. The head is felt by balloting in the fundus of the uterus. The heartbeat is heard above the umbilicus. The back is on the left where the smoothness was felt, and the limbs are on the right where it was more irregular.

Abdominal examination specific to obstetrics

Observe the woman to assess her overall well-being. Specifically, you are looking for discomfort, which may suggest labour or abdominal pain, jaundice, itching, pallor, oedema and an estimate of maternal weight. Observations can be viewed as a maternal early warning score (MEWS): assess blood pressure, heart rate, respiratory rate, saturations and temperature.

For abdominal examination, the woman should lie flat in a semi-prone or left lateral tilt to avoid aortocaval compression. She should be exposed from just below her breasts to her symphysis pubis.

Inspection is the first stage and you should look for size of the abdomen, striae and scars. You can often see fetal movements later in pregnancy. *Palpation* helps assess liquor volume and how firm/soft the uterus is. You may also feel fetal movements or contractions if there are any. This will also reveal any uterine tenderness or irritability.

You must determine the *lie* of the fetus – how the fetus is lying in relation to the long axis of the uterus. If the lie is longitudinal, the fetus lies in the midline of the uterus with the head at one end and buttocks at the other. If the lie is transverse, it is at 90° to this, with the head at one side of the mother and the buttocks at the other – the pelvis would be empty in this case. An oblique lie is where the head or buttocks are palpable in either of the iliac fossae.

Next feel into the pelvis to *determine the presenting part* and if there is any *engagement*. To do this, turn to face the pelvis (i.e. with your back to the woman's head and using two hands on each side of the uterus at the level of the umbilicus to gently work your way towards the pelvis with dipping motions in and out to try to palpate a presenting part). Once you have found a presenting part, try to assess if it is a head or a bottom. A head will feel harder and can generally be balloted between your hands if it is free. A bottom will feel softer, is harder to define and cannot be balloted. If you are unsure of the presenting part, Pawlik's grip can be used (grasp the presenting part between the thumb and forefinger). However, this is painful for the woman and should be avoided if possible. Engagement of the presenting part should be assessed at this point. This is described in 'fifths of the head palpable' abdominally. A head is said to be engaged if it is less than two-fifths palpable as this describes a position in which the widest diameter of the head has descended into the pelvis.

Finally, *find the fundus* using the ulna side of the left hand, and measure the distance from the fundus to the symphysis pubis with a tape measure to get the symphysis–fundal height. After 24 weeks, this should correlate to the gestational age of the fetus in weeks ±2 cm. This can be used as a screening test for a 'large or small for dates' baby and then can be referred for a scan if indicated.

Auscultation is the next stage: Pinard stethoscopes or a sonicaid (handheld ultrasound transducer) are used to hear and measure the heartbeat. The fetal heart can usually be heard if you listen over the anterior shoulder, which can normally be found between the head and the umbilicus. When you are first learning, it may be an idea to tell the woman this so she does not become anxious that you cannot find the heartbeat!

2. BLEEDING IN PREGNANCY (3)

A – Bloody show

The 'show' is a bloody mucus-like vaginal loss that is associated with preparation for labour. The cervical mucus plug is lost due to pre-labour cervical changes. Contractions may commence in the following days. If there is any concern about the amount of bleeding, a speculum examination can be done to check that this is not excessive.

3. ACUTE PELVIC PAIN (3)

D – Pelvic inflammatory disease

This woman has pelvic inflammatory disease (PID): infection of the pelvic organs from ascending infection through the genital tract, normally via sexual contact. Common presentations include constant lower bilateral abdominal pain, a purulent discharge *per vagina*, dyspareunia (pain on intercourse), postcoital or irregular bleeding and menorrhagia or dysmenorrhoea. Fever, vomiting, anorexia and malaise are also seen in women with more severe active infection. Lower abdominal bilateral tenderness, cervical excitation, adnexal tenderness and pyrexia are seen on examination. High vaginal and endocervical swabs must be taken, and a urine sample should be sent for culture. Negative cultures do not exclude the diagnosis of PID as the infection may be higher up into the pelvis. Immediate treatment is with antibiotics (e.g. ceftriaxone, doxycycline and metronidazole), analgesia and admission to hospital in severe cases. There should be follow-up with the genitourinary medicine services to enable education, a full sexual health screen and contact tracing. Patients should be advised to avoid any sexual intercourse until they and their partners have completed the treatment. Advice should be given about avoiding infection by using barrier contraception. Complications include tubo-ovarian abscesses, Fitz-Hugh–Curtis syndrome (perihepatitis leading to perihepatic adhesions), tubal infertility, ectopic pregnancy and chronic pelvic pain.

PID is most common in 18- to 25-year olds, with chlamydia, gonorrhoea and atypical anaerobes being the most common offending pathogens. The rate of chlamydia infections is rising dramatically, particularly in this age group, and empirical antibiotic treatment should be offered to young sexually active women with the symptoms of PID.

4. CARDIOTOCOGRAPHY (2)

D – Sleep pattern of fetus
See Practice Paper 1, Question 5 (cardiotocography) for a description of CTGs.

5. CHRONIC PELVIC PAIN (2)

D – Functional pain
This woman probably has functional abdominal pain. This can only be a diagnosis of exclusion once every other pathology has been ruled out. Sometimes the finding of no pathology can be very reassuring for women and can cause resolution of symptoms. However, in some cases, this can add to the frustration and worry, as there is no pathology to treat. If no pathology is found, the woman should be questioned about sexual and social circumstances as there may be an underlying problem such as relationship difficulties, sexual abuse or fears about sexuality or fertility. When managing such cases, it is difficult to ensure you do not miss any newly developing pathology. Conversely, if investigations continue being performed, this may reinforce the concept that there may be something wrong and the patient may continue to worry about the pain. You must also think about the increased risk of each investigation, such as the increasing risk of bowel injury with repeated laparoscopies.

6. MECHANISMS OF LABOUR (3)

B – Extension
See the Practice Paper 1, Question 14 (mechanisms of labour) for an explanation.

7. CONTRACEPTION (2)

D – 98% effective

Condoms are 98% effective if used correctly, which means that two women in 100 will get pregnant in a year. This of course is dependent on age, frequency of sexual intercourse and correct usage. It is useful to compare this with using no contraception, where 80 to 90 sexually active women out of 100 will become pregnant in a year.

It is important to discuss advantages and disadvantages of condoms and alternative forms of contraception. The advantages of condoms are that they are only used during sexual intercourse, they reduce the risk of some sexually transmitted infections including HIV, there are no side effects, they are suitable for most people and they are easily available. However, the disadvantages are that putting them on can interrupt sex, they can split or slip off and there is a risk of latex allergy and spillage of semen. Condoms are made less effective if the penis touches any area close to vagina before application, if the condom splits, is damaged or slips off, or if oil-based products are used (such as baby lotions), which can damage latex condoms.

Alternative forms of contraception include the combined oral contraceptive pill (COCP), progesterone-only pill, coils (copper or hormonal), progesterone implants, progesterone injections and male or female sterilization.

8. SCREENING (2)

A – Amniocentesis

A screening test gives the risk of a condition being present; for Down syndrome, a high-risk result is said to be a risk of 1 in 150 or more. In these cases, a diagnostic test is offered and, at this gestation, amniocentesis is the correct method.

Amniocentesis is known as a diagnostic test as it gives a definite diagnosis rather than suggesting a risk of a condition. It is performed from 15 weeks' gestation as there is increased risk of miscarriage and talipes if performed earlier. Risk of miscarriage is 0.5% to 1%. Amniotic fluid is extracted using a transabdominal needle under ultrasound guidance. Fetal cells shed from the gut and skin, contained in amniotic fluid, are cultured for chromosome analysis to be performed. A full karyotype takes 2 to 3 weeks; however, polymerase chain reaction (PCR) or fluorescent *in situ* hybridization (FISH) can be used for a more rapid result for a number of conditions such as trisomies, triploidy and Turner syndrome. Indications for chromosomal analysis include for diagnosis in a positive Down syndrome screening test or for a pregnancy that is known to be high risk for chromosomal disorders, DNA analysis for genetic diseases, enzyme assays for inborn errors of metabolism, fetal infection and for information about rhesus iso-immunization via bilirubin. Anti-D is given in RhD –ve women.

Chorionic villus sampling also gives a definite answer but this is performed between 11 and 14 weeks (see Practice Paper 1, Question 19).

Routine anomaly scan is the ultrasound scan performed between 18 and 21 weeks to assess fetal anatomy, to detect structural abnormalities and to site the placenta. Approximately two-thirds of babies with Down syndrome will have normal appearances on this scan. Minor defects will be seen on the other one-third, but these only show an association and are not diagnostic. The accuracy of this scan is affected by fetal position and maternal obesity.

The nuchal translucency (NT) test would not be suitable for this couple as it is a screening tool. The thickness of the skin-fold over the neck of the fetus is measured during ultrasound scanning (USS). A greater NT (i.e. oedema of the fetal neck) is associated with a higher risk of fetal abnormalities including Down syndrome, cardiac defects and other chromosomal abnormalities such as trisomy 18, 13 and Turner syndrome. Where there is increased NT but no chromosomal abnormality, there is an association with multiple other abnormalities including congenital heart disease, exomphalos, diaphragmatic hernia and skeletal defects.

Fetal tissue sampling is rarely performed. Rare conditions need histological examination of the skin or an assay of the enzymes restricted to the liver for diagnosis. Such tissue sampling is performed under ultrasound guidance.

9. ENDOMETRIAL CANCER

E – Obesity

The majority of uterine cancers arise from the endometrium, which is the epithelial lining of the uterine cavity. It is a single layer of columnar ciliated cells, which form mucus-secreting glands by invaginating into the cellular stroma. Both the glandular and stromal (supporting) parts of this can undergo malignant change. Endometrial cancer is the most common cancer of the female genital tract, occurring most commonly in those over 65. The majority of tumours are adenocarcinomas (>90%).

Risk factors include those related to unopposed oestrogen exposure:

- Increasing age – generally found in postmenopausal women, only 5% in those under 40
- Obesity – due to the production of oestrogens from peripheral androgens by aromatization
- Nulliparity
- Early menarche – before age 12
- Late menopause – after age 52
- Unopposed oestrogen therapy – oestrogen-only hormone replacement therapy (now not used as this risk has been identified)

- Tamoxifen – despite having anti-oestrogen properties for breast cancer it has weak oestrogenic activity on the genital tract
- Oestrogen-secreting tumours (e.g. granulosa/theca cell ovarian tumours), although these are rare, they are associated with endometrial hyperplasia/carcinoma in 10% of cases
- Polycystic ovary syndrome – due to continuous anovulation and therefore unopposed oestrogen
- Personal history of breast or colon cancer
- Family history of breast, colon or ovarian (endometrium type) cancer

The COCP, progesterones and pregnancy are protective. Affected women present with postmenopausal bleeding (in postmenopausals) and irregular/intermenstrual bleeding or menorrhagia (in premenopausals).

Endometrial tumours spread directly through the myometrium to the cervix and upper vagina. Staging is as follows:

- Stage 1   Lesion confined to uterus
- Stage 2   Lesion confined to uterus and cervix
- Stage 3   Tumour invades through cervix/uterus
- Stage 4   Bowel/bladder involvement or distant metastases

Ultrasound scan and hysteroscopy are used for investigations of postmenopausal bleeding and menorrhagia in older women. Endometrial biopsy (e.g. using a Pipelle or at hysteroscopy) helps confirm a diagnosis. Stage 1 and 2 tumours are treated with radical hysterectomy and bilateral salpingo-oophorectomy, with or without lymphadenectomy. Adjuvant radiotherapy is used in addition if there is a high risk of recurrence. Stage 3 disease requires surgical debulking before proceeding with radiotherapy and chemotherapy. Stage 4 tumours are managed palliatively.

Radiotherapy has many side effects, which are easily divided into acute and chronic problems. Acute issues include skin irradiation, dysuria and diarrhoea. More chronic side effects are urinary frequency, vaginal dryness and dyspareunia.

10. CAESAREAN SECTION (2)

C – Persistent wound and abdominal discomfort in the months after surgery

Whoever gains consent must ensure the patient understands what is being done, why it is being done, the consequences of having the treatment, the consequences of not having the treatment and the alternative treatments to the one being offered. The person gaining consent should understand the risks in full. Consent for intimate examinations should be recorded in the notes and performed in the presence of a chaperone. Consent for any operation should be documented on a formal consent form.

Serious risks for caesarean section, as stated by the Royal College of Obstetricians and Gynaecologists, include:

Uncommon. Hysterectomy (0.7%–0.8%), need for further surgery at a later date (0.5%), ICU admission (0.9%), increased risk of uterine rupture in subsequent pregnancies (0.4–0.6%), antepartum stillbirth (0.4–0.6%) and increased risk of placenta praevia or accreta in subsequent pregnancies (0.4%–0.8%).
Rare. Thromboembolic disease (0.04%–0.16%), bladder injury (0.1%) and ureteric injury (0.03%).
Common/very common. Persistent wound and abdominal discomfort in the first few months following surgery (9%), increased risk of further caesarean sections in future pregnancies (25%), readmission to hospital (5%), infection (6%) and fetal laceration (2%).

Other procedures that should be documented on the caesarean consent form include blood transfusion, repair of bladder and bowel damage, surgery on major vessels, ovarian cystectomy/oophorectomy if unsuspected pathology is found and hysterectomy.

11. MENSTRUAL HORMONES (3)

C – Luteinizing hormone

Luteinizing hormone is a glycoprotein produced by the anterior pituitary in response to gonadotrophin-releasing hormones from the hypothalamus.

12. INDUCTION OF LABOUR (3)

B – Caesarean section

This woman would not be a suitable prospect for a normal delivery as the baby is in a transverse position and the membranes are ruptured; therefore, turning the baby into a longitudinal position would not be possible. She would therefore need a caesarean section. Urgency of caesarean section is indicated as follows: *Category 1* – immediate threat to the life of the woman or the fetus; *Category 2* – maternal or fetal compromise that is not immediately life-threatening; *Category 3* – no maternal or fetal compromise but needs early delivery; and *Category 4* – delivery timed to suit woman or staff.

Indications for an elective section include:

- Term singleton breech (if external cephalic version is contraindicated or failed)
- Twin pregnancy with breech first twin
- HIV with co-infection of hepatitis C
- Primary genital herpes in the third trimester
- Grade 3 and grade 4 placenta praevia

A caesarean section should not be routinely offered in:

- Twin pregnancy (if first twin is cephalic at term)
- HIV – well controlled
- Hepatitis B or C infection
- Recurrent genital herpes at term
- Preterm birth
- Small for gestational age babies

13. GAMETOGENESIS (2)

D – 64 days

Spermatogenesis takes place when the adult male reaches puberty, and it occurs under the influence of testosterone. The whole process of spermatogenesis takes 64 days. Primordial germ cells divide by mitosis and differentiate into spermatogonia, which lie immediately beneath the basement membrane of seminiferous tubules. As spermatogenesis progresses, the germ cells move from the basement membrane into the lumen of the seminiferous tubules. Spermatogonia divide by mitosis and differentiate into primary spermatocytes. Primary spermatocytes contain 46 double-structured chromosomes. These divide by meiosis. The primary spermatocytes initially complete the first meiotic division to give secondary spermatocytes. Secondary spermatocytes therefore contain 23 double-structured chromosomes, which complete the second meiotic division to give spermatids. Spermatids contain 23 single chromosomes. Spermatids undergo spermiogenesis (see following) to give spermatozoa.

In summary, every primary spermatocyte eventually gives rise to four spermatid daughter cells, two with 22 + X chromosomes and two with 22 + Y chromosomes. Spermatozoa are the end product of spermatogenesis. They have undergone spermiogenesis, which is the process by which spermatids differentiate into the distinctly shaped spermatozoa. Spermatozoa are made up of a head (within which the nucleus lies) capped by the acrosome (containing hydrolytic enzymes), a middle piece, which provides power for swimming (generated by large helical mitochondria), and a tail (the propulsion system made up of microtubules).

Sperm, from Greek *sperma* = seed.

14. CARDIOTOCOGRAPHY (3)

A – Early decelerations
See Practice Paper 1, Question 5.

15. GENITAL ULCERATION

E – Syphilis
Treponema pallidum, which is spread by sexual contact, is responsible for syphilis. Primary syphilis occurs 10 to 90 days after initial infection when

a dull red papule appears on the site of inoculation. It ulcerates to give a single, painless well-demarcated ulcer known as a chancre. This heals to leave a thin scar within 8 weeks. Diagnosis is by darkfield microscopy from the serum at the base of the chancre or direct immunofluorescence and serology. The patient can go on to develop secondary, latent, gummatous and neurosyphilis. Treatment is with penicillin.

Chancroid is caused by the Gram-negative bacterium *Haemophilus ducreyi* and is found mostly in tropical countries. It is an ulcerative condition of the genitalia (single/multiple painful superficial ulcers), which develops within a week of exposure. Inflammation may lead to a phimosis. Enlargement and suppuration of inguinal lymph nodes may occur, leading to a unilocular abscess (bubo) that can rupture to form a sinus. Diagnosis is by microscopy and culture. Treatment is with appropriate antibiotics (e.g. azithromycin/ceftriaxone).

Lymphogranuloma venereum (LGV) is a sexually transmitted infection caused by serovars L1, L2 and L3 of *Chlamydia trachomatis*. It is mainly found in the tropics. Between 3 and 21 days after infection, one-third of people develop a small painless papule, which ulcerates and heals after several days. The patients then develop lymphadenopathy, which is unilateral in two-thirds of cases. Inguinal abscesses (buboes) may form and develop a sinus. Acute ulcerative proctitis may develop when infection takes place via the rectal mucosa. Diagnosis is by culture or serology. Treatment is with tetracyclines.

Granuloma inguinale (Donovanosis) is a tropical condition caused by *Klebsiella granulomatis*. It predominantly affects the genitalia and is therefore thought to be a sexually transmitted disease, although this has not been proven. After a prepatent period of 3 days to 6 months, there is development of a flat-topped papule that ulcerates painlessly, spreads along skin-folds and eventually heals with scarring. Diagnosis is by Giemsa-stained smear microscopy – the bacteria are seen in mononuclear cells as Donovan bodies. Treatment is usually with tetracyclines.

Genital herpes is caused by the DNA-containing herpes simplex virus (types 1 and 2). The infection remains prevalent due to asymptomatic shedding of the virus. Clinical features of primary infection include dysuria with painful, itchy lesions and occasionally urethral or vaginal discharge. Patients may also complain of constitutional symptoms (fever, headache, malaise and myalgia). Lesions are papular, vesicular or pustular; these crust and heal within 4 weeks. Examination may reveal inguinal lymphadenitis. After primary infection has resolved, there is a period of asymptomatic viral shedding. Herpes simplex virus remains dormant in dorsal root ganglia, and reactivation occurs in 75% of cases. Recurrent attacks tend to be milder, shorter and not associated with systemic features. Diagnosis is by viral swabs (specimen sent in Hanks' viral transport medium) or serology (primary infection only). Treatment is with oral acyclovir, valaciclovir or famiciclovir, particularly in primary infections.

They have less effect in recurrence but can still be helpful particularly if given in the prodrome.

Below is a useful summary table:

Name	Syphilis	Chancroid	Lymphogranuloma venereum	Granuloma inguinale	Herpes simplex
Pathogen	*Treponema pallidum*	*Haemophilus ducreyi*	*Chlamydia trachomatis*	*Klebsiella granulomatis*	*Herpes simplex virus*
Latent period	10–90 days	7 days	3–21 days	3 days to 6 months	N/A
Ulcer	Single well-demarcated	Single or multiple	Small, single	Single, spreads	Numerous
Pain	No	Yes	No	No	Yes
Other symptoms	Can go on to develop further problems	Bubo	Bubo	Heals with scarring	Systemic features
Diagnosis	Darkfield microscopy or direct immuno-fluorescence and serology	Gram smear microscopy and culture	Culture or serology	Giemsa-stained smear microscopy	Culture and viral isolation, serology
Treatment	Penicillin	Azithromycin	Tetracyclines	Tetracyclines	Acyclovir, valaciclovir or famiciclovir

Bubo, from Greek *boubon* = groin or swollen groin. Also gives rise to 'bubonic plague', and allegedly, the American colloquial 'boo-boo', used to describe minor cuts and scrapes.

Venereal, from Latin *venereus* = desire (derived from Venus, the goddess of love).

Charles Donovan, Irish biologist (1863–1951).

16. MALE INFERTILITY

D – Poorly motile sperm

Male infertility can be due to problems with sperm production, sperm function or sperm delivery. The quality of sperm can be investigated using semen analysis. Two semen analyses are needed 3 months apart as sperm count varies and it takes over 2 months for spermatogenesis to be completed. Conditions that may be seen on semen reports are:

- Asthenospermia: poorly motile sperm (i.e. lack the normal forward movement)
- Azoospermia: complete absence of sperm, such as testicular failure
- Oligospermia: reduced sperm count of normal appearance
- Teratospermia: morphologically defective, with abnormalities of head, midpiece or tail
- Leucospermia: infection

Leucospermia and antisperm antibodies can both be associated with agglutination and can affect sperm function.

The World Health Organization (WHO) provides reference ranges for semen analysis (below), although this does not give accurate predictive values about which man will father a child. This semen analysis only has predictive value when morphology is below 15% and motility is below 20%. WHO normal values in semen analysis:

Volume	>1.5 mL
pH	≥7.2
Concentration	>15 × 10^6/mL
Motility	>32% progressive motility
Morphology	>4% normal
Alive	>58%

Astheno-, from Greek *asthenos* = without strength.
Terato-, from Greek *teras* = monster.

17. INFECTION IN PREGNANCY (2)

A – Chickenpox

Chickenpox is caused by the DNA varicella zoster virus (human herpes virus 3) via airborne spread and direct personal contact with vesicle fluid. There is an incubation period of 3 to 21 days. There is a prodromal malaise and fever followed by an itchy rash of maculopapules, which become vesicular and crust over before healing. It is infectious 48 hours before the rash appears and until the vesicles all crust over, which normally takes 5 days. The disease is often seen in children where a mild infection ensues.

Ninety percent of pregnant women are immune due to previous infection and so, if these women come into contact with chickenpox in pregnancy, they can be reassured that they will not contract the disease again. A varicella vaccine is available and should be considered in women wishing to get pregnant who are non-immune. Around 3 in 1000 pregnancies are affected. The sequelae of infection are more serious in pregnant women with a risk of pneumonia (10%), hepatitis, encephalitis and mortality (1%). Diagnosis is clinical and treatment supportive with advice to avoid other pregnant women.

If a non-immune woman has contact with chickenpox, then she should be offered varicella zoster immunoglobulins within 10 days of exposure if she is not already immune. If chickenpox develops, she should be advised to avoid other pregnant women and should be given oral acyclovir if she is seen within 24 hours of the onset of the rash. Some women do not know if they are immune or not, and this can be easily checked by calling the lab, who will be able to test the booking bloods.

The fetus is at risk of developing fetal varicella syndrome, particularly if infection occurs before 16 weeks, which includes dermatomal skin scarring, neurological defects, fetal growth retardation, limb hypoplasia, eye defects and hydrops fetalis.

Salmonella is a Gram-negative bacterium and is found in raw or partially cooked eggs, raw meat and chicken. Incubation time is 12 to 72 hours. Pregnancy increases the incidence and severity of symptoms of gastroenteritis. There are no adverse effects of maternal gastroenteritis on the fetus as long as the mother remains well hydrated.

Cytomegalovirus affects 3 in 1000 live births. It is transmitted through urine, saliva and other bodily products. The maternal infection is usually asymptomatic after a 3- to 12-week incubation period. Maternal primary infection can be seen by IgM in the blood, and maternal immunity can be detected by IgG in the blood. Ten to fifteen percent of fetuses will be affected and this can occur at any gestation. Infection can be diagnosed using amniocentesis or cordocentesis. Eighty percent of infected fetuses will be normal at birth but develop symptoms later in life such as mental handicap, visual impairment, progressive hearing loss or psychomotor retardation. Signs of infection at birth include hydrops, intrauterine growth restriction, exomphalos, microcephaly, hydrocephalus, hepatosplenomegaly and thrombocytopenia.

18. VAGINAL BLEEDING (2)

E – Uterine fibroids

Fibroids (leiomyomata) are whorls of smooth muscle cells interspersed with collagen. They are benign tumours of the myometrium. Fibroids are present in 20% of women of reproductive age and are largely asymptomatic. They are more common in nulliparous and Afro-Caribbean women. They can be multiple and vary widely in size. Presentation depends on the size and location of fibroids as some are microscopic and others have been known to be over 5 kg! The most common presentation is menorrhagia and abdominal swelling. Pressure on the bladder can lead to frequency of micturition or hydronephrosis, due to ureteric compression. Other presenting features include infertility, miscarriage or pelvic discomfort. Fibroids can be distinguished on ultrasound as intramural (within the uterine wall), subserous (beneath the serosal surface of the uterus) or submucosal (beneath the mucosal surface of the uterus). Treatment is not required if fibroids are asymptomatic.

Medical treatment includes those that are used for menorrhagia (tranexamic acid, progesterone, COCP) and the use of gonadotrophin-releasing hormone agonists preoperatively. Surgical options include myomectomy (abdominally, laparoscopically or hysteroscopically), uterine artery embolization and hysterectomy. A new treatment, ulipristal acetate, which is a selective progesterone receptor modulator (SPRM), acts on fibroid tissue to block progesterone activity, thus inhibiting cell proliferation and inducing apoptosis. It induces amenorrhoea by acting at the pituitary level, reduces endometrial bleeding directly and can be used preoperatively for 3 months.

Leiomyomata, from Greek *leios* = smooth + *myos* = muscle + *oma* = tumour.

19. OBSTETRIC EMERGENCIES (4)

E – Uterine rupture

Uterine rupture can occur gradually as labour progresses or more suddenly. A complete rupture is where the uterine cavity communicates directly with the peritoneal cavity and the fetus enters the abdominal cavity. This often results in fetal death (75%) and is life-threatening to the mother due to massive intra-abdominal haemorrhage, particularly if the rupture extends into the uterine arteries or the broad ligament plexus of veins. Incomplete uterine rupture is where the uterine cavity is separated from the peritoneal cavity by the visceral peritoneum of the uterus alone.

Uterine rupture is extremely rare in primigravida and in women who have had one normal delivery. An increased risk is seen in women with any previous uterine surgery. There is a 0.4–0.6% risk of rupture occurring at the scar site of a previous caesarean section in a woman attempting a vaginal birth after caesarean (VBAC). This risk is increased further if prostaglandins or oxytocin are used. The risk is increased to almost one-third if the previous section was a classical section (midline uterine incision rather than the normal lower segment transverse incision), and most obstetricians would advise against labour in these women, instead offering delivery by elective caesarean section.

A uterine rupture presents with CTG abnormalities, abdominal pain, maternal shock, fetal parts being palpable on abdominal examination and vaginal bleeding (although much bleeding is intraperitoneal). Prior to this, the patient may experience scar tenderness in between contractions, cessation of contractions, haematuria, vaginal bleeding or evidence of shock from hypovolaemia.

Management is initially the same for any obstetric emergency – shout for help and assess and manage ABC. Stop any oxytocin infusion. An immediate laparotomy is needed to deliver the baby and arrest bleeding. The uterus should be repaired if possible; otherwise, an emergency hysterectomy must be performed.

Antepartum risk factors for uterine rupture include external trauma, classical and lower segment caesarean section, other uterine surgery and certain congenital malformations of the uterus, such as the pregnancy developing in a rudimentary horn. Intrapartum risks include prostaglandins or oxytocin use in women with a previous section, oxytocin use in a multiparous woman and obstructed labour.

Just because there is an increased risk of scar rupture, it does not mean that everyone who has had a previous section needs a repeat one. It is generally considered that a trial of vaginal delivery is safer than a further section; however, it must be closely monitored and prostaglandins and oxytocin are used with caution. A woman who has had two or more caesarean sections would normally be advised to have a further section due to the higher risk of scar rupture.

20. FETAL ULTRASOUND (2)

E – Head circumference

Ultrasound scanning (USS) is a means of monitoring pregnancy and to date is without proven maternal or fetal risk. Scans can be performed abdominally or transvaginally.

The head circumference or biparietal diameter is used to date a fetus over 14 weeks. Because the fetus becomes more flexed in shape after this point, the crown–rump length, which is used before 14 weeks, is less accurate. As gestation increases, the accuracy of dating the pregnancy by ultrasound decreases; therefore, it is very difficult to give 'late bookers' an accurate EDD, which creates problems for planning an induction of labour if spontaneous labour does not occur by 41 weeks.

The second trimester scan is generally done at 20 weeks as this allows time for anatomy to have developed but still gives time for a termination to be planned before 24 weeks (i.e. without the added complication of fetocide) if any abnormality is detected and termination is requested. A detailed fetal structural anatomical survey is performed. If any abnormality is detected, the parents are referred to the fetal medicine unit. Fetal growth and liquor volume are measured at this scan, although it is very rare that intrauterine growth restriction or oligohydramnios would be seen this early. If parents wish to know the sex of the baby, then most units will provide this information; however, due to misuse of this information by some cultures, it is not offered by all centres and it is never 100% guaranteed correct. The placental site is determined and, if it is covering the os, or near to the os, then a re-scan must be completed at 34 weeks to exclude placenta praevia.

Reasons for follow-up scans include:

- Measuring small (intrauterine growth restriction) for date fetuses in the third trimester. Serial scans show trends of growth in abdominal circumference, head circumference and femur length, and these are plotted on centile graphs. A differentiation can be made between a small but well-grown fetus and a growth-restricted fetus. The growth of the latter will tail off, but the former will continue along the centile lines, even if it is a low centile line. In a growth-restricted fetus, the head will continue to grow normally at the expense of abdominal growth. The scans should be done at least 2 weeks apart.

- Amniotic fluid volume can be assessed, if there is clinical suspicion of oligohydramnios or polyhydramnios, by measuring the deepest pool of liquor seen that does not contain limbs or cord. Reasons for oligohydramnios include ruptured membranes, fetal renal abnormalities or placental insufficiencies. Polyhydramnios can result from diabetes, multiple pregnancies or fetal swallowing problems such as oesophageal atresia.
- Follow-up of any structures not seen or any abnormalities detected on the 20-week scan.
- Real-time USS is used to assess fetal well-being by Doppler assessment of blood flow in the umbilical artery and other fetal vessels or by biophysical profile. Biophysical profile measures breathing movements, gross body movements, fetal tone, heart rate activity and amniotic fluid volume. The absence or reversal of end diastolic flow in umbilical artery Doppler studies suggests fetal deterioration and delivery should be considered.
- Fetal echocardiography is offered to women with a high risk of fetal cardiac abnormalities, which includes women with congenital cardiac disease themselves, previous children with congenital cardiac disease and some women with epilepsy and diabetes.
- Uterine artery Doppler flow studies are done to assess the resistance in the maternal uterine arteries. A high resistance is seen in those at increased risk of pre-eclampsia, abruption and growth restriction.
- To confirm breech presentation.

21. POSTPARTUM HAEMORRHAGE (3)

C – Infection
Infection (i.e. endometritis) is the most common cause of secondary postpartum haemorrhage and can be due to retained products of conception, such as the placenta. The woman may complain of malodorous prolonged vaginal bleeding associated with fever and sweating. Examination reveals tenderness in the lower abdomen. A speculum examination should be performed and a high vaginal swab taken. A full blood count is taken to look for anaemia and infection. Antibiotics (e.g. cefuroxime and metronidazole) are the first-line treatment. If this does not settle the bleeding, an ultrasound can be done to rule out retained products of conception, which may require surgical evacuation.

22. PAIN IN PREGNANCY (3)

D – Symphysis pubis dysfunction
Women with symphysis pubis dysfunction describe pain and discomfort in the pelvic area, which can radiate to the upper thighs or perineum. The pain worsens as the pregnancy progresses due to the increasing weight of the uterus. Pain is generally exacerbated by walking and may

be severe enough to limit mobility. The diagnosis is clinical and can be confirmed by increased pain on pressure over the symphysis pubis or by compression of the pelvis. Treatment is supportive with analgesia, pelvic support braces and crutches. Symphysis pubis dysfunction is seen in 3% of pregnancies.

Labour is defined as painful regular contractions associated with dilation and effacement of the cervix and downward progression of the presenting part. It is important to remember that labour may be triggered by pathological causes of abdominal pain. The round ligament of the uterus runs from the uterine horns down through the deep inguinal ring to terminate in the labia majora. It supports the uterus. During pregnancy, stretching of the round ligament due to the increasing size of the uterus and the action of progesterone can cause non-specific abdominal pain.

Braxton Hicks contractions are sometimes described as false labour or practice contractions. The uterus contracts sporadically from early pregnancy and, as labour approaches, the frequency and amplitude of these contractions increase. These are easily confused with labour, but Braxton Hicks contractions are characteristically relieved by time, rest, a warm bath or shower, drinking water or changing activities.

John Braxton Hicks, British obstetrician (1823–1897).

23. MANAGEMENT OF INCONTINENCE (2)

D – Pelvic floor exercises with a trained physiotherapist
This woman is suffering from stress incontinence. The first-line treatment is at least 3 months of supervised pelvic floor muscle training.

Stress incontinence is the most common type of incontinence in women and is seen with coughing, laughing, sneezing and running, and any other condition that causes raised intra-abdominal pressure. Other causes of incontinence include overactive bladder (OAB), retention with overflow, fistula and congenital abnormalities. Incontinence associated with urgency is known as urge incontinence and is part of the overactive bladder picture. Bedside examination includes examination of the genital area and asking the patient to cough, looking for leakage of urine. A neurological examination is needed, particularly of roots S2 to S4 (supply of the urinary and anal sphincters).

Predisposing factors to stress incontinence are pregnancy and multiparity, prolapse, menopause, collagen disorder, increasing age and obesity.

Treatment can be conservative or surgical depending on the patient's wishes with regard to future pregnancies, severity of symptoms and presence of other pathology. First-line treatment should be at least 3 months of supervised pelvic floor muscle training. This should consist of at least eight contractions, three times a day, and if it is beneficial this should be continued. If this does not improve symptoms then surgical options should be discussed.

24. MENOPAUSE

A – Follicle-stimulating hormone

The menopause is defined as the permanent cessation of menstruation due to failure of ovarian follicular development in the presence of adequate gonadotrophin stimulation. The average age of the menopause in the UK is 51 years. Premature menopause (primary ovarian failure) is diagnosed as the onset of menopause below 40 years and can be idiopathic or as a result of oophorectomy or radiotherapy. The perimenopausal period, or climacteric, is of variable duration as the menstrual cycle lengthens and anovulation ensues.

In simple terms, menopause occurs when the supply of oocytes is exhausted. Most oocytes are lost spontaneously due to aging, but some will have been used for ovulation. The permanent cessation of periods is due to loss of ovarian follicular activity. Oestradiol production by the granulosa cells of developing follicles is reduced as menopause approaches, anovulatory cycles become more common and progesterone production reduces. There is increased production of follicle-stimulating hormone (FSH) and luteinizing hormone by the pituitary due to lack of negative feedback from the diminishing oestrogen levels. (Other pituitary hormones are not affected.)

The symptoms attributed to the menopause are largely due to oestrogen deficiency. Immediate effects of the menopause include vasomotor symptoms (hot flushes, night sweats, sleep disturbance, palpitations and dizziness) and psychological symptoms (low mood, irritability, poor memory, loss of libido). Intermediate effects, which take a couple of years to develop, are atrophy of the vagina and vulva (→ atrophic vaginitis, manifesting in dryness, itching, dyspareunia), atrophy of pelvic tissues (→ prolapse) and atrophy of the urethral epithelium (→ dysuria, frequency and urgency). There is a 30% reduction in skin collagen. Long-term effects of the menopause include osteoporosis with subsequent pathological fracture (common sites include the distal radius, femoral neck and vertebrae) and an increase in the risk of atherosclerotic cardiovascular disease.

The diagnosis of menopause is made retrospectively after 12 months of amenorrhoea, with or without symptoms of the menopause. Investigations are only required if there are diagnostic difficulties. FSH should be >30 u/L postmenopausally; however, this can be raised for months or years prior to cessation of menstruation.

Menopause, from Greek *men* = month + *paussis* = cessation.

25. PHYSIOLOGICAL CHANGES IN PREGNANCY

A – All normal physiological results for pregnancy

A healthy range of haemoglobin for pregnant women over 30 weeks' gestation is between 10.5 and 14.5 g/dL due to changes in blood volume and haemodilution. A level under 10.5 g/dL requires addition of parenteral iron, and very low levels may need further investigation.

White cells are raised during pregnancy. It may have been thought that there is a urinary infection due to the increased urinary frequency with raised white blood cells; however, it is common to have increased frequency of urine due to the anatomical changes in pregnancy; the lack of dysuria and of evidence on urine dipstick would make a urinary infection unlikely.

Platelets are known to fall during pregnancy, but a very low level is worrying particularly in the presence of pre-eclampsia. A level below 100×10^9/L would be more worrying. Alkaline phosphatase is produced by the placenta so, in the absence of other liver function test (LFT) abnormalities and symptoms, this can be regarded as physiological. Albumin is decreased in pregnancy and does not indicate a nutritional deficit. Sodium and potassium should be unchanged during pregnancy.

During pregnancy, renal blood flow increases from an average of 1.2 to 1.5 mL/min, which is associated with an increase in glomerular filtration rate and leads to a decrease in blood urea (from an average of 4.3 to 3.1 mmol/L) and in blood creatinine (from 73 to 47 umol/L). This is important as, if there is a slightly increased – or even normal – urea and creatinine during pregnancy, it could indicate significant renal disease.

	Increase	Unchanged	Decrease
Respiratory	Tidal vol + 200 mL Inspiratory capacity + 100 mL Oxygen consumption (+20%–33%)	Respiratory rate Peak flow	Total lung capacity −200 mL Residual volume −200 mL Expiratory reserve −100 mL Inspiratory reserve −100 mL Functional residual capacity −300 mL
Cardiovascular system (CVS)	Plasma vol (45% by 32 wk) Red cell mass (25%) Cardiac output (40%) Heart rate (10%) Stroke volume (30%) Blood flow Uterus 400 mL Renal 300 mL	Mean arterial pressure Central venous pressure Pulmonary wedge pressure	Mid-trimester BP Systemic and pulmonary vascular resistance

Continued

	Increase	Unchanged	Decrease
Haematology	Mean cell volume Plasma vol (50%) WCC TIBC	Mean cell Hb concentration	Hb concentration Haematocrit (dilutional) Platelet count Serum ferritin, iron
Gastrointestinal (GI)	Weight 10 kg (variable) Nutritional requirements Gastric reflux Gallstones	Amylase	GIT motility Stomach pH
Liver	Alkaline phosphatase (placental) Plasma cholesterol Triglycerides	Bilirubin	Albumin, AST, ALT
Immunology	ESR C3, C4, complement	CRP	Circulating immune complexes

Endocrinology	Total T3 + T4
	Thyroid-binding
	  globulin
	Insulin
	ACTH, CRH, cortisol
	Prolactin
	1,25-dihydroxy-vit D
		Free T3 + T4
		Synacthen
		Adrenaline,
		  noradrenaline
		Calcitonin, free
		  ionized calcium
			Fasting glucose
			Glucose tolerance
			Thyroid-stimulating
			  hormone
			Total serum
			  calcium, albumin,
			  parathyroid
			  hormone

Renal	Renal blood flow (25%)
	Creatinine clearance
	  (40%)
	Kidney length 1–1.5 cm
	Bladder capacity
	Renin, angiotensin II
	Aldosterone
		Daily voided volume
		Plasma Na, K, Cl
			Plasma Ur, Cr,
			  bicarb,
			  phosphorus

26. PLACENTAL ABNORMALITIES

D – Placenta percreta

Placenta accreta broadly describes placental invasion into the uterine wall and is divided more specifically into placenta increta and placenta percreta (below). It is caused by over-invasion by the fetal trophoblast through the maternal decidual barrier when implantation occurs in the first trimester. Risk factors include previous retained placenta, previous caesarean section, a history of previous dilation and curettage (D&C) or suction termination, placenta praevia, high parity, advanced maternal age and previous postpartum endometritis.

Placenta increta invades the myometrium only. *Placenta percreta* invades the myometrium and the outer serosal layer of the uterus. It can invade adjacent structures including the bladder and bowel.

Normally, the placenta separates from the uterus following contraction of the uterus during the third stage of labour. In the aforementioned conditions, there is no physiological cleavage plane so the placenta cannot shear off.

The placenta should be delivered within 30 minutes after delivery of the baby. If this does not occur, a manual removal of the placenta may be needed in theatre. This involves insertion of a hand through the cervix into the uterus to find the plane between the uterus and the placenta and the careful separation of the placenta from the uterus, using the fingers. Separation would not be possible with placenta accrete, and massive haemorrhage can ensue. If massive haemorrhage occurs, a hysterectomy may be needed to control the bleeding. If the bleeding is minimal, suction curettage or conservative measures can be used. Suction curettage should only be used with caution as the uterus is very soft following pregnancy and there is a high risk of perforation. Conservative treatment involves leaving the placenta *in situ*, where it is eventually absorbed.

Placenta praevia is where the placenta lies close to or covers the internal cervical os. A caesarean section is normally used for delivery.

Placenta, from Greek *plakoeis* = flat cake.
Accreta, from Latin *ad* = towards + *crescere* = to grow.

27. MENORRHAGIA (1)

D – Intrauterine or systemic progestogens

A levonorgestrel-releasing intrauterine system (LNG-IUS) is the first-line treatment for menorrhagia according to the NICE guidance. Progestogens are the most appropriate treatment as they offer her contraception and reduction in bleeding. She is not suitable for the COCP due to the combination of age and smoking habits; the other treatments listed do not provide contraception.

Subjective menorrhagia is when women complain of heavy periods. Objective menorrhagia is >80 mL blood loss per cycle. Only 50% of women who complain of heavy bleeding actually have more than 80 mL of blood loss, but subjective menorrhagia must still be treated. Sixty percent of women with objective menorrhagia develop anaemia. The main causes for menorrhagia are dysfunctional uterine bleeding, uterine pathology such as fibroids and, rarely, medical conditions including clotting disorders.

There are many different ways of treating heavy menstrual bleeding and, while this is covered by NICE guidance, it is also a matter of personal choice. An intrauterine device that delivers progestogen directly to the lining of uterus is available (LNG-IUS, Mirena). It can be kept *in situ* for 5 years and can reduce bleeding by 95%, giving amenorrhoea in many women, and also provides excellent contraception. Irregular bleeding can be a problem particularly in the first 6 months, and this must be explained to women prior to insertion; otherwise, there is a high removal rate. If an LNG-IUS does not work, tranexamic acid or NSAIDs can be used. Other options are the COCP or an oral formulation of a progesterone-only pill: norethisterone (15 mg) daily from days 5 to 26. Progestogens can also be administered by injection every 8 or 12 weeks, which can eventually lead to amenorrhoea if used for long enough; however, these can also produce irregular and heavy bleeding for the first few months of use.

Menstrual flow is reduced or stopped by destroying the endometrium by ablation. Hysteroscopic procedures include laser ablation, resection or coagulation using an electric roller ball. Microwave ablation, heat ablation and electrocautery are all non-hysteroscopic procedures. Pregnancy is contraindicated after ablation. These options would help with the treatment of menorrhagia but would offer no contraception, and the patient in this scenario may want more children. Hysterectomy is the last resort.

28. MANAGEMENT OF SMEAR RESULTS (2)

A – Colposcopy

The fact that there is a pre-malignant phase for cervical cancer makes it suitable for screening, so the pre-malignant disease can be treated before the invasion occurs. Cervical screening aims to detect the precancerous lesion (cervical intraepithelial neoplasia [CIN]) on the cervix prior to it developing into cancer.

This patient should be referred for colposcopy as there is high-grade dyskaryosis; therefore, it is very likely that there will be a histological abnormality with this grade of cytological abnormality. It is only with low-grade dyskaryosis that human papillomavirus (HPV) testing is required.

Treatment options for CIN

Local ablation should only be used if the squamocolumnar junction can be seen completely on examination, there is no suggestion of invasive disease, there are no glandular abnormalities and the patient will attend regular follow-up. Many ablation techniques exist. Laser vaporization is where tissue is destroyed using a CO_2 laser in an outpatient procedure. There is no tissue for pathology but the depth of tissue destruction is known. 'Cold' coagulation is where the tissue is heated to 100°C (as an outpatient procedure). Radical electrotherapy involves using a monopolar high-frequency current to perform cervical cautery, which can easily be done as an outpatient procedure. Cryotherapy involves freezing the cervix using a nitrogen probe, again this can easily done as an outpatient procedure. The limitations of cold coagulation, radical electrotherapy and cryotherapy are that there is no tissue available for histological testing and the depth of tissue destruction is not known. If these techniques are used, a diagnostic biopsy for histological assessment must be taken from abnormal areas.

Excision techniques, rather than ablative ones, are recommended in CIN II and III, so a definite tissue diagnosis can be made and incision margins can be confirmed. Loop excision of the transition zone involves a high-frequency current being passed through a wire loop that is used to take tissue away. This provides tissue for histological examination, and it is an easy outpatient procedure. There is, however, a small risk of cervical incompetence and stenosis. Cone biopsy describes surgical excision of cervical tissue often under anaesthesia. This provides a large specimen for pathology but is associated with cervical incompetence and stenosis.

Screening starts at 25 years, as invasive cervical cancer is rare below this age and the body is still developing. The cervices of young women often give an abnormal smear result when there is nothing wrong, which can lead to overtreatment with invasive measures where these lesions are very likely to regress with no treatment. Overtreatment exposes women to unnecessary risks such as pain, bleeding, infection and, rarely, fertility problems. If a woman has never been sexually active, then the chance of her developing cervical cancer is very low (never impossible) so she may choose to decline cervical screening.

29. RHESUS DISEASE (3)

B – Give antenatal anti-D prophylaxis 500 IU at 28 weeks
Even though this woman has received previous anti-D, it is not in a great enough amount to protect her throughout the whole pregnancy; therefore, she must receive a further dose as described (see Practice Paper 1, Question 25).

30. SCREENING (3)

E – Serum quadruple test
The *triple test* is a screening test for Down syndrome and spina bifida. A number of serum markers are used in combination to give a risk of Down syndrome. Increasing maternal age is the strongest risk factor. The serum markers used in the triple test are α-fetoprotein (AFP), oestriol and human chorionic gonadotrophin β-subunit (βhCG), with inhibin being added to make the quadruple test. This is available from 15 to 20 weeks (optimal at 15–16 weeks) with results available 2 weeks after the test. High βhCG, low AFP and low oestriol are associated with Down syndrome. False positives occur in around 5% of cases. A 'positive' result is defined as a risk of greater than 1 in 150. In these cases, a diagnostic test would be offered; at this gestation, amniocentesis would be most appropriate. A finding of raised AFP alone is associated with a break in fetal skin often indicating neural tube defects such as spina bifida and anencephaly. As there is a large overlap with the normal and abnormal levels of AFP, further testing is needed for firm diagnosis, such as a scan for spina bifida.

Amniocentesis and CVS would not be offered as an initial test as they are invasive and have a 0.5% to 1% risk of miscarriage. They are only offered for high-risk screening results. CVS is performed between 11 and 14 weeks, and amniocentesis is used in later gestations. Nuchal translucency is the measurement of thickness of the back of the fetal neck with a higher measurement correlating with fetal abnormalities. In the first trimester, this measurement is assessed in conjunction with certain maternal blood tests as the combined screening test.

Fetal echocardiography is used for women with a high risk of fetal cardiac abnormalities and is done in the second trimester. Indications are women with congenital heart disease, diabetes or epilepsy, those with a previous child with congenital heart disease or abnormal or inadequate views of the heart at routine second trimester scans, or a high-risk nuchal translucency result. This has no role in the screening for Down syndrome, although affected babies are at increased risk of cardiac abnormalities. Therefore, they may have this test subsequently if the diagnosis is confirmed.

31. TWINS (2)

A – Dizygotic dichorionic diamniotic

Dizygotic twins are the most common type of twins (60%). They develop due to fertilization of two different ova, from the same or opposite ovaries, by two different sperm, so are not identical. They can be of different sexes and are no more genetically similar than siblings would be. They implant separately into the decidua and have their own circulation. They are always dichorionic and diamniotic, which means each fetus has its own chorion, amnion and placenta. Placental tissue may appear continuous due to close implantation sites, but there will be no significant vascular communications.

Chorionicity is best determined by ultrasound in the first trimester. Dichorionic twins have widely separated first trimester sacs or clearly separate placentae and a dividing membrane thicker than 2 mm.

32. MENORRHAGIA (2)

D – Myomectomy

Following dysfunctional uterine bleeding, uterine pathology is the next most common cause for menorrhagia. Pathology can be benign such as uterine fibroids, endometrial polyps, adenomyosis or pelvic infection, or it is rarely malignant such as endometrial cancer (see Question 18).

Myomectomy allows conservation of a patient's fertility. This is either an abdominal or a laparoscopic procedure. The pseudo capsule of the fibroid is incised, the bulk of the tumour is enucleated and the resulting defect is sealed. Risks of this procedure include uncontrolled bleeding requiring hysterectomy, recurrence of fibroids and adhesion formation leading to reduced fertility. Hysteroscopic resection is not an option in this case as they are not submucosal.

A hysterectomy is the only treatment that will ensure amenorrhoea. Surgical approach is vaginally or abdominally, although generally with large fibroids an abdominal approach is more appropriate. Risks of this procedure are bleeding, infection, pain, damage to bowel or urinary tracts, postoperative thromboembolism and vaginal prolapse in later life. Hysterectomy is not suitable in this case as the patient wishes to retain her fertility.

Uterine artery embolization is performed by radiologists. An arterial catheter is passed into the femoral artery and through the uterine artery where a coil or piece of foam is deposited to stop the blood supply to the fibroid. Fibroids can shrink by 50%, but the normal myometrium is unaffected as there is collateral circulation via the ovarian and vaginal vessels. Risks include pain, bleeding, infection, fibroid expulsion and damage to ovaries due to ionizing radiation. Hysteroscopic resection of fibroids is possible with only submucosal fibroids. This treatment may lead not only to reduction of bleeding but improvement of fertility with submucosal fibroids.

Menorrhagia, from Greek *meniaios* = monthly + *rhoia* = flowing.

33. PREMATURE LABOUR (2)

D – Erythromycin

Preterm pre-labour rupture of membranes (PPROM) is where the membranes rupture without contractions before 37 weeks, and this occurs in 2% to 3% of pregnancies. The woman describes a gush of fluid *per vagina* associated with a subsequent continuous trickle. Diagnosis is made on sterile speculum examination to visualize the amniotic fluid draining from the cervical os, and the patient is asked to cough during examination to elicit a gush of fluid from the cervix. A vaginal swab, urine specimen and liquor specimen are taken to test for infection. A digital examination should *not* be performed due to the risk of introducing infection. Other investigations that may help in diagnosis are the nitrazine test, which measures the pH of the vagina. Amniotic fluid is more alkaline than normal vaginal secretions; however, there are false positives with blood, urine, semen or antiseptic cleaning agents. An ultrasound may be performed to check for reduced liquor if there is a convincing history but no liquor seen on examination.

If PPROM occurs at term, the majority of women labour within 24 to 48 hours. Women should be counselled and offered either immediate or delayed induction (at 24 hours). However, if rupture of membranes occurs preterm, the risks of continuing the pregnancy (such as maternal and fetal infections) have to be weighed against the risks of prematurity; therefore, the management is usually conservative before 34 weeks and the woman is observed for signs of chorioamnionitis. Concerning features suggesting infection or chorioamnionitis include maternal pyrexia and tachycardia, foul-smelling liquor or meconium, uterine tenderness or fetal tachycardia. Blood tests for white cell count and CRP are non-specific and no longer recommended. Ultrasound scans can be performed but have limited value in predicting fetal infection.

The patient should receive prophylactic antibiotics, specifically erythromycin, to treat or prevent ascending infection, prolong the latency period, to prevent chorioamnionitis and reduce neonatal sepsis. The mother should also receive steroids to reduce the incidence of neonatal respiratory distress, necrotizing enterocolitis and intraventricular haemorrhage.

Risk factors for PPROM include increased uterine volume such as polyhydramnios and multiple pregnancies, low socioeconomic status, infectious causes such as amnionitis and cervicitis, fetal anomalies, subchorionic haemorrhage, substance abuse (including smoking) and maternal trauma.

Co-amoxiclav (augmentin) is *not* used due to the high incidence of necrotizing enterocolitis after delivery. Gentamicin, an aminoglycoside, should be avoided in pregnancy unless essential due to the risk of auditory or vestibular nerve damage.

34. CONTRACEPTION (3)

A. No – hypertension
Any hypertension (even controlled disease) is a category 3 condition where the risks generally outweigh the benefits (see Practice Paper 1, Question 44).

35. GAMETOGENESIS (3)

C – Spermatid
See Practice Paper 2, Question 13.

36. INFECTION IN PREGNANCY (3)

C – Group B streptococcus
Up to one-quarter of women have vaginal colonization by group B streptococcus (GBS) at some stage of pregnancy. Infection is asymptomatic to the mother, so it is detected using culture of vaginal swabs, which are taken opportunistically when a mother is to be examined for any reason. GBS is associated with neonatal sepsis. Fifty percent of babies born to GBS-positive women will become colonized during vaginal delivery, but only about 1% develop infection. Neonatal GBS sepsis causes 1 in 65 neonatal deaths. If it is picked up on routine swabs, the woman should deliver on an obstetric unit so antibiotics can be given in labour to reduce neonatal infection.

Intrapartum antibiotic prophylaxis should be given if GBS is detected incidentally in the vagina or urine in the *current* pregnancy or if a woman has had a previous baby with neonatal GBS infection. There is no need for antibiotics if GBS was detected in the previous pregnancy with no ill effects to the baby. There is no need for GBS antibiotics if the woman is having an elective caesarean section, but the normal prophylactic antibiotics should still be used. Intravenous benzylpenicillin is the antibiotic of choice, given as soon as possible after the onset of labour and at least 2 hours before delivery.

There is no national screening programme for GBS as initial positive results may become negative without treatment. Also there is no evidence for antenatal treatment for vaginal colonization as infection may quickly return following treatment. However, women with a positive urine culture of GBS ($>10^5$ cfu/mL) should receive treatment at the time of diagnosis.

Toxoplasma gondii is a parasite that comes from unwashed fruit and vegetables, raw/cured/poorly cooked meat, unpasteurized goat milk or from contaminated soil or cat faeces. Health education is therefore very important for prevention. It is rare for mothers to display clinical features, although some develop flu-like symptoms. Treatment is with spiramycin. Fetal infection occurs in 40% of cases, with the majority occurring at higher gestations (severity is greatest at lower gestations). Fetal effects of toxoplasmosis infection are miscarriage, stillbirth or the classic triad of hydrocephalus, chorioretinitis and intracranial calcifications. Fetal infection can be diagnosed by amniocentesis or cordocentesis.

Herpes simplex virus affects either the oral or the genital area. Primary infection during pregnancy should, as with any primary infection, prompt a referral to the GUM clinic to ensure accurate diagnosis and appropriate screening for other sexually transmitted infections. It is treated with oral acyclovir. If primary infection occurs within 6 weeks of the expected delivery date, a caesarean section should be recommended due to high transmission rates at this time. Neonatal infection is associated with high mortality due to severe systemic disease including encephalitis. Recurrent infection with genital herpes is not an indication for caesarean delivery, but admission to hospital for delivery would probably be advisable.

37. MENORRHAGIA (3)

D – Total hysterectomy

This patient is clearly distressed and requires more than just medical treatment. She is requesting a hysterectomy and, as long as she has been fully counselled for this and the other options, it is reasonable for this patient to go ahead with it. She has a normal BMI, which means there are no additional risks for the surgery. If this had been simple menorrhagia without the complication of the cervical abnormalities, it would have been more advisable to suggest endometrial ablation as a lower risk option. However, in patients with colposcopic abnormalities and a strong desire for a hysterectomy, it is appropriate to proceed with the hysterectomy as it can also be considered as a treatment for cervical abnormalities, in effect to 'kill two birds with one stone'. The patient may still be followed up with vault smears due to the previous abnormalities.

A hysterectomy is the only treatment that will ensure amenorrhoea. Obviously, in this case, a total hysterectomy, which removes the uterus and cervix, would be performed; otherwise, this would not treat the cervical abnormalities. This could be undertaken vaginally or abdominally. A total hysterectomy with bilateral salpingo-oophorectomy also removes (*ectomy*) the tubes (*salpingo*) and ovaries (*oophor*). The uterus alone is removed in a subtotal hysterectomy and the tubes, ovaries and cervix are retained. Risks of hysterectomy include bleeding, infection, pain, damage to bowel and urinary tracts, postoperative thromboembolism and vault prolapse in later life. Subtotal hysterectomies tend to be quicker with less risk of damage to the urinary tract and bowel.

38. OBSTETRIC EMERGENCIES (5)

C – Placental abruption

Placental abruption describes separation of the placenta from the uterus prior to the third stage of labour. Mild abruption, where there is minimal separation, may present with little pain or bleeding and with minimal consequence to fetus or mother. Major abruptions present with sudden-onset constant, sharp, severe low abdominal or back pain, maternal shock and variable amounts of vaginal bleeding. The uterus is irritable and tender and may become hard due to tonic contraction. The tense uterus means it is difficult to palpate fetal parts and there is often loss of fetal movements. Intrauterine death from hypoxia is common unless action is taken. The clinical condition of the mother and degree of shock may not correlate well with the amount of blood loss seen vaginally as bleeding can be contained behind the placenta (concealed abruption).

In this case, the epidural was effective for the level of pain from contractions but the increased level of pain from the abruption was such that it was registered by the mother despite the epidural. Delivery must be expedited and, in this case, a caesarean section is required. If the cervix had been fully dilated, an instrumental delivery could have been considered.

Risk factors for abruption are hypertension, pre-eclampsia, sudden decompression after membrane rupture in polyhydramnios or multiple pregnancies, previous abruption (10% recurrence), trauma to the abdomen and tobacco or cocaine abuse, although the cause is unknown in many cases. The incidence is 0.5% to 2%.

An amniotic fluid embolus has a poor prognosis. It is unclear what the exact pathophysiology is, but it is suggested that there is an anaphylactic reaction to fetal antigens entering the maternal circulation. The majority occur in labour but can occur at caesarean section or at any time during the pregnancy. It is more common in multiparous women. There is often a trigger such as placental abruption, abdominal trauma, intrauterine death or iatrogenic causes such as external cephalic version, suction or medical termination of pregnancy, and amniocentesis. This must be considered in all collapsed obstetric patients, but characteristic presentation is in late stages of labour or immediately postpartum where a woman starts to gasp for air, may fit and may go on to have cardiac arrest. Disseminated intravascular coagulation can develop leading to massive haemorrhage, coma and death. If the mother survives, diagnosis can be made by finding fetal squames in bronchial washings or in a sample of blood from the right ventricle. If the mother dies, diagnosis is at postmortem.

Uterine hyperstimulation can occur when using prostaglandin or oxytocin for induction of labour. It can lead to significant fetal distress as there is inadequate time to allow adequate blood flow to the fetus between contractions. Oxytocin should be stopped and tocolytics can be used if needed.

39. MENORRHAGIA (4)

A – Tranexamic acid and mefanamic acid

This woman is suffering from menorrhagia (heavy cyclical menstrual bleeding over several consecutive cycles) and primary dysmenorrhoea (excessively painful periods). The first-line treatment according to NICE is with the LNG-IUS; however, insertion would be problematic in a young woman who has never been sexually active. Also, her mother has expressed a wish to avoid hormones. Therefore, the next option is to use tranexamic acid and mefanamic acid. Antifibrinolytics (e.g. tranexamic acid) inhibit the breakdown of a formed clot. These are only to be taken during the heavy days of menstruation. Menstrual loss is reduced due to increased clot formation in the spiral arteries by reducing fibrinolytic activity (by inhibiting plasminogen activator). For this reason, they must not be used by women with a predisposition to thromboembolism. This can reduce blood loss by 50%. NSAIDs (mefanamic acid) act as prostaglandin synthesis inhibitors to reduce pain and also to reduce blood loss by up to 25%. Side effects are mainly gastrointestinal.

If this does not provide sufficient relief of symptoms, further options can be considered and the hormonal option may need to be revisited.

The COCP can reduce the amount of pain and bleeding experienced during menstruation by 50%. It can also regulate periods if there is an erratic cycle. This has to be discussed sensitively as it is a form of contraception and there can be social issues and confusion with young women using contraception. Progestogens can reduce bleeding and also act as contraception. They are useful if the patient is not suitable for the COCP due to contraindications such as weight, age and smoking habits.

Gonadotrophin-releasing hormone (GnRH) analogues are not first-line treatments for menorrhagia or dysmenorrhoea. They are used in dysmenorrhoea caused by endometriosis or can be used to shrink fibroids prior to definitive treatment. GnRH analogues cause amenorrhoea by down-regulating the pituitary hormones, leading to inhibition of ovarian activity. There are consequences of the hypoestrogenic state (similar to menopause) including hot flushes and vaginal dryness. Loss of bone mineral density is also a problem with use for more than 6 months; therefore, they should only be used short-term or with add-back therapy such as tibolone (a synthetic steroid often used as hormone replacement therapy).

40. PRE-ECLAMPSIA (2)

D – Magnesium sulphate

In addition to raised blood pressure (BP) and proteinuria, clinical features of pre-eclampsia are headaches, visual disturbances, restlessness or agitation, fluid retention with reduced urine output, epigastric pain, vomiting, hyperreflexia or signs of clonus (signs of cerebral irritability), papilloedema, retinal oedema or haemorrhages, liver tenderness, low platelets $<100 \times 10^6$/L, abnormal liver enzymes or any signs of HELLP (haemolysis, elevated liver enzymes and low platelets) syndrome. However, there may be no signs before convulsions occur.

If a woman develops severe pre-eclampsia, she must have regular observations of blood tests and strict fluid balance. Bloods include FBC, U & E, LFTs, albumin and coagulation. The fetus should also be monitored using CTG or USS as indicated.

Managing seizures

Prophylactic administration of magnesium sulphate is used for a woman at risk of convulsions and is continued 24 hours after delivery or 24 hours after the last fit. Fluid balance, reflexes, respiratory rate and oxygen saturation must be monitored as magnesium toxicity can have a depressant effect on the central nervous system.

A convulsion is an obstetric emergency, and the full team should be involved. First, call for help and summon the senior obstetrician, senior midwife and anaesthetist. Resuscitation should be initiated as with any person who is convulsing by first checking it is safe for you to approach, limiting injury to the patient and then initiating management with ABC. The woman should be placed in the left lateral position to avoid aortocaval compression and to keep the airway open. An airway should be used if needed and high-flow oxygen should be administered. After a convulsion, the baby should only be delivered once the mother's condition is stable and the appropriate people are present. Delivery should not be performed if it is not safe to do so as the mother's life has priority over the baby's. Magnesium sulphate is also used for the treatment of fits in pregnancy.

41. PREMATURE LABOUR (3)

A – Atosiban

Premature labour is labour before 37 weeks. Labour is suggested by the presence of painful regular contractions associated with cervical change, although there may just be some lower abdominal pain or silent dilation of the cervix.

Tocolytics inhibit smooth muscle in the uterus to delay rather than stop labour, to allow time for steroids to take effect and to allow transfer of the mother to a hospital that has adequate facilities for neonatal resuscitation, if needed. They are only given for 48 hours as this is how long the steroids need to work. Contraindications to allowing 48 hours for steroids to work include maternal conditions requiring immediate delivery, intra-uterine infection or fetal compromise.

Atosiban works by competitive inhibition of oxytocin and binds to myometrial receptors causing an inhibition of intracellular calcium release leading to muscle relaxation. There are minimal maternal side effects, but it is very expensive.

β-Sympathomimetics stimulate β-receptors (some are β_2 selective) on myometrial cell membranes to reduce intracellular calcium levels and therefore inhibit the actin–myosin interaction that would normally lead to uterine smooth muscle contraction. They are not popular due to the high number of side effects, which include tachycardia, hyperkalaemia, skin flushing, nausea, vomiting, visual disturbances and hyperglycaemia. More severe consequences such as hypotension, pulmonary oedema, severe maternal bradycardia and other arrhythmias have been seen – and even maternal death. Due to these side effects, it is important to be sure of the diagnosis before administering these. Examples are ritodrine, terbutaline and salbutamol.

Calcium channel blockers reduce the influx of intracellular calcium ions into myometrial cells, promoting relaxation of the uterine muscle. Side effects are due to peripheral vascular dilation and include dizziness, flushing and headache. No obvious fetal adverse effects have been seen. Nifedipine is widely used, although not licensed in UK as a tocolytic.

Cyclooxygenase inhibitors (including NSAIDs) inhibit cyclooxygenase, thus blocking prostaglandin production. Maternal side effects are minimal but include gastrointestinal irritation, peptic ulceration, thrombocytopenia, allergic reactions, headaches and dizziness. A more concerning effect is on the fetus as it has been shown that the patency of the ductus arteriosus is dependent on prostaglandins, and ductal constriction can occur with these drugs. It has also been shown that the NSAID indomethacin can reduce the fetal urine output.

42. MENSTRUAL HORMONES (4)

D – Oestradiol

Oestradiol is a steroid hormone that is mainly secreted by the ovary. Levels of oestrogen and progesterone are low during the initial stages of the follicular phase due to the regression of the corpus luteum from the previous cycle. Primary follicles develop in the ovary under the influence of follicle-stimulating hormone (FSH) and luteinizing hormone (LH), and this causes the level of oestrogen to rise due to increased production by the granulosa cells of these developing follicles. The increased level of oestrogen leads to negative feedback, producing a decline in LH and FSH concentrations. The level of oestrogen reaches its peak 18 hours prior to ovulation, and this *very* high level of oestrogen is thought to be responsible for the mid-cycle surge in LH (positive feedback), which initiates ovulation. Immediately prior to ovulation, oestrogen levels fall and there is a rise in progesterone production. After ovulation, the corpus luteum is formed from the remainder of the follicle, and this is the main source of oestrogen and progesterone post-ovulation. Oestrogen and progesterone are maintained at a high level for the luteal phase and only fall when the corpus luteum degenerates and the next cycle starts. Therefore, during menses, levels of oestrogen are low. If conception and implantation occur, the corpus luteum is maintained by gonadotrophin released by the trophoblast.

The latter half of the follicular phase (up to day 14) of menstrual cycle correlates to the proliferative phase of the endometrium. The high concentration of oestrogen seen at this time promotes rapid regeneration of the endometrium that has been shed during the recent menses. It stimulates proliferation of glandular and stromal elements of the endometrium to give tubular glands arranged in a regular pattern, parallel to each other with little secretion. Oestrogen also stimulates production of increased amounts of thin, clear, stringy cervical mucus, which is easily penetrable by sperm; a feature known as 'spinnbarkeit'.

Spinnbarkeit, from German *spinnbarkeit* = having the ability to be spun.
Oestr-, from Greek *oistros* = insane desire or frenzy.

43. RHESUS DISEASE (4)

D – Give postnatal anti-D and take Kleihauer test
See Practice Paper 1, Question 25.

44. MISCARRIAGE (2)

C – Inevitable miscarriage

This scenario describes an inevitable miscarriage where there is cramping, abdominal pain, vaginal bleeding and dilation of the cervical os. The fetus may still be alive, but miscarriage *will* occur, as the cervical os is open.

It is important to counsel women appropriately when they have had recurrent miscarriages. This woman will have had three consecutive miscarriages but, as long as she does not have any specific recurring cause, she still has a 60% to 75% chance of a successful pregnancy. However, because she has had three consecutive miscarriages, she should be investigated.

There are a number of reasons why miscarriages may happen; however, 50% of miscarriages, both sporadic and recurrent, have no identifiable cause. Fetal chromosomal abnormalities are seen in half of the first trimester miscarriages including autosomal trisomy (50%), polyploidy (20%) and 45XO (20%). This incidence decreases to 20% with second trimester miscarriages. Endocrine factors include polycystic ovary syndrome and poorly controlled diabetes. Immunological causes include autoimmune disease and alloimmune disease. Uterine anomalies may contribute to miscarriages, such as bicornuate or septae uteri and fibroids. Infection in the mother during pregnancy can lead to poor outcomes for the fetus. Specific infections such as rubella and cytomegalovirus can cross the placenta and cause miscarriage.

The investigations that are carried out include karyotyping from the parents, maternal blood tests for lupus anticoagulant and anticardiolipin antibodies (suggestive of antiphospholipid syndrome), a thrombophilia screen and possible hysterosalpingogram and/or pelvic ultrasound.

45. OVARIAN CYSTS

D – Teratoma

The presentation is of torsion of an ovarian cyst and the operation findings suggest a teratoma. Germ cell tumours are all very different from each other. They include dysgerminoma, endodermal sinus or yolk sac tumour, choriocarcinoma and teratoma. These are more commonly seen in young women and children. They comprise 20% to 25% of ovarian tumours, but only 4% are malignant.

Teratoma (dermoid cyst) is a common benign cyst, which contains elements of all three embryonic germ cell layers. Teratomas are thought to occur when the ovum develops without fertilization, known as parthenogenesis. They are generally seen in women in their 20s. Epithelium, hair and even teeth can be found in mature teratomas. They are usually small, bilateral and often asymptomatic but do cause pain if there is torsion or rupture. Malignant change is rare (<1%) and is generally seen in squamous cells and in postmenopausal women. They can be hormonally active and secrete hCG, α-fetoprotein and thyroxine.

Endodermal sinus or yolk sac tumour is the second most common malignant germ cell tumour of the ovary. The median age of onset is 19 years, and it is rarely seen over 40 years. Patients present with sudden-onset pelvic symptoms and a pelvic mass. There is a normal hCG but increased α-fetoprotein serum levels. Twenty percent of patients have coexistent teratomas.

Dysgerminomas are the most common malignant germ cell tumour and the most common ovarian malignancy found in young women, with 75% occurring in women aged 10 to 30 years. It is the most commonly seen ovarian malignancy in pregnancy. Ten percent are bilateral. There may be an increased serum hCG level.

Sex cord/stromal tumours are rare and represent only 5% of all ovarian tumours. These include granulosa cell tumours, thecomas, fibromas and Sertoli/Leydig cell tumours.

Granulosa cell tumours are usually slow-growing malignant tumours. They commonly secrete sex hormones, primarily oestrogen, which can, depending on the age of presentation, lead to precocious pseudopuberty, irregular menstrual bleeding or postmenopausal bleeding. This is useful when screening for recurrence using serum oestradiol levels. On histological examination, pathognomonic 'gland-like' spaces, Call–Exner bodies and 'coffee bean' nuclei are seen.

Fibroma tumours contain fibroblastic-type cells and are rarely malignant. Fibromas may present with non-malignant ascites and pleural effusion, which resolve after tumour removal (Meigs syndrome).

The most common types of ovarian carcinoma are epithelial, such as serous, mucinous, endometrioid, clear cell and Brenner tumours.

Non-epithelial tumours such as the one in this question are often seen in younger women, so preservation of fertility is more important. Extremely good results are seen with chemotherapy and limited surgery. While 5-year survival for all ovarian cancer is 43%, this is much improved for germ cell tumours, which can see 5-year survival rates of 75%.

Joe Vincent Meigs, American gynecologist (1892–1963).

46. TWINS (3)

D – Monozygotic dichorionic diamniotic

Monozygotic dichorionic diamniotic twins occur if division occurs at less than 3 days after fertilization (eight-cell stage). The two embryos can implant at separate sites and each has a separate chorion, amnion and placenta. They will have the same structural appearance *in utero* as dizygotic twins but will be identical twins.

47. OVARIAN CANCER (3)

D – Mucinous tumour

Investigations for pelvic masses include blood tests for routine haematological and biochemical measurements and tumour markers. Tumour markers are useful in diagnosis, response to treatment and recurrence. Eighty percent of malignant ovarian masses have an increased CA-125, although a raised CA-125 may also be seen with peritoneal trauma and a normal CA-125 does not rule out cancer. Around 65% of ovarian germ cell tumours have an increased serum hCG, α-fetoprotein or both.

An ultrasound or CT is useful to look for benign explanations for the pelvic mass such as simple ovarian cysts and uterine fibroids, and this will also assess spread to some extent. Malignant cysts tend to have a solid appearance, a thickened cyst wall, presence of septae within the cyst, bleeding within cyst and bilateral cysts. A chest X-ray is needed to rule out pulmonary metastases and to look for pleural effusions. Disease extent is only fully confirmed by laparotomy and biopsy at the time of definitive surgery. Ovarian cancer is staged as follows:

- Stage 1   Disease macroscopically confined to ovaries
- Stage 2   Disease is beyond ovaries but confined to pelvis
- Stage 3   Disease is beyond pelvis but confined to abdomen
- Stage 4   Disease is beyond the abdomen

Mucinous tumours comprise 20% of ovarian tumours. Mucinous tumours are generally large multiloculated cysts containing mucinous fluid. Benign tumours are unilateral, and malignant tumours are bilateral in only 20% of cases. Less than 10% of these tumours are malignant, and they are associated with tumours of the appendix and gallbladder. In 5% of cases, the mucin-filled cyst ruptures with dissemination of mucin-secreting cells, leading to a build-up of mucinous fluid in the abdomen (pseudomyxoma peritonei).

Endometrioid tumours are uncommon and usually malignant. Histological findings are similar to endometrial cancer and 15% to 30% have a coexistent primary in the endometrium. Clear cell tumours are uncommon, and nearly all are malignant with a poor prognosis. They are thin-walled unilocular tumours with cells that have clear cytoplasm (hence the name). There is an association between this tumour and endometriosis. Urothelial-like tumours (Brenner tumours) are uncommon, small, usually unilateral and rarely malignant. The main component is ovarian stroma, but they do contain urothelial-type epithelium.

48. PATHOGENESIS OF CERVICAL CANCER (2)

E – Human papillomavirus 16 and 18

Cervical cancer is the fourth most common malignancy in women worldwide. The two peaks of diagnosis are 35 to 39 years and 60 to

64 years. There are a small number of women who are diagnosed with early cervical cancer from smear tests; however, the vast majority of women diagnosed with invasive carcinoma have never had screening. Most (80%) are symptomatic, and presentation can be with abnormal *per vaginam* bleeding (postcoital, intermenstrual or postmenopausal) or a chronic vaginal discharge (purulent, blood-stained, watery, mucoid or malodorous). Late disease is often indicated by pain, including backache or referred leg pain, leg oedema, altered bowel habit, haematuria, malaise and weight loss.

Human papillomavirus (HPV) is a sexually transmitted DNA virus of which there are more than 80 types. There is a strong association between HPV serotypes 16, 18 and 33 and pre-invasive and invasive cervical cancer. HPV is thought to act by producing proteins E6 and E7, which influence the action of the p53 tumour suppressor gene. There is a vaccine for HPV, which is given to girls in the UK aged 12 to 13, to provide immunity for at least 20 years. Immunocompromised patients may still be infected despite a completed course. It is hoped that using the vaccine will reduce cervical and vulval dysplasia and genital warts. Currently, about one-third of all women in their 20s carry the HPV.

The majority (up to 90%) of cervical cancers are squamous, and these can be divided into keratinizing (most common), large cell, non-keratinizing and small cell subtypes. Ten percent are adenocarcinomas, and these tend to have a worse prognosis because of late presentation. Spread is by direct extension into adjacent structures such as the ureters, bladder or rectum and can also occur via lymph vessels. Blood-borne spread is rare. Staging of cervical carcinoma is as follows:

- Stage 0   Carcinoma *in situ*
- Stage 1   Lesions confined to cervix
- Stage 2   Invasion into upper vagina but not pelvic wall
- Stage 3   Invasion of lower vagina/pelvic wall or causing ureteric obstruction
- Stage 4   Invasion of bladder or rectal mucosa

Stage 1 is further divided into 1a(i) (tumour <3 mm deep and <7 mm across), 1a(ii) (<5 mm deep and <7 mm across), 1b(i) (tumour <4 cm) and 1b(ii) (tumour >4 cm). Stage 2 is split into 2a (invasion of upper two-thirds of vagina but not parametrium) and 2b (invasion of parametrium). Stage 4b is given in cases with distant metastases.

Treatment varies from simple excision at Stage 1a, which can be by cone biopsy, to preserve fertility, with close cytological follow-up. If fertility is not required, then a total hysterectomy should be done. With all other stages of cervical cancer, treatment is radical surgery and/or radiotherapy depending on the condition of the patient and the stage of disease.

HPV 6b and 11 are commonly related to genital warts and are not oncogenic. Hepatitis B and C viruses are not related directly to cervical cancer but may predispose to it if the patient is severely immunocompromised. Herpes simplex virus causes herpes.

49. EARLY PREGNANCY (3)

B – Ectopic pregnancy

The most likely diagnosis in this patient is an ectopic pregnancy, despite the patient having no pain; with a βhCG result of 2365 IU, a gestational sac should have been visualized if it were intrauterine. A laparoscopy should be considered to look for the ectopic fetus. A repeat βhCG can be taken in 48 hours if the patient is asymptomatic but there is a high clinical suspicion for ectopic pregnancy. If the result of the βhCG had been lower than 1000 IU and no gestational sac had been seen, the βhCG should be rechecked in 48 hours to assess whether it was doubling, reaching a plateau or falling, as it is much more likely in this case to be too small to visualize using ultrasound.

50. VAGINAL DISCHARGE (2)

C – Ultrasound scan ± hysteroscopy and endometrial biopsy

This woman is at high risk of endometrial cancer and should be urgently referred for an ultrasound scan ± hysteroscopy and endometrial biopsy, the gold standard for investigation. This can be done as an outpatient procedure or under general anaesthetic, if the woman prefers or if there are other medical problems.

Dilation and curettage used to be the gold standard but is now known to miss 10% of endometrial cancers. This is performed under general anaesthetic.

Endometrial biopsy can be performed at an outpatient clinic via a Pipelle or Vabra aspirator. The Pipelle biopsy only samples 4% of the endometrial surface and will miss one-third of tumours. The Vabra device picks up more tumours as it samples around 40% of endometrial surface but is more painful and more expensive. Endometrial biopsy alone should only be used for patients with very low risk of carcinoma due to the low pick-up rates. At first presentation, it is acceptable to take a Pipelle biopsy as long as the patient is also referred by fast track for hysteroscopy with endometrial biopsy. If the Pipelle biopsy shows malignancy, then hysteroscopy will be avoided and referral can be made straight to gynaecology oncology for staging.

Transvaginal ultrasound is used to measure the thickness of the endometrium in postmenopausal women. Endometrial cancer is unlikely if the thickness is less than 4 mm. Malignancy is much more likely if fluid is seen in the endometrial cavity. Ultrasound can be used as a non-invasive screening test, especially if surgical measures are not tolerated.

Practice Paper 3: Questions

1. CONGENITAL HEART DISEASE

You are called acutely to the postnatal ward to see a 48-hour-old baby girl. She was seen the day before by your colleague, who performed her baby check and found no abnormalities. On arrival, you find a baby who is grunting and cyanotic. All pulses are palpable, and there is no murmur on auscultation of the chest. You transfer her to the neonatal unit where you find her oxygen saturations are 55% in air.

Which of the following congenital cardiac lesions would be consistent with these findings?

A. Coarctation of the aorta
B. Eisenmenger syndrome
C. Patent ductus arteriosus
D. Tetralogy of Fallot
E. Transposition of the great arteries

2. BLOOD GASES (1)

A 12-year-old boy with a history of type 1 diabetes is seen in the emergency department. He has been vomiting for the last 24 hours. His blood sugar is high, and he is breathing much harder than usual. You cannulate him to give him some fluid and take a venous blood gas.

pH	7.19
$PaCO_2$	2.8 kPa
Base excess	−9
HCO_3	14

Normal reference ranges for venous blood gases:

pH	7.36–7.44
$PaCO_2$	4.7–6.0 kPa, 35–45 mmHg
Base excess	± 2
HCO_3	20–25

Which of the following is your interpretation of this blood gas?

A. Metabolic acidosis (uncompensated)
B. Metabolic acidosis with some respiratory compensation
C. Mixed metabolic and respiratory acidosis
D. Respiratory acidosis (uncompensated)
E. Respiratory acidosis with some metabolic compensation

3. CAUSES OF PRECOCIOUS PUBERTY

A 7-year-old girl is referred to the paediatrician as she has started showing signs of puberty. On examination, she has some breast tissue and sparse pubic hair, as well as axillary hair. She is growing well and her growth chart shows her height was tracking along the twenty-fifth centile, but her new height is now above the fiftieth centile. Her mother is worried as no one else in her class has any signs of puberty and she is being teased. She has not started to menstruate yet. She has no other symptoms, and there is nothing else of note on examination.

What is the most likely cause of her precocious puberty?

A. Congenital adrenal hyperplasia
B. Hypothyroidism
C. Idiopathic
D. McCune–Albright syndrome
E. Pituitary tumour

4. DEHYDRATION

A 9-month-old boy presents to the emergency department with a three-day history of diarrhoea and vomiting. He is still taking his bottles of milk but vomits them straight back. On examination, he is tachycardic, has a normal capillary refill time, a slight reduction in skin turgor and dry mucous membranes. He is not wetting his nappies as much as usual.

What percentage of weight do you expect to be lost from dehydration in this case?

A. 0%
B. 5%
C. 10%
D. 15%
E. 20%

5. DEVELOPMENTAL MILESTONES (1)

A 3-year-old boy is in his asthma review clinic. His older brother is known to have developmental delay. Your consultant asks you to assess the patient's development.

Assuming he has normal development, which of the following would you expect him *not* to be able to do?

A. Build a tower of five bricks
B. Copy a circle
C. Feed with a fork
D. Hop on one leg
E. Know his first and last name

6. ELECTROLYTE DISTURBANCE (1)

A 4-year-old boy presents to the emergency department with a cough, rapid breathing and a fever. He has been vomiting and is passing only small amounts of dark urine. On examination, he is not clinically dehydrated and looks slightly puffy around his eyes. He has crackles on the right side of his chest. He is unable to tolerate oral antibiotics so you insert a peripheral cannula. Because he is vomiting, you perform routine electrolyte studies while inserting the cannula.

You receive the following blood results:

Na	129	(135–145 mmol/L)
K	4.2	(3.5–5.0 mmol/L)
Urea	3.2	(1.5–4.5 mmol/L)
Creatinine	83	(40–110 µmol/L)
pH	7.37	(7.35–7.45)
Glucose	4.2	(3.4–5.5 mmol/L)

Which of the following is the most likely cause of the electrolyte disturbance?

A. Conn syndrome
B. Diabetes insipidus
C. Hypovolaemic hypernatraemia
D. Hypovolaemic hyponatraemia
E. Syndrome of inappropriate ADH secretion

7. THE CHOKING CHILD

You are at a wedding, sitting next to your 4-year-old nephew. He was eating a sausage and suddenly starts coughing vigorously. He is very agitated and continues to cough. He has been coughing for over a minute, and he is now crying between coughs.

You suspect an inhaled foreign body; which of the following would be your next course of action?

A. Encourage coughing
B. Five back blows
C. Five chest thrusts
D. Heimlich manoeuvre
E. Rescue breaths

8. INVESTIGATION OF FAILURE TO THRIVE

A 6-month-old girl born in Bangladesh is referred to you by her general practitioner as she is not growing along the centiles. She was born on the fiftieth centile and has now dropped below the second centile, despite a good intake. She has had two chest infections but has never needed to be hospitalized. On examination, she looks thin but is not pale. Her abdomen is not distended and is soft on palpation.

What investigation is most likely to give you a cause for her failure to thrive?

A. Full blood count
B. Coeliac screen
C. Dietary review
D. Sweat test
E. Thyroid function test

9. BREASTFEEDING

A 28-year-old woman who is breastfeeding has asked the community midwife for some advice regarding nutrition. She is a vegetarian but eats a balanced, varied diet. She wants to know what supplements, if any, she should take.

Which of the following supplements is recommended for breastfeeding mothers?

A. Vitamin A
B. Vitamin D
C. Folic acid
D. Iron (for vegetarians)
E. No supplements needed if eating a healthy diet

10. DIAGNOSIS OF ACUTE ASTHMA

A 12-year-old boy presents to the emergency department with worsening shortness of breath and a wheeze for the last 24 hours. On examination, he has a respiratory rate of 35/min and has bilateral wheeze on auscultation. You suspect he has a severe exacerbation of asthma.

What would you expect his peak flow to be?

A. 75%–100%
B. 50%–75%
C. 33%–50%
D. <33%
E. <20%

11. INVESTIGATION OF BRUISING

A 4-year-old boy, who was previously fit and well, developed some petechial spots on his legs after climbing a tree. A few days later, the rash had spread over his entire body. He had not been any more lethargic than normal and was eating well. On examination, you note a large bruise on his hip and a black eye, for which his mother could not give any explanation.

Which of the following investigations would be likely to confirm the diagnosis?

A. Bone marrow biopsy
B. Clotting screen
C. Full blood count
D. Skeletal survey
E. No investigation required

12. JUVENILE IDIOPATHIC ARTHRITIS

A 5-year-old girl has suffered from arthritis for the last 6 months. It only affects her knees and elbows, and she has never had sacroiliac tenderness or nail problems. She has no rash or fever, but she does have regular ophthalmology follow-up due to her increased risk of developing uveitis. Blood tests reveal that she is antinuclear antibody positive but rheumatoid factor negative.

What type of arthritis is she most likely to have?

A. Enthesitis
B. Oligoarticular juvenile idiopathic arthritis
C. Polyarticular juvenile idiopathic arthritis
D. Psoriatic arthritis
E. Systemic juvenile idiopathic arthritis

13. ABDOMINAL PAIN (1)

An 8-year-old boy presents to the emergency department with abdominal pain, fever, nausea and some diarrhoea. The pain is poorly localized, although on palpation you feel he is most tender in the right lower quadrant, and he demonstrates guarding over this area. There are no obvious swellings.

What is the most likely cause for his abdominal pain?

A. Appendicitis
B. Gastroenteritis
C. Inguinal hernia
D. Mesenteric adenitis
E. Torsion of the testis

14. ACUTE RENAL FAILURE

A 3-year-old girl presents to the emergency department with a 3-day history of diarrhoea and vomiting. Her mother is worried as she has blood in her stool. On examination, she appears mildly dehydrated and pale but is otherwise well. You perform some blood tests and a urine dipstick.

Bloods:

Hb	7.2 g/dL
WCC	8.0 g/dL
Platelets	69×10^9/L
Na	145 mmol/L
K	6.1 mmol/L
Urea	32 mmol/L
Creatinine	219 µmol/L

Urine dipstick:

Protein	3+
Blood	Negative
Leucocytes	Negative
Nitrites	Negative

What is the most likely diagnosis?

A. Glomerulonephritis
B. Haemolytic uraemic syndrome
C. Henoch–Schönlein purpura
D. Leukaemia
E. Pyelonephritis

15. GUTHRIE CARD

A newborn baby has a heel-prick blood test taken for Guthrie card screening.

Which of the following is *not* screened for on the newborn Guthrie card?

A. Congenital hypothyroidism
B. Cystic fibrosis
C. Galactosaemia
D. Phenylketonuria
E. Sickle cell disease

16. INVESTIGATION OF HEAD INJURY

A 10-year-old boy falls from a lower branch of a tree while playing with his brother at home. There was no loss of consciousness at the time, but he now has a headache and is feeling sick. He is brought to the emergency department 20 minutes later. On examination, there is no focal neurology.

Which of the following is an indication for an immediate CT scan?

A. Amnesia of the event and the preceding 4 hours
B. Glasgow Coma Score of 14 on admission
C. Obvious tender swelling to the side of the head
D. One episode of vomiting in the department
E. Previous head injury 2 years earlier

17. FEBRILE ILLNESS (1)

A 13-month-old boy presents to the general practitioner. He has a 24-hour history of irritability. His mother reports he has been 'tugging' at his left ear. His temperature is 38.2°C. On examination of the left ear, there is a bulging red tympanic membrane.

Which of the following describes the appropriate management of this case?

A. Five-day course of oral antibiotics
B. Insertion of oil to the external ear canal
C. No action required
D. Oral analgesia
E. Oral antihistamine

18. INVESTIGATION OF CHRONIC COUGH (1)

A 4-year-old boy is referred to the outpatient clinic with a 10-month history of cough. This occurs most nights, and he is usually symptom-free during the day. He has had two episodes of wheeze: the first at 9 months of age associated with bronchiolitis, the second at age 3 when he had a viral upper respiratory tract infection.

Which of the following would you like to perform?

A. Chest X-ray
B. Peak expiratory flow rate before and after bronchodilator
C. pH study
D. Sweat test
E. Trial of therapeutic bronchodilators

19. MANAGEMENT OF DIABETES

Kevin is a 10-year-old boy with type 1 diabetes. He is on a multi-dose regime of 8 units of Lantus in the evening, and he uses novarapid when he eats. He takes his novarpid just before he eats and uses 1 unit per 15 g of carbohydrate. He comes for a 3-month review at the diabetic centre. From his capillary glucose monitoring diary, you can see he does frequent measurements, though they seem to be all over the place. Generally, his capillary glucose readings are between 6 and 8 in the morning but rise to between 16 and 20 after any meal he eats. What advice could you give him to improve his glucose levels?

A. Change his novarpid so he takes it just after he has had his food rather than before
B. Change his novarapid to 1 unit per 10 g carbohydrate
C. Change his novarapid to 1 unit per 20 g carbohydrate
D. Increase his Lantus to 9 units in the evening
E. Move his Lantus to the morning

20. SHOCK

A 5-year-old boy presents to the emergency department with a red, non-blanching rash over his trunk and peripheries. His mother says that he has been complaining of a headache. He is crying but is limp in his mother's arms. He is cool to touch and has a central capillary refill time of 4 seconds. He is taken to resus and the nurse puts an oxygen mask on him. You arrive to assess him.

Which of the following would be your first course of action?

A. Give a bolus of antibiotic
B. Give a fluid bolus of 10 mL/kg
C. Give a fluid bolus of 20 mL/kg
D. Intubation and ventilation
E. Perform a lumbar puncture

21. THE VOMITING INFANT (1)

A 4-month-old boy presents to the emergency department with vomiting, poor feeding and excessive crying for the last 8 hours. He has previously been a well boy with normal development and growth but was born prematurely. On examination, he looks unwell and appears in pain particularly when you press in the lower right quadrant. He is chubby, but you think you can feel a mass in his groin.

What is the most likely diagnosis?

A. Appendicitis
B. Inguinal hernia
C. Intussusception
D. Pyloric stenosis
E. Volvulus

22. SYNDROME RECOGNITION (1)

A midwife asks you to review a baby on the postnatal ward as she is worried it is hypotonic. The baby is indeed hypotonic, and you also notice he has an unusual looking face. He has a flat nasal bridge, almond-shaped eyes with prominent epicanthic folds and low set ears. His genitalia are normal.

What is the most likely cause of this child's signs?

A. Down syndrome
B. Fetal alcohol syndrome
C. Hypothyroidism
D. Prader–Willi syndrome
E. Turner syndrome

23. CEREBRAL PALSY

A 3-year-old girl is being assessed in the child development centre by the physiotherapists. She has increased tone of her lower and upper limbs. Her legs are affected more than her arms, and she has exaggerated reflexes in both her legs. You note that she has an abnormal gait, walking on her tiptoes with her knees and hips both flexed. She was born at 25 weeks' gestation, and she had a stormy course during the neonatal period.

What type of cerebral palsy is this girl most likely to have?

A. Ataxic cerebral palsy
B. Athetoid cerebral palsy
C. Diplegic cerebral palsy
D. Hemiplegic cerebral palsy
E. Quadriplegic cerebral palsy

24. INVESTIGATION OF SHORT STATURE

A 4-year-old girl is referred to the paediatric clinic due to poor growth. She weighed 3.5 kg at birth and initially grew along the fiftieth centile for weight, length and head circumference. Since her first birthday, her growth has tailed off and her height is now well below the fourth centile with her weight on the ninth centile. The only other history of note was that she was admitted to the neonatal unit when she was born because of low blood sugars and jaundice.

What investigation is most likely to reveal her underlying problem?

A. Bone age
B. Chromosomal analysis
C. Growth hormone test
D. Mid-parental centile
E. Thyroid function tests

25. MANAGEMENT OF ACUTE ASTHMA

You are asked to see a 7-year-old boy in the emergency department who has a history of asthma. He says he had a cold yesterday and now presents with a 6-hour history of 'feeling tight'. On arriving, he tells that he is disappointed to be here as he was going to see Leeds United this afternoon. On examination, he has equal air entry bilaterally associated with a loud polyphonic wheeze. His saturations are 93% in air and his peak expiratory flow rate is 60% of his best in clinic. His heart rate is 110/min and his respiratory rate is 28/min.

Which of the following would be your most immediate step?

A. Give a β-agonist via a nebulizer
B. Give a β-agonist via a spacer
C. Give oral steroids
D. Start oxygen via a face mask
E. Take no action

26. RESPIRATORY DISTRESS

A term baby is born by elective caesarean section as the baby is in a breech presentation. The mother has been well during the pregnancy and a vaginal swab from a previous pregnancy was clear. A few hours after birth you are called to see the baby as he is 'working hard'. On examination he has a respiratory rate of 100/min, is afebrile and well perfused. The chest is clear with equal air entry.

Which of the following is the most likely diagnosis?

A. Congenital pneumonia
B. Pneumothorax
C. Respiratory distress syndrome
D. Sepsis
E. Transient tachypnoea of the newborn

27. INVESTIGATION OF DIARRHOEA

A 2-year-old girl is referred by her GP with a 6-week history of foul-smelling diarrhoea, associated with weight loss. On examination, her abdomen looks full and slightly distended.

Which of the following is the most appropriate first-line investigation that would identify the cause?

A. Antigliadin IgA
B. Large bowel biopsy
C. Small bowel biopsy
D. Stool sample
E. Tissue transglutaminase IgA

28. STRUCTURAL HEART DISEASE

A 4-year-old boy is brought to the general practitioner with a cold. On auscultating the chest, a loud murmur is heard. The murmur occurs at the beginning of systole and is heard loudest at the upper left sternal edge. It radiates to the back and is associated with a thrill.

Which of the following is the most likely diagnosis?

A. Aortic stenosis
B. Coarctation of the aorta
C. Mitral regurgitation
D. Pulmonary stenosis
E. Ventricular septal defect

29. FEBRILE ILLNESS (2)

An 18-month-old girl presents to the general practitioner with fever and a runny nose. On examination, there are no signs of a serious illness, though she has a temperature of 38°C. The mother is concerned as she had a febrile convulsion 4 months ago.

Which of the following statements is true regarding this febrile child?

A. Do not routinely give antipyretics to solely reduce body temperature
B. Give ibuprofen and paracetamol simultaneously to maximize effect
C. Strip the child to her nappies
D. Tepid sponging is recommended
E. She should be given antipyretics to prevent a febrile convulsion

30. INVESTIGATION OF DELAYED PUBERTY

A 14-year-old female is referred to paediatric outpatient as she has not entered puberty yet. She has no breast development or pubic hair. On examination, she is well and a full neurological examination is normal. She is short for her age but has no dysmorphic features. Her mother says that she herself 'developed late' but cannot remember exactly when she went through puberty.

Which investigation should be done initially?

A. Gonadotrophin levels
B. Karyotyping
C. Ovarian ultrasound
D. Pituitary CT
E. No investigation required

31. MANAGEMENT OF SEIZURES

You are called to the emergency department where a 4-year-old boy is having a seizure. He is known to have epilepsy and is on regular phenytoin. He was brought in by ambulance and the paramedic has given buccal midazolam *en route*. The emergency doctor has cited a cannula from which a sample of blood has revealed a blood sugar of 4.8 mmol/L. He is still fitting 10 minutes after the buccal midazolam.

Which of the following would be your next step in management?

A. Bolus 10% dextrose
B. Intravenous lorazepam
C. Intravenous phenytoin
D. Intubation and ventilation
E. Rectal paraldehyde

32. NEONATAL RESUSCITATION

You are working in the emergency department when you are called to an ambulance. A mother has just delivered her baby a few seconds before arriving. As you enter the ambulance, the paramedic is clamping the cord. The baby is not breathing and looks floppy and pale.

Which of the following would be your most immediate action?

A. Administer five rescue breaths
B. Cardiac compressions
C. Evaluate breathing
D. Manage airway
E. Warm and dry the baby

33. SCROTAL PAIN

An 8-year-old boy presents with a 3-hour history of a painful, swollen testicle. The pain started gradually overnight and he now scores it as 6/10. He has no nausea and has not vomited. On examination, his abdomen is soft but there is an obvious swelling and redness of the left scrotum. There is mild tenderness in the upper area of the testicle. His cremasteric reflex is present.

What is the most likely diagnosis?

A. Epididymitis
B. Hydrocele
C. Inguinal hernia
D. Torsion of the hydatid of Morgagni
E. Torsion of the testicle

34. SPLENOMEGALY

A 3-year-old girl is brought to her general practitioner. She has been treated for a chest infection with antibiotics for 10 days but is still no better. Her mum has noticed that she is pale and lethargic. On examination, the girl appears unwell, and the doctor is able to palpate the spleen. He also notices a number of bruises over her arms and body, for which mum is unable to account.

What is the most likely diagnosis?

A. Acute lymphoblastic leukaemia
B. Acute myeloid leukaemia
C. Cystic fibrosis
D. Glandular fever
E. Neglect and physical abuse

35. EPILEPSY SYNDROMES

A 9-year-old boy suffers from epilepsy. His mother describes his seizures as infrequent. She normally hears a strange noise in the night from her son's room and then finds the right-hand side of his mouth and face are twitching. He is usually drooling and is unrousable. This lasts for a few minutes, and the child has no recollection of the event. A subsequent EEG shows high amplitude spikes in the left centrotemporal region.

What is the most likely type of epilepsy this boy has?

A. Absence seizures
B. Benign rolandic epilepsy
C. Juvenile myoclonic epilepsy
D. Lennox–Gastaut type epilepsy
E. Tonic–clonic epilepsy

36. IMMUNIZATION

A 2-month-old boy is brought to the general practitioner by his mother for routine immunizations.

Which of the following immunizations should *not* routinely be given at 2 months of age?

A. Diphtheria
B. *Haemophilus influenzae*
C. Meningitis C
D. Pneumococcus
E. Rotavirus

37. MANAGEMENT OF CARDIAC DISEASE

A 5-month-old infant was found to be failing to thrive. On examination, a quiet murmur is heard at the lower left sternal edge throughout systole. Over the past 2 months, he has become short of breath during feeding. His weight has now fallen down two centile lines.

Which of the following would be your first step in management?

A. ACE inhibitor
B. Digoxin
C. Diuretics
D. Insertion of a feeding nasogastric tube
E. Surgical correction

38. OPHTHALMIA NEONATORUM

An anxious mother attends the general practice as her 7-day-old newborn has sticky eyes. Both eyes have a mucopurulent exudate. You take swabs including a scraping and advise the mother to clean the eyes four times a day with cooled, boiled tap water. Three days later you are informed that an intracellular organism has grown from the samples you sent.

Which of the following organisms is responsible for the infection?

A. *Chlamydia trachomatis*
B. *Neisseria gonorrhoeae*
C. *Pseudomonas aeruginosa*
D. *Staphylococcus aureus*
E. *Streptococcus pneumoniae*

39. COUGH

A 3-year-old boy from Syria presents to the general practitioner with a 2-month history of cough. It started with a cold, but that has since resolved. Currently, he has severe bouts of coughing, occasionally followed by vomiting. On examination, he has bilateral equal air entry and no crepitations.

Which of the following is the most likely diagnosis?

A. Asthma
B. Bronchiolitis
C. Inhaled foreign body
D. Pneumonia
E. Whooping cough

40. DIAGNOSIS OF SEIZURES

A 7-year-old boy is brought to the emergency department by ambulance following a 10-minute seizure. He has now stopped fitting but remains drowsy. He has a 3-year history of headaches, nausea and lethargy, which is present only in the winter months. He lives with his family in a poorly maintained council flat with gas heating.

Which of the following would confirm your diagnosis of seizures?

A. Arterial pO_2
B. Carboxyhaemoglobin levels
C. Chest X-ray
D. ECG
E. Oxygen saturations

41. GENETIC INHERITANCE

Following is a list of genetic conditions.

Which of these conditions has an autosomal dominant inheritance pattern?

A. Haemophilia A
B. Incontinentia pigmenti
C. Klinefelter syndrome
D. Oculocutaneous albinism
E. Tuberous sclerosis

42. MANAGEMENT OF ECZEMA

A 12-year-old boy has a prolonged history of atopic eczema. The extensor surfaces of his limbs are dry, excoriated and inflamed. He says that the rash is incessantly itchy.

Which of the following would be appropriate adjuncts to his topical emollient and steroids?

A. Bandages
B. Phototherapy
C. Systemic steroids
D. Tacrolimus
E. All of the above

43. SYNCOPE

A 2-year-old girl is bought into the emergency department by her mother following a fit. She had been playing with her brother when mum heard her cry briefly. She then went quiet, looked extremely pale and then fell to the ground and was unrousable. Mum noticed her body shake for about 10 seconds before she then came round and was back to her normal self, playing within minutes. Her brother says she had trapped her finger in the door just prior to the event.

What is the most likely cause for her loss of consciousness?

A. Absence seizure
B. Breath-holding attack
C. Cardiac arrhythmia
D. Epileptic fit
E. Reflex anoxic seizure

44. INVESTIGATION OF JAUNDICE (1)

A health visitor refers a 3-week-old baby to the assessment unit as she is concerned he is jaundiced. He has gained weight and is generally well. On examination, you confirm that he is jaundiced but, other than this, there is no abnormality to be found.

Which of the following is the most important investigation to perform at this point?

A. Direct antibody test
B. Split bilirubin
C. TORCH screen
D. Unconjugated bilirubin
E. No investigation required

45. MANAGEMENT OF URINARY TRACT INFECTION

A 4-year-old girl presents with a fever, lethargy and vomiting. She complains of dysuria and has 2+ leucocytes and nitrites on urine dipstick. There are no signs to find on examination, and she is alert and well hydrated. You make the diagnosis of a urinary tract infection and send her urine for culture.

What treatment should she receive?

A. A 3-day course of oral antibiotics
B. A 7-day course of oral antibiotics
C. Intravenous antibiotics
D. No treatment required
E. No treatment until microscopy and culture result is obtained

46. PURPURIC RASH

A 4-year-old girl attends the emergency department with a 2-day history of a palpable purpuric rash over her lower limbs and buttocks. She is systemically well but recently had a cold. You make the diagnosis clinically.

Which of the following is *not* a complication of this condition?

A. Abdominal pain
B. Arthritis
C. Conjunctivitis
D. Recurrence
E. Renal failure

47. SKIN RASH (1)

A 13-year-old male has been unwell for a number of days with a sore throat. Three days after the onset of the illness, he developed a widespread rash over his torso and proximal extremities. The rash is made up of numerous scaly papules, each 0.5 to 2 cm in size. On examination of his oropharynx, you note bilaterally inflamed tonsils with exudates.

Which of the following is the most likely diagnosis?

A. Atopic eczema
B. Measles
C. Meningococcal sepsis
D. Psoriasis
E. Scarlet fever

48. APGAR SCORE

You are working in the emergency department when you are called to an ambulance. A mother has just delivered her baby a few seconds before arriving. The baby is one minute old with a good cry, is breathing regularly and has a heart rate of 120/min. She is not limp but has reduced tone. She is pink centrally but the peripheries are blue.

What is the Apgar score for this baby?

A. 6
B. 7
C. 8
D. 9
E. 10

49. HEADACHE

A 14-year-old female presents with a one-day history of severe throbbing headache. She is feeling nauseated but has not vomited. There is no blurring of vision or flashing lights, but she has some photophobia. She had a similar headache, which lasted a day about 3 months ago. She is on the oral contraceptive pill. Neurological examination is unremarkable, and there is no papilloedema on fundoscopy.

What is the most likely explanation for her headache?

A. Cluster headache
B. Idiopathic intracranial hypertension
C. Intracranial tumour
D. Migraine
E. Tension headache

50. MANAGEMENT OF CONSTIPATION

A 3-year-old girl is seen in the outpatient clinic due to her long-standing history of constipation. For the last 6 months, she has not passed a normal stool. She is straining, in pain and only passing very small 'rabbit-like droppings'. Her mum is also worried as she is continually soiling her pants and has not managed to take her out of nappies.

What is the most important initial step in treating this child's constipation?

A. Encourage increased dietary fibre
B. Enema disimpaction regimen
C. Lactulose twice a day
D. Make sure child is placed on the toilet after every meal
E. Movicol disimpaction regimen

Practice Paper 3: Answers

1. CONGENITAL HEART DISEASE

E – Transposition of the great arteries

This neonate is clearly unwell. With these features, you should be very suspicious of congenital sepsis or pneumonia so your priority would be to perform blood cultures, CRP, FBC and chest X-ray. Empirical antibiotics (e.g. amoxicillin and gentamicin) should be commenced without delay.

These features are also suspicious of a cardiac lesion. In transposition of the great arteries, the great vessels are reversed (transposed) with the aorta coming off the right ventricle and the pulmonary artery off the left ventricle. Affected children are therefore dependent on the ductus arteriosus to supply oxygenated blood to the systemic circulation ('duct dependent'). As the duct closes after birth, the baby will become profoundly cyanotic and acidotic. Chest X-ray shows a characteristic narrow mediastinum with an egg-on-side appearance of the heart shadow. The 'switch operation' (surgical swapping of the pulmonary artery and aorta) is required as definitive management.

Coarctation of the aorta also often presents when the ductus closes, but this is not a cyanotic disease. The baby would usually present with shock, poor perfusion of the limbs distal to the lesion and absent femoral pulses. Tetralogy of Fallot would usually not present so early in life and would usually be associated with a pulmonary stenosis murmur. Eisenmenger syndrome is a cyanotic heart lesion that occurs later in life with reversal of flow across septal defects due to right ventricular hypertrophy. A patent ductus arteriosus presents with a loud machinery-like murmur in a child with heart failure.

An algorithm of interpretation of cardiovascular examination findings follows (adapted from *Clinical Paediatrics for Postgraduate Examinations*).*

Etienne-Louis Fallot, French physician (1850–1911).
Victor Eisenmenger, Austrian physician (1864–1932).

---

* Stephenson T, Wallace H, Thomson A. *Clinical Paediatrics for Postgraduate Examinations*. 3rd ed. London: Churchill Livingstone, 2003.

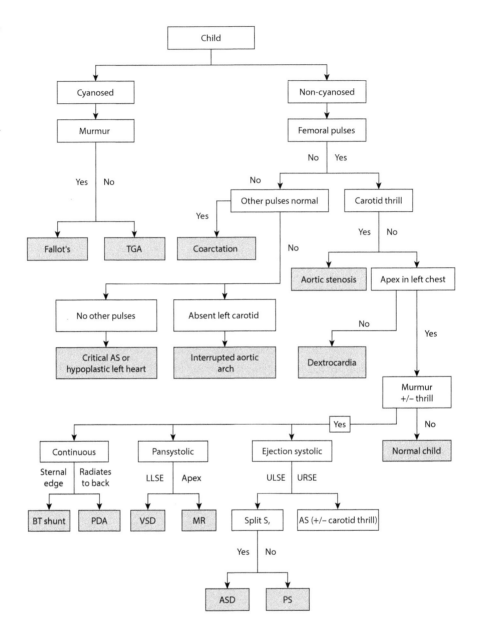

2. BLOOD GASES (1)

B – Metabolic acidosis with some respiratory compensation

This boy is most likely in diabetic ketoacidosis (DKA) and has a metabolic acidosis with some respiratory compensation. However, you do not have a result for ketones; therefore, you cannot technically diagnose DKA. He will need aggressive management as DKA is a life-threatening complication of type 1 diabetes.

Interpretation of blood gas results

The power of hydrogen (pH) is an inverse logarithmic scale. That is, rather than following a linear pattern, each unit of pH is a 10-fold representation of H^+ concentration. Therefore, a shift from 7.5 to 6.5 is a 10-fold increase in H^+ concentration. The body normally controls serum pH within a tight range. A normal intracellular pH is required for the functioning of many enzyme systems. When blood becomes profoundly acidotic (pH <7), cellular function becomes impossible and death ensues.

Answering three questions should give you the interpretation of any blood gas.

1. What is the pH?
   Assess the pH. Is it acidotic or alkalotic? This is the overall status of the patient, regardless of compensation.

2. What is the $PaCO_2$?
   It is known that if you mix carbon dioxide (CO_2) with water, acid (H^+) will be produced (see equations below). CO_2 is a good indicator of 'ventilation' and, if the pH corresponds with the pCO_2, the anomaly is caused by a respiratory problem (i.e. a high pCO_2 with a low pH is a respiratory acidosis). If the CO_2 does not account for the pH, then it is compensating for a metabolic abnormality.

3. Confirm your findings by assessing the base excess/bicarbonate.
   The base excess (i.e. an excess of bicarbonate, HCO_3^-) indicates the metabolic status. If the base excess provides a cause for the abnormal pH, this is a metabolic picture (i.e. a high pH and positive base excess is a metabolic alkalosis).

As a final tip, always remember to assess the conditions of the blood gas (i.e. what inspired oxygen concentration was the patient using, what type of sample was it – arterial, venous, capillary), was it taken correctly and do the results fit with the patient's condition. Also, remember that you can have a 'mixed' blood gas, i.e. a mixed metabolic/respiratory acidosis where both the CO_2 and the bicarbonate are low (a compensated respiratory acidosis would have a high bicarbonate).

$$H_2O + CO_2 \rightarrow H_2CO_3$$

$$2H_2CO_3 + H_2O \rightarrow 4H^+ + 2HCO_3^-$$

Interpretation	pH	pCO$_2$	Base excess
Normal	7.36–7.44	4.7–6.0 kPa	>−2, <+2
Metabolic acidosis	↓	Normal	<−2
Metabolic acidosis with respiratory compensation	↓ or normal	↓	<−2

Continued

Interpretation	pH	pCO$_2$	Base excess
Metabolic alkalosis	↑	Normal	>+2
Metabolic alkalosis with respiratory compensation	↑ or normal	↑	>+2
Respiratory acidosis	↓	↑	>−2, <+2
Respiratory acidosis with metabolic compensation	↓ or normal	↑	>+2
Respiratory alkalosis	↑	↓	>−2, <+2
Respiratory alkalosis with metabolic compensation	↑ or normal	↓	<−2
Mixed metabolic and respiratory acidosis	↓	↑	<−2

FURTHER READING

1. Advanced Life Support Group. *Advanced Paediatric Life Support: The Practical Approach.* 5th ed. London: Wiley-Blackwell, 2011.

3. CAUSES OF PRECOCIOUS PUBERTY

C – Idiopathic

This 7-year-old girl is showing signs of puberty: a growth spurt, breast development and pubic and axillary hair. She has true precocious puberty, and it is most likely to be idiopathic. Precocious puberty is defined as the start of puberty in girls under the age of 8 and in boys under the age of 10. It can be divided into true and pseudo.

In true precocious puberty, the course of puberty occurs in a normal synchronous manner (as in this case), suggesting an intact hypothalamic–pituitary axis. It is more common in girls and is idiopathic in 80% to 90% of cases. Other causes of true precocious puberty include: intracranial pathology such as tumours (although pituitary tumours are more likely to be associated with delayed puberty), haemorrhage, hydrocephalus, neurofibromatosis, cerebral palsy and primary hypothyroidism. Although true precocious puberty is less common in boys, if it does occur, there is more likely to be a central cause; therefore, it should be investigated. This would normally involve a brain MRI, gonadotrophin levels and sex steroid levels.

In pseudo (false) precocious puberty, the course of puberty occurs in an abnormal manner. For example, axillary and pubic hair with a growth spurt is seen in females, but there is no breast budding. Boys may show features of puberty but still have prepubertal-sized testes. Pseudo precocious puberty is gonadotrophin-independent and usually extracranial. Causes include adrenal virilizing tumours, congenital adrenal hyperplasia, Cushing syndrome, testicular or ovarian malignancy and gonadotrophin-secreting tumours (e.g. hepatoblastoma).

McCune–Albright syndrome is a sporadic genetic condition characterized by precocious puberty (due to primary ovarian cysts secreting oestradiol), café-au-lait spots and polyostotic fibrous dysplasia (where normal bone is replaced by cystic bone growth).

Premature pubarche (presence of pubic hair with no other signs of puberty) and premature thelarche (the appearance of breast tissue, without thickening and pigmentation of the nipples in girls with no other signs of puberty) can both occur and are seen as normal variants. However, it is important to ensure there is no excess androgen production suggestive of an underlying pathological cause.

The phases of puberty are described by the Tanner staging.

Tanner staging of pubic hair (male and female):

- Tanner 1 → no pubic hair (<10 yr)
- Tanner 2 → small amount of downy hair (10–11.5 yr)
- Tanner 3 → hair becomes more coarse and curly (11.5–13 yr)
- Tanner 4 → adult hair quality extending across pubis but not the thigh (13–15 yr)
- Tanner 5 → hair extends to medial surface of thighs (>15 yr)

Tanner staging of genitals (male only):

- Tanner 1 → prepubertal, testicular volume <1.5 mL (<9 yr)
- Tanner 2 → testicular volume 1.6–6 mL, scrotal skin thins (9–11 yr)
- Tanner 3 → testicular volume 6–12 mL, scrotum enlarges (11–12.5 yr)
- Tanner 4 → testicular volume 12–20 mL, scrotal skin enlarges further (12.5–14 yr)
- Tanner 5 → testicular volume >20 mL, adult scrotum and penis (>14 yr)

Tanner staging of breasts (females only):

- Tanner 1 → no glandular tissue, areola follows skin contours on chest (<10 yr)
- Tanner 2 → breast bud forms, areola begins to widen (10–11.5 yr)
- Tanner 3 → breast elevates and extends beyond borders of areola (11.5–13 yr)
- Tanner 4 → increased breast size, areola/nipple form a secondary mound (13–15 yr)
- Tanner 5 → breast reaches adult size (>15 yr)

Thelarche, from Greek *thele* = nipple + *arche* = beginning.
Puberty, from Latin *pubertas* = adulthood.
Fuller Albright, American endocrinologist (1900–1969).
Donovan James McCune, American pediatrician (1902–1976).
James Mourilyan Tanner, British paediatrician (1920b).

4. DEHYDRATION

C – 10%

Approximately 70% to 80% of a child's body is made up of water. Children who are unwell with fever, vomiting, diarrhoea or not taking fluids should be assessed for signs of dehydration, such as*:

- Prolonged capillary refill time
- Abnormal skin turgor

---

* National Collaborating Centre for Women's and Children's Health. *Diarrhoea and Vomiting in Children under 5* (NICE guideline). London: NICE, 2009. Available at: http://guidance.nice.org.uk/CG84/NICEGuidance/pdf/English

- Abnormal respiratory pattern
- Weak pulse
- Cool extremities

Assessment of degree of dehydration*:

	Mild (3%–5%)	Moderate (6%–9%)	Severe (≥10%)
General condition	Thirsty, alert, restless	Thirsty; restless/listless, lethargic	Drowsy, limp, cold, cyanotic extremities, may be comatose
Pulse	Normal	Tachycardia	Tachycardia
Palpable pulses	Normal	Normal or weak	Weak or absent
Blood pressure	Normal	Orthostatic hypotension	Hypotension
Respirations	Normal	Deep, may be rapid	Deep and rapid
Cutaneous perfusion	Normal	Normal/cool	Cold, mottled and/or acrocyansosis
Skin turgor	Normal	Slight reduction	Reduced
Fontanelle	Normal	Slightly depressed	Sunken
Mucous membrane	Moist	Dry	Very dry
Tears	Present	Present or absent	Absent
Urine output	Normal	Oliguria	Anuria and severe oliguria

Dehydration itself does not cause death; shock does. Shock can be present even when a child is not dehydrated. Shock requires aggressive intravascular fluid therapy, whereas the treatment of dehydration requires gradual fluid replacement. Overhydrating can potentially be more dangerous than the dehydration that is being treated.

5. DEVELOPMENTAL MILESTONES (1)

D – Hop on one leg
A 3-year old would be expected to be able to pedal a tricycle but not be able to hop until they are 4 years old. In fine motor and vision development, a 3-year old should be able to copy a circle and build a tower of nine bricks. Language-wise they would be speaking in at least three-word sentences and would know their first and last names. They would not be expected to be able to count until they were 4. Socially, 3-year olds play make-believe, can eat with a fork and can brush their teeth. They should be being potty-trained and be dry during the day.

* Kliegman RM, Marcdante KJ. *Nelson Essentials of Paediatrics*. Oxford: Elsevier, 2006.

Developmental milestones:

Age	Gross motor	Fine motor and vision	Hearing and language	Social
6 weeks	Symmetrical limb movements	Fixes and follows to 90°	Coos, startles to noise	Smiles
3 months	No head lag	Plays with hands	Turns to sound	Laughs
6 months	Sits with support Rolls	Palmar grasp and transfers	Babbles	Not shy
9 months	Pull to stand	Points Early pincer grip	Double babble (non-specific)	Plays peek-a-boo Stranger anxiety
12 months	Cruises furniture	Neat pincer grip	Says a few words	Waves bye-bye Finger feeds
15 months	Walks (broad gait)	Tower of 2 bricks Straight scribble	2–6 words Obeys commands	Uses cup and spoon
18 months	Runs, squats Walks with toy	Tower of 3 bricks Circular scribble	Knows 3 body parts 6–20 words	Domestic mimicry Takes shoes off
2 years	Kicks a ball Up and down stairs	Tower of 6 bricks Copies straight line	2–3 word sentences	Feeds with fork Temper tantrum
3 years	Pedals tricycle	Tower of 9 bricks Copies circle	Knows first and last names	Brushes teeth Make-believe play
4 years	Hops	Steps of bricks Copies cross	Counts to 10	Able to undress

6. ELECTROLYTE DISTURBANCE (1)

E – Syndrome of inappropriate ADH secretion

This child has pneumonia associated with the syndrome of inappropriate antidiuretic hormone (SIADH). Though he is producing small volumes of concentrated urine, this is because of water retention rather than hypovolaemia. In addition, if he was dehydrated, we may expect a raised urea.

A normal plasma sodium concentration is 135 to 145 mmol/L. Hyponatraemia is usually defined as plasma Na^+ <130 mmol/L, and hypernatraemia is defined as plasma Na >150+ mmol/L.

Causes of hyponatraemia include:

- Gain of H_2O in excess of Na^+ gain
- Excess water intake (e.g. psychogenic polydipsia)
- Acute renal failure
- SIADH secretion
- Loss of Na^+ in excess of H_2O loss
- Renal losses
- Extrarenal losses (e.g. dehydration secondary to gastroenteritis)

Causes of hypernatraemia include:

- Loss of H_2O in excess of Na^+ loss
- Renal losses
- Extrarenal losses with appropriate oliguria (concentrated urine)
- Gastrointestinal loss
- Increased insensible H_2O loss (e.g. pyrexia)
- Inadequate water intake
- Gain of Na^+ in excess of H_2O gain
- Iatrogenic – excess hypernatraemic intravenous infusions and/or drugs
- Incorrect infant formula reconstitution
- Accidental or deliberate salt poisoning

Any imbalances in sodium must be corrected slowly and re-evaluated regularly. SIADH secretion should always be considered if a child is hyponatraemic. It is quite often seen in a child with pneumonia. Causes of SIADH include lung disease (pneumonia, ventilation, acute asthma), central nervous system disease (trauma, meningitis, tumour), postoperative pain and drugs (carbamazepine, morphine). In order to make the diagnosis, it is important to rule out hypovolaemia. Typically, a small amount of concentrated urine is produced. Treatment involves restricting the amount of fluid given to the child to approximately two-thirds of their normal maintenance input.

Conn syndrome is caused by an aldosterone-secreting tumour within the adrenal cortex. Patients with hyperaldosteronism usually present with a prolonged non-specific illness associated with polyuria and polydipsia. Aldosterone causes the retention of sodium at the distal tubule of the nephron at the expense of potassium ions, which are lost in the urine. The retained sodium causes water reabsorption resulting in fluid retention, hypervolaemia and hypertension. The typical biochemical picture in hyperaldosteronism is hypernatraemia with hypokalaemia in the presence of a normal renal function. Diagnosis can be confirmed by finding a raised plasma aldosterone and suppressed plasma renin levels (the renin–aldosterone ratio is typically less than 0.05).

Jerome Conn, American endocrinologist (1907–1981).

7. THE CHOKING CHILD

A – Encourage coughing
You may not become a paediatrician, but an inhaled foreign body in a child is relatively common. As a general practitioner, parent or wedding guest, you could instantly become a hero! The vast majority of deaths occur in preschool-aged children. Food is the most common object, but almost anything can cause an obstruction.

If a foreign body is directly visible and accessible within the mouth, then it can be removed, but great care has to be taken not to push it further into the airway. Blind finger sweeps should never be performed.

When considering how to act the first question to ask yourself is 'is the child coughing effectively'?

If yes, then they should be encouraged as a spontaneous cough is more likely to be effective at relieving the obstruction than externally imposed manoeuvres. No further intervention should be made unless the cough becomes ineffective. An effective breath is defined as one in which the child is able to speak, cry or take breaths between coughs. Though appearing much more distressing, it at least confirms a partially open airway. Performing any kind of procedure may move the foreign object, making a partial obstruction a complete obstruction. If the child is coughing, then they should be continuously reassessed and never left alone. If the cough becomes ineffective, then interventions should begin, as described in the algorithm below:

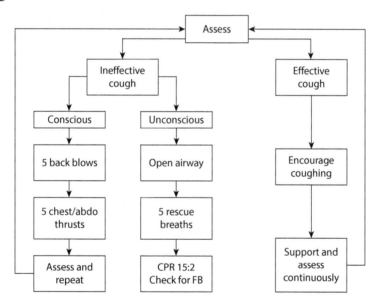

If the child is not coughing effectively and they remain conscious, then they should be given cycles of 5 back blows followed by 5 chest/abdominal thrusts. Each cycle should be followed by a reassessment. If the child is unconscious (and therefore by definition not coughing effectively), then one should open the airway and commence basic life support.

FURTHER READING

1. Advanced Life Support Group. *Advanced Paediatric Life Support: The Practical Approach*. 5th ed. London: Wiley-Blackwell, 2011.

8. INVESTIGATION OF FAILURE TO THRIVE

D – Sweat test

This girl is likely to have cystic fibrosis, which is diagnosed with a sweat test. She was not born in the UK and so would have missed out on the neonatal screening. Newborn screening for cystic fibrosis is being introduced worldwide but currently is not done in Bangladesh. A common presentation of cystic fibrosis is failure to thrive (FTT) along with a history of chest infections. FTT can be caused by numerous problems.

Non-organic FTT results from various environmental and psychosocial factors:

- Inadequate provision or intake of food
- Family dysfunction, lack of support and difficult parent–child interactions
- Children who are subject to neglect

Organic FTT:

- Prenatal causes
- Premature babies, intrauterine growth retardation
- Maternal infection
- Fetal alcohol syndrome
- Chromosomal abnormalities
- Inadequate intake
- Lack of appetite, seen in iron deficiency anaemia and chronic infection
- Mechanical problems such as a poor suck or swallow secondary to hypotonia
- Excessive vomiting caused by metabolic, renal or neurological disease, or gastroesophageal reflux leading to oesophagitis, can lead to food refusal
- Poor absorption or utilization of metabolites
- Cystic fibrosis due to the lack of pancreatic enzymes
- Coeliac disease causes malabsorption but is unlikely in this case as there are no other signs such as a distended abdomen or diarrhoea. Also the child is unlikely to have been exposed to gluten yet at 6 months of age
- Hypothyroidism, diabetes mellitus, inborn errors of metabolism, renal failure
- Increased metabolic demand
- Hyperthyroidism, congenital heart disease, chronic lung disease, renal failure
- Malignancy

FTT must be distinguished from constitutionally delayed growth, a variation of normal growth. Children with short stature resulting from constitutional delay have a deceleration of growth in the first 2 years that can be confused with FTT, but then they grow parallel to but below the third percentile. In reality, children with FFT would have more than one investigation, and you would most likely include a full blood count, thyroid function tests and a coeliac screen. However, in this case, a sweat test is most likely to reveal the cause as there are no other signs of hypothyroidism, coeliac disease or iron deficiency anaemia.

9. BREASTFEEDING

B - Vitamin D

While breastfeeding women are advised to have a healthy diet, it is now recommended for pregnant and breastfeeding women to take vitamin D supplementation (10 mg per day). This helps increase both the mother's and the baby's vitamin D stores and reduces the baby's risk of developing rickets. It is particularly important for the women at greatest risk of deficiency, which include those who are obese, have limited skin exposure to sunlight or who are of South Asian, African, Caribbean or Middle Eastern descent.

Folic acid is important to take while pregnant to help prevent neural tube defects but is not needed after 12 weeks of pregnancy. Iron supplementation is not routinely recommended for breastfeeding. Vitamin A is also not recommended; in fact, there is a risk of birth defects associated with vitamin A; supplementation should be avoided during pregnancy.

All mothers should be encouraged to breastfeed. The advantages of breastfeeding to the baby are a reduced risk of infections (as breast milk provides secretory IgA, lactoferrin, peroxidases and lysozymes), reduced risk of sudden infant death syndrome and less diarrhoeal illnesses. Advantages to the mother include the fact that it is free, it aids the bonding process, it provides a contraceptive effect (due to high prolactin levels) and there is a reduced risk of premenopausal breast and ovarian cancers. Babies fed with artificial feeds are more at risk of necrotizing enterocolitis, urinary tract infections, gastrointestinal infections, respiratory infections, ear infections, asthma, eczema and type 1 diabetes.

10. DIAGNOSIS OF ACUTE ASTHMA

C – 33%–50%

The peak expiratory flow rate (PEFR) is often used to help guide diagnosis and management of asthma. The clinical signs to guide the level of severity of acute exacerbations of asthma are:

Moderate asthma	A patient with moderate asthma is able to talk in sentences. PEFR >50% of best or predicted. SpO$_2$ ≥92%. Heart rate: ≤140 bpm (2–5 years), ≤125 bpm (>5 years). Respiratory rate: ≤40 rpm (2–5 years), ≤30 rpm (>5 years). No features of acute severe asthma

Continued

Severe asthma	A patient with severe asthma cannot complete sentences in one breath or is too breathless to talk or feed
	• PEFR 33%–50% of best or predicted
	• SpO_2 <92%
	Heart rate:
	• 140 bpm (2–5 years)
	• 125 bpm (>5 years)
	Respiratory rate
	• 40 rpm (2–5 years)
	• 30 rpm (>5 years)
Life-threatening asthma	A patient with life-threatening asthma will have any one of the following:
	• PEFR <33% best or predicted
	• SpO_2 <92%
	• Silent chest
	• Cyanosis
	• Feeble respiratory effort
	• Hypotension
	• Exhaustion
	• Confusion or
	• Coma

FURTHER READING

1. British guideline on the management of asthma. A national clinical guideline 2014 (Table 14: Levels of severity of acute asthma attacks in children).

11. INVESTIGATION OF BRUISING

C – Full blood count

This boy most likely has idiopathic thrombocytopenia (ITP), which is diagnosed by a very low platelet count (<40 × 10⁹/L) with no evidence of anaemia and a normal white cell count. Unexplained or extensive bruising in any child is worrying.

Causes of bruising include:

- Trauma (accidental or non-accidental)
- Clotting disorders
- Platelet disorders
- Malignancy

Non-accidental injury cannot be fully ruled out in this case as the bruises are not accounted for and a thorough history would need to be taken. It is unusual to have a widespread petechial rash with physical abuse, although one may be seen over the face and neck from strangulation. A diagnosis of non-accidental injury should certainly not be made until other causes have been ruled out.

Leukaemia and other malignancies can present with unexplained bruising; however, the child in this case is very well and there are no other signs and symptoms that would suggest an underlying malignancy, such as organomegaly or lymphandopathy. Haematology departments usually perform a blood film, which would confirm the presence of any abnormal cells such as in leukaemia. A bone marrow biopsy would subsequently be performed to confirm the diagnosis.

Clotting disorders are rare, especially at this age. They would normally present with bruising, without petechiae, as well as the possibility of obvious haemorrhage from mucous membranes, intra-articular or iatrogenic sites. A platelet disorder is the most likely answer in this case, and ITP would be the most common one. ITP is defined as isolated thrombocytopenia with normal bone marrow where no other cause has been found. Pathogenesis involves the peripheral destruction of platelets, and it is often seen a few weeks after a viral illness, presenting with petechiae and superficial bruising. ITP can also present with bleeding from the nose or gums and a rare but serious complication is intracranial haemorrhage (<1%). No treatment is required in most cases and spontaneous remission occurs within 2 months. In life-threatening haemorrhage, a platelet transfusion may be needed.

Causes of thrombocytopenia can be divided into those with decreased platelet production or those with decreased platelet survival. Decreased production is seen in congenital causes such as thrombocytopenia/absent radii syndrome (TAR), in illnesses (mainly viral) and leukaemia. Decreased survival is seen with ITP, systemic lupus erythematosus (SLE), haemolytic uraemic syndrome and is associated with certain drugs. Thrombocytopenia can be dilutional and is seen when large transfusions are given (stored blood loses functional platelets and coagulation factors).

12. JUVENILE IDIOPATHIC ARTHRITIS

B – Oligoarticular juvenile idiopathic arthritis
Juvenile idiopathic arthritis (JIA) is defined as arthritis of unknown aetiology beginning before the sixteenth birthday and persisting for at least 6 weeks where other known conditions are excluded. JIA is categorized into:

- Systemic JIA
- Oligoarticular JIA
- Polyarticular JIA
- Psoriatic arthritis
- Enthesitis-related arthritis

Oligoarthritis affects four joints or fewer, accounts for 60% of all JIA and is seen most commonly in girls under 6 years of age. It affects the medium-sized joints such as the elbows and knees, and it is associated with anterior uveitis (inflammation of the middle eye) as well as having the highest association with antinuclear antibody (ANA).

Polyarticular JIA affects five or more joints and often affects the small joints of the hands and feet. This girl is unlikely to have polyarticular arthritis as it is seen more commonly in older girls, and rheumatoid factor is often positive. The cervical spine and temporomandibular joints can also be affected.

Systemic JIA is the association of arthritis with a fever and salmon pink rash. The fever is 'quotidian' (peaks daily) and should be present for 2 weeks. The rash is a fluctuating macular erythematous rash that mainly affects the trunk and proximal limbs. There may also be splenomegaly, hepatomegaly, lymphadenopathy as well as serositis (pericarditis, pleurisy).

Psoriatic arthritis describes arthritis related to psoriasis. It can affect a few or many joints. The distal interphalangeal joints are often affected, and there can be associated nail dystrophy, pitting and onycholysis (separation of the nail from the nail bed). The association with psoriasis may be limited to a family history, or the psoriatic rash may not develop until years later.

Enthesitis is the inflammation of an enthesis – where a tendon or ligament inserts into bone. There is often tenderness in the sacroiliac joint; this form of arthritis is associated with HLA-B27 as well as anterior uveitis.

Enthesis, from Greek *en* = in + *tithemi* = to place ('an insertion').
Quotidian, from Latin *quotidie* = daily.

13. ABDOMINAL PAIN (1)

A – Appendicitis
Appendicitis is common in children and is caused by inflammation and swelling of the appendix. The lumen to the appendix becomes blocked and the appendiceal wall subsequently becomes oedematous and inflamed. Initially, the pain is poorly defined and periumbilical but moves to the right iliac fossa (RIF) due to inflammation of the peritoneum over the appendix. Nausea, anorexia, vomiting and a low-grade fever may also be present. The child with appendicitis typically lies still, and there is usually tenderness and guarding over the McBurney's point (one-third of the way between the anterior superior iliac spine and the umbilicus). There are a number of other signs that suggest peritoneal irritation in the RIF:

Rovsing's sign	→	pain in the RIF in response to left-sided palpation
Cough sign	→	pain in the RIF after a voluntary cough
Obturator sign	→	pain on internal rotation of the flexed right thigh caused by an inflammatory mass overlying the psoas muscle

Perforation is a complication of appendicitis and is more common in younger children because of the non-classical presentation and late diagnosis. Appendicitis can present differently to the symptoms given here. The pain may be elsewhere in the abdomen or, in children who are very young, abdominal pain is often not obvious. Loose stools occur in 10%

of cases due to a pelvic or retro-caecal appendix. Urinary symptoms may also be present if the appendix is in the pelvis. Dysuria occurs in 10% of cases with an excess of leucocytes in the urine.

Mesenteric adenitis often presents with RIF pain, but there is no guarding. Inguinal hernias can present with right-sided abdominal pain, but there is an associated swelling in the inguinal or scrotal region. Testicular torsion is a surgical emergency and can present with abdominal pain. A swollen, painful testis or scrotum is apparent on examination. It is therefore an absolute must to examine the genitalia of any child who presents with abdominal pain.

Charles McBurney, American surgeon (1845–1913).
Niels Thorkild Rovsing, Danish surgeon (1862–1927).

14. ACUTE RENAL FAILURE

B – Haemolytic uraemic syndrome

This 3-year-old girl is anaemic, thrombocytopenic and is in acute renal failure. The most likely diagnosis is haemolytic uraemic syndrome (HUS).

HUS is characterized by acute renal failure, microangiopathic anaemia and thrombocytopenia (with a normal clotting time). It is commonly seen after gastroenteritis caused by *Escherichia coli* (the verotoxin-producing O157:H7 strain), *Salmonella*, *Shigella* or *Campylobacter*. Children present with vomiting and diarrhoea (which is often bloody); acute renal failure occurs soon after. This form of HUS is known as the epidemic/typical version and is seen more commonly in younger children and in the summer months. It usually has a good outcome, and permanent renal damage is uncommon. However, the rarer type ('sporadic type') is seen in older children, and renal damage is more severe. Drugs and malignancy can also all cause HUS, and there is a hereditary form. A blood film is diagnostic, showing a microangiopathic haemolytic anaemia.

Complications of HUS include abdominal pain, myocarditis, encephalitis-like features, hepatitis, pancreatitis and retinal haemorrhages. Renal damage can lead to hypertension. Treatment is conservative and symptomatic and includes careful fluid and electrolyte balance, treatment of renal failure with dialysis and transfusion of blood and platelets as required.

Henoch–Schönlein purpura (HSP) is a vasculitis that affects the whole body. It classically presents with a purpuric rash over the back of the legs and buttocks. It is not associated with anaemia or thrombocytopenia but can lead to nephritis and thus haematuria and proteinuria. Arthritis is a common feature, and HSP can also affect the abdomen, leading to abdominal pain and occasionally melaena. Glomerulonephritis may present in a number of ways: nephrotic or nephritic syndrome, acute renal failure or asymptomatic haematuria and/or proteinuria. It does not normally present with anaemia and thrombocytopenia. Leukaemia is unlikely in this situation as, although the child has anaemia and thrombocytopenia, she is otherwise well. Acute renal failure can be a presenting feature of malignancies if there is tumour lysis syndrome, but it is unlikely in a child that is otherwise well.

15. GUTHRIE CARD

C – Galactosaemia

The national newborn screening programme was introduced in the UK 1969 for phenylketonuria (PKU), and in 1981 congenital hypothyroidism (CHT) was added.

Currently all babies in the UK will have a Guthrie card to screen for:

- PKU
- CHT
- Cystic fibrosis
- Sickle cell disease and thalassaemia
- MCADD (medium chain acetyl Co-A dehydrogenase deficiency)

MCADD is an inborn error of metabolism where fat cannot be broken down, resulting in low energy and hypoglycaemic episodes. It is the most recent disease to have been added to the newborn screening programme.

The Wilson–Jungner criteria describe the features of a good screening tool:

- The condition should be an important health problem
- The natural history should be understood
- There should be a recognizable latent or early symptomatic stage
- There should be an accepted treatment recognized for the disease
- Treatment should be more effective if started early
- There should be a policy on who should be treated
- Diagnosis and treatment should be cost-effective

The test/tool should be:

- Easy to perform and interpret
- Acceptable
- Accurate, reliable, sensitive and specific
- Case-finding should be a continuous process

Galactosaemia is a rare metabolic disorder in which the sugar galactose cannot be broken down. It can be a life-threatening illness in the newborn period, and the cardinal features are hepatomegaly, cataracts and jaundice. Babies often also have feeding difficulties, vomiting and lethargy. Although it could be screened for on the newborn blood spot, it is usually picked up clinically before the results would be back; therefore it is not included in the UK newborn screening programme.

Robert Guthrie, American microbiologist (1916–1995).

16. INVESTIGATION OF HEAD INJURY

A – Amnesia of the event and the preceding 4 hours

Initial assessment of any head injury follows ABC. Cervical spine evaluation is performed in conjunction with airway assessment. C-spine immobilization is appropriate if any of the following apply: Glasgow Coma Scale (GCS) <15, neck tenderness or pain, any focal neurological deficit, paraesthesia or other clinical suspicion of a cervical spine injury. Immobilization should be maintained until a full-risk assessment including clinical assessment (and imaging if necessary) indicates removal is safe.

If GCS <8, an anaesthetist should secure the airway by means of tracheal intubation and ventilation. A full skeletal survey should also be performed to assess any other injuries.

Indications for CT head scanning in patients under 16 years of age are as follows:

- Clinical suspicion of non-accidental injury
- Post-traumatic seizure but no history of epilepsy
- Age >1 year: GCS <14 on assessment in the emergency department
- Age <1 year: GCS (paediatric) <15 on assessment in the emergency department
- GCS <15 at 2 hours after the injury
- Suspicion of open or depressed skull injury or tense fontanelle
- Sign of basal skull fracture
- Haemotympanum (blood behind the tympanic membrane)
- Raccoon eyes
- Cerebrospinal fluid otorrhoea/rhinorrhoea
- Battle's sign (blood at the mastoid)
- Focal neurological deficit
- Age <1 year: presence of bruise, swelling or laceration >5 cm on the head

If the child has more than one of the following risk factors, then a CT head should also be performed:

- Dangerous mechanism of injury (high-speed road traffic accident either as a pedestrian, cyclist or vehicle occupant, fall from >3 m, high-speed injury)
- Witnessed loss of consciousness lasting >5 minutes
- Abnormal drowsiness
- Three or more discrete episodes of vomiting
- Amnesia (anterograde or retrograde) lasting >5 minutes

For more information, see the NICE guidelines for imaging in head injury.*

---

* National Collaborating Centre for Acute Care. *Head Injury* (NICE Clinical Guideline 176). London: NICE, 2014. Available at: http://guidance.nice.org.uk/CG176/NICEGuidance/pdf/English

17. FEBRILE ILLNESS (1)

D – Oral analgesia

Acute otitis media (AOM) is a purulent middle ear process. Earache is the single most important symptom. Other ear-related symptoms include tugging and rubbing of the ear, irritability, restless sleep and fever. Non-specific symptoms such as cough and rhinorrhoea may also be present. Examination with an otoscope may reveal a bulging tympanic membrane with loss of the normal landmarks, a change in colour (red or yellow) and poor mobility.

In this case, it would be entirely reasonable to use paracetamol for control of discomfort and as an antipyretic.

General management of AOM would include:

- Children with AOM should not routinely be prescribed antibiotics as the initial treatment.
- Consider antibiotics in children if:
  - Children younger than 2 years of age with bilateral AOM
  - Perforation and/or discharge in the ear canal (otorrhoea) associated with AOM
- If an antibiotic is to be prescribed, the conventional 5-day course is recommended at dosage levels indicated in the paediatric British National Formulary.
- Delayed antibiotic treatment (antibiotic to be collected at parents' discretion after 72 hours if the child has not improved) is an alternative approach, which can be applied in general practice.
- Parents should give paracetamol for analgesia and be advised of the potential danger of overuse.
- Children with AOM should not be prescribed decongestants or antihistamines.
- Insertion of oils should not be prescribed for reducing pain in children with AOM.

FURTHER READING

1. Clinical knowledge summary (CKS) for otitis media. Available at: http://cks.nice.org.uk/otitis-media-acute

18. INVESTIGATION OF CHRONIC COUGH (1)

E – Trial of therapeutic bronchodilators

Chronic cough is a common problem in paediatrics and general practice. The differential diagnosis includes:

- Asthma (cough exacerbated by exercise, frequent nocturnal cough, atopic family history)
- Gastroesophageal reflux (associated with feeding reflux symptoms)
- Inhaled foreign body

- Inhaled irritants
- Allergic rhinitis (sneezing, itchy eyes, watery rhinorrhoea)
- Sinusitis (prolonged nasal discharge)
- Post-infectious cough syndrome
- Habit cough (a cough not responsive to treatment that only occurs during waking hours)
- Tuberculosis
- Cystic fibrosis (now picked up more frequently on Guthrie card and so many do not develop symptoms before the diagnosis is made)
- Immune deficiency (frequent upper respiratory tract infections)
- Bronchiectasis

Asthma is the most common cause of recurrent cough in children. It is usually associated with wheeze and/or breathlessness and is triggered by exercise, cold or dust. In many children, a nocturnal cough may be the only presenting clinical feature. Asthma is defined as a chronic inflammatory disorder of the airways in susceptible individuals. Inflammatory symptoms are usually associated with widespread but variable airflow obstruction and an increase in airway response to a variety of stimuli. Obstruction is often reversible, either spontaneously or with treatment.

The diagnosis of asthma can usually be made from the history and examination, though you may wish to perform some investigations. A chest X-ray may show hyperinflation, but with mild symptoms it would be hard to justify exposing the child to radiation. Peak expiratory flow rate (PEFR) is very useful in asthma as it is easy to perform. PEFR becomes even more useful if a diary is maintained documenting morning, evening and pre/post bronchodilator PEFRs. However, most children under 5 years of age are unable to perform this coordinated test, so a trial of bronchodilators would be the most useful diagnostic test. If the cough persisted despite this, further investigation is warranted.

Asthma, from Greek *asthma* = panting.

19. MANAGEMENT OF DIABETES

B – Change his novarapid to 1 unit per 10 g carbohydrate

This boy is on a basal–bolus insulin regimen. He takes a long-acting insulin (Lantus) and a short-acting one (novarapid). The long-acting insulin is taken in the evening and the short-acting insulin is taken with food. Carbohydrate counting is used to calculate how much insulin he should take with his food. He works out how much carbohydrate he is going to eat and then takes 1 unit of insulin for every 15 g of carbohydrate. When a child is initially diagnosed, an estimate of 0.5 to 1.0 units/kg/day insulin is often used to start with. This is usually split with a third as the long-acting insulin in the evening and the remaining two-thirds as the short-acting insulin taken with food. Monitoring of diabetes is done by measuring blood sugars daily. Preprandial (before food) blood glucose should be 4 to 8 mmol/L and postprandial readings should be around 10 mmol/L. When morning glucose levels are high, this suggests the long-acting evening insulin needs to be increased. If postprandial glucose levels are high, the short-acting insulin needs to be increased.

It is best to only adjust one insulin dose at a time and allow a few days to assess the outcome. It is also useful to check blood sugars more regularly when changing insulin regimens.

In this case, Kevin's glucose level is good in the morning but high after his meals. This would imply his evening Lantus is at a correct dose, but we need to increase the amount of insulin he takes with his food. If we change his carbohydrate counting to 1 unit for every 10 g of carbohydrate eaten, this will increase the dose he takes with his meals. Insulin should always be given before a meal for tighter control; therefore, changing his insulin to after eating would not help with his blood sugars. In younger children and infants, insulin is sometimes given after they have eaten as it is often difficult to know exactly what and how much the child will eat. To prevent hypoglycaemia, the amount of insulin that needs to be given is calculated once the child has eaten.

FURTHER READING

1. NICE guidelines. Available at: http://www.nice.org.uk/guidance/CG15/chapter/1-Guidance#/

20. SHOCK

C – Give a fluid bolus of 20 mL/kg

In children under 3 years of age, the classical signs of neck rigidity, photophobia, headache and vomiting are often absent making clinical diagnosis of meningitis harder.

Signs of possible meningitis in children under 3 years are:

- Coma
- Drowsiness
- High-pitched cry or irritability
- Poor feeding
- Unexplained pyrexia
- Convulsions with or without fever
- Apnoea or cyanotic attacks
- Purpuric rash

A purpuric rash in an ill child with a headache should raise a strong suspicion of meningitis associated with sepsis. The most common organism responsible for causing septicaemia in infants and children is meningococcus (*Neisseria meningitidis*). Group B streptococcus is also common in infants. The *Advanced Paediatric Life Support* manual (the gold standard for acute care) states that all children who are acutely unwell should be approached in an ABC fashion. This includes meningitis. In this case, the patient is crying; therefore, we know that the airway is intact and the child is breathing. It would be useful to assess the respiratory rate, monitor blood saturations and apply some facial oxygen to minimize tissue hypoxia. Though intubation and ventilation may become necessary, they are not required at this point.

Capillary refill time (CRT) is a measure of perfusion. It is performed by applying cutaneous pressure on the centre of the sternum (central) or digit (peripheral) for 5 seconds. The 'refill' or return of colour should occur within 2 to 3 seconds. CRT is a very useful sign in early septic shock when the child may be otherwise well. In this case, as the perfusion is poor, your first action would be to site a peripheral cannula (taking a blood sugar, blood culture, full blood count, C-reactive protein and venous blood gas) and then give a fluid bolus (20 mL/kg is the recommended first bolus). This is done to improve the perfusion for maximizing the distribution of antibiotics, which should be given immediately after the fluid bolus. Antibiotics should not be delayed for a lumbar puncture.

21. THE VOMITING INFANT (1)

B – Inguinal hernia

This child presents with an inguinal hernia. Inguinal hernias in children are most commonly indirect (passing down the inguinal canal into the scrotum, lateral to the inferior epigastric vessels) and are the result of a patent processus vaginalis. Indirect inguinal hernias have an incidence of 5% and are more common in premature babies, males and on the right-hand side (due to delayed descent of the right testis). Children often present with an intermittent swelling in the groin, which is more prominent after crying. An incarcerated hernia (this case) presents with poor feeding, vomiting, crying and a painful lump. Incarcerated hernias are a medical emergency as they can quickly lead to bowel strangulation and perforation. All uncomplicated inguinal hernias should have an elective herniorrhaphy to prevent incarceration.

Pyloric stenosis is due to hypertrophy and hyperplasia of the muscular layers of the pylorus, causing a functional gastric outlet obstruction. It usually presents between 3 and 8 weeks of age with non-bilious vomiting that becomes projectile. Affected babies are extremely hungry but have poor weight gain and may appear dehydrated. Pyloric stenosis is diagnosed by giving the baby a 'test feed'. When the baby is given milk, visible gastric peristalsis may be seen over the epigastrium and the pylorus is felt as an olive-shaped mass in the upper abdomen; if the diagnosis is in doubt, an ultrasound can be performed. Investigations reveal a hypochloraemic, hypokalaemic metabolic alkalosis. Infants often need to be rehydrated before definite surgical treatment (Ramstedt's pyloromyotomy – the muscle of the pylorus is cut longitudinally down to the mucosa). The baby can tolerate milk feeds a few hours after the operation.

Intussusception describes the invagination of a proximal portion of bowel (the intussusceptum) into a distal segment (the intussuscipiens), most commonly at the ileocaecal junction. This telescoping of the bowel leads to bowel wall oedema, ischaemia and eventually necrosis. It is most common between 6 and 18 months of age. The typical presentation is of a previously healthy baby experiencing bouts of colicky abdominal pain and vomiting. There is often diarrhoea, which eventually looks like 'red currant jelly' (engorgement and ischaemia of the intestinal mucosa cause bleeding and an outpouring of mucus). A sausage-shaped mass may be palpable in the right upper quadrant. Management is by resuscitation followed by reduction of the intussusception by a rectal air enema. If this is ineffective (25% of cases), then operative reduction is required.

Appendicitis presents classically with poorly defined periumbilical pain that shifts to the right lower quadrant due to the inflammation of the peritoneum over the appendix. A mass is not normally felt, though nausea, vomiting and a low-grade fever are associated.

Volvulus is defined as the complete twisting of a loop of bowel around its mesenteric stalk. It is associated with malrotation of the bowel and most commonly presents in the neonatal period, but it can be seen in children up to 12 months old. The hallmark features are bilious vomiting and abdominal pain; but in older children, symptoms may be vague (chronic intermittent vomiting, abdominal pain, constipation and failure to thrive).

Inguinal, from Latin *inguinalis* = groin.

22. SYNDROME RECOGNITION (1)

A – Down syndrome

Down syndrome (trisomy 21) is estimated at 1 per 800 to 1000 births. As maternal age increases so does the incidence of Down (1:385 risk at 35 years, 1:30 at 45 years). However, more children with Down syndrome are born to younger mothers. The triple test is used to give the level of risk to the mother and is not a diagnosis. Amniocentesis or chorionic villus sampling needs to be done for a definite diagnosis.

There are numerous physical features of Down syndrome, and not all children will have all the signs. There is usually brachycephaly (short head) and a short neck. In the face, there are upslanting palpebral fissures, a flat nasal bridge, low set ears and almond-shaped eyes caused by an epicanthic fold on the medial aspect of the eye; Brushfield spots (white spots on the iris) are seen. The hands of children with Down syndrome have a single palmar crease (in 50% of cases), a high number of ulnar loop dermatoglyphs (fingerprint loop patterns that start on the ulnar side), clinodactyly (incurving of the little finger) and a single flexion furrow of the fifth finger. A sandal gap (large space between the big and second toes) is seen in the feet. Hypotonia is often seen as well as short limbs and excessive joint laxity.

Nearly all children with Down syndrome have some form of learning disability ranging from mild (IQ 50–70) to moderate (IQ 35–50). A small percentage of children have severe to profound learning difficulties. Children with Down syndrome have an increased risk of certain medical conditions, including congenital heart defects (atrioventricular septal defect [AVSD] and ventricular septal defect [VSD]), gastroesophageal reflux, hypothyroidism, cataracts and strabismus, recurrent otitis media, obstructive sleep apnoea, leukaemia, atresias (especially duodenal) and Hirschsprung disease.

Hypotonia is seen in hypothyroidism, but affected children usually have coarse facial features. In Prader–Willi, hypotonia and almond-shaped eyes are also seen, but there is often cryptorchidism and genital hypoplasia. Babies with fetal alcohol syndrome are not particularly hypotonic and have characteristic facies with a thin top lip, short nose and small eyes with hypertelorism (increased distance between the eyes). Turner syndrome is seen only in girls and is not associated with hypotonia.

Thomas Brushfield, British psychiatrist (1858–1937).
John Langdon Down, British physician (1828–1896).

23. CEREBRAL PALSY

C – Diplegic cerebral palsy

Cerebral palsy (CP) describes a group of disorders affecting movement caused by a permanent, non-progressive lesion in the developing brain. It is primarily a disorder of movement but is often coupled with other neurological problems. Although it is non-progressive, the clinical picture can change as the child grows and develops. Diagnosis is clinical. During the first year of life, there is abnormal tone (initial hypotonia, which eventually leads to spasticity). There is usually delay in gross motor development or abnormal movements. Often the primitive reflexes, such as the Moro and grasp reflexes, persist longer than they should. Associated problems include learning difficulties (ranging from mild to severe), epilepsy, visual impairment, hearing loss, speech disorders, behavioural disorders and respiratory problems.

CP can be divided into different forms:

- Spastic (70%)
- Hemiplegic
- Diplegic
- Quadriplegic
- Ataxic
- Dyskinetic
- Mixed

The girl in this scenario most likely has diplegia as both her legs and arms are involved but the upper limbs are less severely affected. These children often demonstrate scissoring of the legs due to excessive adduction of the hips and have a characteristic gait: the feet are equin-ovarus (plantarflexed and turned inward), the hips and knees are flexed and they walk on tiptoes. This form of CP is seen in association with periventricular leukomalacia (white-matter injury near the cerebral ventricles, seen on ultrasound or MRI) often found in ex-premature babies. Affected children often do not have severe learning difficulties or epilepsy.

Hemiplegia affects one side of the body only and it is the arm that is often more affected than the leg. They have a typical gait that is accentuated when running – the affected leg is extended at the knee and circumduction occurs (the foot needs to make a semicircle with the toe scraping the ground in order to move forward); the arm is also in a typical position (elbow and wrist flexed with finger extension). Quadriplegia is the most severe form of CP, where all limbs are significantly involved. It is often associated with learning difficulties, epilepsy, swallowing problems and gastroesophageal reflux. Affected children often develop flexion con-tractures by late childhood.

24. INVESTIGATION OF SHORT STATURE

C – Growth hormone test

Growth velocity is far more important than an isolated measurement of height. This child is most likely to have growth hormone deficiency. This leads to short stature (about half the normal growth velocity) associated with a markedly delayed bone age. There is a normal rate of growth until 6 to 12 months of age, then the growth velocity tails off. It is also associated with neonatal hypoglycaemia, jaundice and a doll-like face. Hypothyroidism is also associated with short stature, but there is often weight gain and other signs of thyroid disease such as dry skin, constipation and bradycardia. Routine Guthrie testing assesses for thyroid function and would rule out the majority of cases of hypothyroidism.

In familial short stature, the child will grow along the centiles, there will be no delay in bone age and the parental heights will be low. It is therefore important to know the parents' heights and calculate the mid-parental height. This child is not growing along the centiles and therefore is unlikely to have familial short stature.

In constitutional short stature, the child has poor initial growth cross-ing centiles. However, this is temporary and growth then normalizes. Puberty is normally delayed, and the growth spurt occurs later, result-ing in a normal adult height. There is a delay in bone age (often between 1 and 4 years), but serial measurements will show advancement parallel to the child's age and in line with their height. There is no diagnostic investigation, and it is a diagnosis of exclusion.

Chronic disease and poor nutrition can both lead to poor growth and short stature. Again, there is delayed bone age but, unlike constitutional delay, these children will not grow to their full potential if the underlying disease is left untreated. Cushing and precocious puberty both lead to short stature due to advancement in bone age, which leads to an initial increase in height velocity, but premature fusion of epiphysis leads to a reduced final height.

Many syndromes are associated with short stature, including Turner, Prader–Willi (excess weight gain, delayed puberty, short stature, infertility and learning disability), Noonan (low set ears, wide set eyes, growth retardation, scoliosis, learning disability and heart defects), Down, Russell–Silver (triangular-shaped face, curvature of the little finger [clinodactyly], precocious puberty, body asymmetry and poor growth), achondroplasia (normal-sized trunk but shortened limbs) and spondyloepiphyseal dysplasia (shortened trunk with normal limbs). These are nearly always associated with a normal bone age as there is a primary cause for the short stature. Where there is a suspicion of any of the aforementioned, chromosomal and DNA analysis can be useful.

Bone age is useful when assessing a child with short stature. This investigation is a good way of defining a child's age from the amount of ossification seen in their bones. It is usually assessed using radiographs of the carpel bones and scoring each of the centres of ossification, which is then converted into a bone age.

25. MANAGEMENT OF ACUTE ASTHMA

B – Give a β-agonist via a spacer
The symptoms may not sound bad but this is by definition a moderate acute exacerbation of asthma. Do not treat it lightly! Moderate attacks can soon become severe if adequate bronchodilation is not established rapidly. The British Thoracic Society guidelines are the gold standard for managing asthma, covering diagnosis through to management. In this case, using a β-agonist (such as salbutamol) should help open up the airways. This boy will also need a course of oral steroids, but that would not be your first step. It is difficult to know how to administer β-agonists during an acute exacerbation, especially as using a nebulizer is practically a lot easier. However, a recent Cochrane Review did show that children using a spacer would spend less time in A&E than if a nebulizer was used.*

---

* Cates CJ, Welsh EJ, Rowe BH. Holding chambers (spacers) versus nebulisers for beta-agonist treatment of acute asthma. *Cochrane Database of Systematic Reviews* 2013, Issue 9. Art. No.: CD000052. DOI: 10.1002/14651858.CD000052.pub3

Once a β-agonist has been administered, the child should be reviewed after an hour. Prior to discharge it is good practice to:

- Give oral prednisolone for 3 days
- Review the need for regular treatment and the use of inhaled steroids
- Review the inhaler technique
- Provide a written asthma action plan for treating future attacks
- Arrange follow-up according to local policy

26. RESPIRATORY DISTRESS

E – Transient tachypnoea of the newborn

Transient tachypnoea of the newborn (TTN) is due to a delayed clearance of fluid from the fetal lungs. This makes TTN much more common in babies born by elective caesarean section. During vaginal delivery, adrenaline levels rise in the baby due to stress, which causes active uptake of fetal lung fluid via sodium channels. As there is no stress during an elective caesarean, the adrenaline-mediated response does not occur, leaving fluid in the newborn's lungs. Babies with TTN can have respiratory rates as high as 100 to 120/min. A chest X-ray should be performed to rule out congenital pneumonia. In TTN, the chest X-ray will show hyperinflation, oedema and fluid in the fissures. Most infants with TTN will not require any treatment other than oxygen.

It is not possible to differentiate TTN from early-onset sepsis, so empirical antibiotics should be started until infection has been entirely ruled out. There are no risks for sepsis in this scenario (negative swab, no prolonged rupture of membranes) so sepsis is unlikely.

Maternal factors that increase the risk of sepsis and congenital pneumonia include:

- Prolonged rupture of membranes (>18 hours)
- Maternal group B streptococcus on high vaginal swab or urine
- Maternal fever (>38°C)
- *In utero* fetal tachycardia >160/min
- Maternal antibiotics (for suspected sepsis)

Respiratory distress syndrome is caused by a deficiency of surfactant in the lungs and primarily occurs in preterm infants.

27. INVESTIGATION OF DIARRHOEA

E – Tissue transglutaminase IgA

This girl has coeliac disease, an autoimmune gluten-related enteropathy of the small bowel. When the patient consumes gluten (a protein found in wheat, rye and barley), a T-cell-mediated autoimmune reaction occurs, causing damage to the intestinal mucosa. It affects 1 in 1000 people, and children can present with failure to thrive, diarrhoea, steatorrhoea, fatigue, abdominal distension and pain, muscle wasting and iron deficiency anaemia.

The first-line investigation for coeliac disease is IgA anti-TG2 (tissue transglutaminase type 2). It must be remembered that those who are IgA deficient may have a falsely negative test and therefore should have IgA levels measured at the same time. Those with IgA deficiency should have at least one additional test (IgG anti-TG2 and IgG EMA [anti-endomysal antibody]).

Children who have a positive IgA anti-TG2 usually go onto have a duodenal or jejunal biopsy taken during endoscopy.

Characteristic histological findings in coeliac disease are:

- Partial to total villous atrophy
- Crypt hyperplasia and lengthening
- Intraepithelial lymphocytes

Other causes of villous atrophy include temporary gluten intolerance secondary to gastroschisis, kwashiorkor, tropical sprue, cows' milk intolerance, giardiasis and severe combined immunodeficiency.

A biopsy is the gold standard for diagnosing coeliac disease. However, children who have very high titres of anti-TG2 and signs and symptoms of coeliac disease do not necessarily need a biopsy. These children can have further blood tests to make the diagnosis without a biopsy. These include IgG EMA and human leucocyte antigen (HLA) testing. Ninety-five percent of children with coeliac disease are HLA-DQ2 or HLA-DQ8 positive.

Coeliac disease is treated with a strict lifelong gluten-free diet. There is an increased risk of enteropathy-associated T-cell lymphoma and non-Hodgkin lymphoma, as well as an association with other autoimmune diseases such as vitiligo and thyroid disease. *Dermatitis herpetiformis* (an intensely itchy, blistering papulovesicular rash found on the extensor surfaces) is associated with coeliac disease and may respond to gluten-avoidance or dapsone.

FURTHER READING

1. Husby S, Koletzko S, Korponay-Szabo IR, et al. European Society for Pediatric Gastroenterology, Hepatology, and Nutrition guidelines for the diagnosis of coeliac disease. *J Pediatr Gastroenterol Nutr* 2012;54:136–160.

28. STRUCTURAL HEART DISEASE

D – Pulmonary stenosis

Heart murmurs are a relatively common finding in children, and many pathological lesions have distinct patterns of murmurs. Murmurs are caused by turbulent blood flow, usually through valves but also through vessels and heart chambers. Most murmurs are innocent, such as vibratory murmurs and venous hums. Innocent murmurs are generally asymptomatic, systolic, are louder during fever and exercise and vary with respiration and posture.

Heart murmurs are graded on their intensity:

Grade I	Faint murmur, usually only cardiologists can hear
Grade II	Quiet murmur
Grade III	Moderate intensity, no thrill
Grade IV	Loud murmur, with a thrill
Grade V	Very loud murmur with a thrill, still requires a stethoscope to hear
Grade VI	Very loud murmur with thrill, can be heard close to chest wall without a stethoscope

The thrill in this case makes this a Grade IV murmur. The position at the upper left sternal angle makes pulmonary stenosis likely. Pulmonary stenosis is associated with syndromes such as Noonan and Alagille (autosomal dominant syndrome comprising jaundice, xanthomas, congenital heart defects, butterfly-shaped vertebrae and dysmorphic facies). It is also one of the features of the tetralogy of Fallot.

Tetralogy of Fallot is the most common congenital cyanotic heart disease. A chest X-ray may show a characteristic boot-shaped heart. The tetralogy is made up of a large ventricular septal defect (VSD), pulmonary stenosis, an aorta that overrides the VSD and right ventricular hypertrophy.

29. FEBRILE ILLNESS (2)

A – Do not routinely give antipyretics to solely reduce body temperature

The following points should be considered when treating a child with a fever:

- Tepid sponging is not recommended
- Do not over- or under-dress a child with fever
- Consider either paracetamol or ibuprofen as an option if the child appears distressed
- Take the views and wishes of parents and carers into account when considering the use of antipyretic agents
- Do not routinely give antipyretic drugs to a child with fever with the sole aim of reducing body temperature
- Do not administer paracetamol and ibuprofen at the same time but consider using the alternative agent if the child does not respond to the first drug
- Do not use antipyretic agents with the sole aim of preventing febrile convulsions

A traffic light system has been recommended for the identification of acutely unwell febrile children. This is based on assessments of colour, activity, respiratory function, hydration and other signs of serious illness (see NICE guidelines*).

30. INVESTIGATION OF DELAYED PUBERTY

A – Gonadotrophin levels

Delayed puberty is defined as the absence of pubertal development by the age of 13 in females and 14 in males or the failure of progression over a 2-year period. Pubertal delay is seen more commonly in males but is more likely to have an underlying cause in a female. This 14-year-old female warrants investigation.

Gonadotrophins are a useful first-line tool to determine which further investigations are needed as delayed puberty can either be associated with low or high gonadotrophin secretion.

The most common cause of delayed puberty in males is constitutional delay, and there is often associated growth delay and a family history of pubertal delay. However, this is a diagnosis of exclusion, and there are other important causes of delayed puberty that need to be ruled out, especially in females. Examination should include pubertal staging, accurate height and weight measurements and a bone age.

Constitutional delay causes pubertal delay secondary to low gonadotrophin (luteinizing hormone and follicle-stimulating hormone) secretion. Chronic illness such as cystic fibrosis, asthma, Crohn and anorexia can also lead to low gonadotrophin secretion. Other causes include disorders of the hypothalamic–pituitary axis including hypothyroidism, panhypopituitarism, Kallmann syndrome (inability to smell [anosmia], decrease in gonadotrophin-releasing hormone, developmental delay) and intracranial tumours. Visual field examination should be performed and, where there is suspicion of a pituitary tumour, a CT needs to be performed. Thyroid and pituitary function tests help assess the function of the hypothalamic–pituitary axis.

Raised gonadotrophin levels with defective gonads can also lead to delayed puberty. This is seen in Turner syndrome (XO) and Klinefelter syndrome (XXY). If examination is suspicious, karyotyping (chromosomal analysis) should be requested. Damage to the gonads can also be secondary to chemotherapy, radiotherapy, surgery or torsion. Imaging of the gonads can be performed when there is doubt.

Henry Turner, American endocrinologist (1892–1970).
Harry Fitch Klinefelter, American endocrinologist (1912b).

---

* National Collaborating Centre for Women's and Children's Health. *Feverish Illness in Children*, NICE Clinical Guideline 160. London: NICE, 2013. Available at: http://guidance.nice.org.uk/CG160/NICEGuidance/pdf/English

31. MANAGEMENT OF SEIZURES

B – Intravenous lorazepam

Managing a seizure is an acute emergency. Benzodiazepines are the backbone of seizure management and will be successful in the termination of most seizures if given correctly and promptly. Manage all seizures in an ABC (DEFG – don't ever forget glucose) fashion. Managing the airway and assessing breathing is paramount as many seizures will terminate themselves and one needs to only ensure adequate oxygenation. If the seizure continues, one member of the team should continue to assess and manage the airway, breathing and circulation.

Check the blood sugar as hypoglycaemia is a common and easily managed cause of convulsions (using 5 mL/kg 10% dextrose).

If a patient has intravenous access, the order of management is:

1. ABC (DEFG)
2. Lorazepam intravenously (two doses)
3. Draw up and give phenytoin intravenously (unless already on phenytoin, in which case give phenobarbitone)
4. Give paraldehyde rectally if directed by senior staff after the start of the phenytoin infusion
5. Intubation and ventilation with thiopental

This algorithm does not cover all cases, as some children with documented epilepsy may respond to certain drugs; often an individual protocol can be more appropriate. One would usually wait 10 minutes between steps; however, preparing the next medication would be common practice. During this period, the child should have their airway maintained while breathing and circulation are monitored. This is particularly important once benzodiazepines have been given as they can cause respiratory depression. An anaesthetist should be called early if you suspect that intubation and ventilation are likely.

FURTHER READING

1. Advanced Life Support Group. *Advanced Paediatric Life Support: The Practical Approach.* 5th ed. London: Wiley-Blackwell, 2011.

32. NEONATAL RESUSCITATION

E – Warm and dry the baby

The resuscitation council have given guidance on the best steps to take during resuscitation of a newborn. The resuscitation of a newborn is the only emergency of which we are aware that requires a step before 'airway'. Warming and drying the baby is vitally important as cold babies are more likely to develop acidosis, hypoglycaemia and reduced surfactant production.

In practice, warming and drying the baby, opening the airway and assessing the newborn all form one swift movement for an experienced paediatrician. The steps in neonatal resuscitation can be summarized as:

- Clamp the cord
- Warm and dry the baby
- Open and clear the airway
- Evaluate breathing, heart rate, colour and tone
- Five inflation breaths
- Continuing ventilation
- Cardiac compressions

In this case, once the baby has been warmed and dried, it is likely it will need active resuscitation as it is not breathing and is pale and floppy. Opening the airway and aerating the lungs is usually successful in most cases. This is done by placing the head in the neutral position (not head-tilt–chin-lift) and giving five inflation breaths.

33. SCROTAL PAIN

D – Torsion of the hydatid of Morgagni

This boy is most likely to have torsion of the hydatid of Morgagni (a small embryological remnant at the upper pole of the testes), which is the most common cause of an acute scrotum in children. It is a benign condition but needs to be distinguished from testicular torsion, which is a surgical emergency.

Torsion of a testis refers to the twisting of the spermatic cord in or just below the inguinal canal. Strangulation of the gonadal vessels can lead to testicular necrosis and atrophy. Testicular torsion is more common in adolescents, whereas torsion of the hydatid is seen in younger children, typically 7 to 12 years. The pain in torsion of the hydatid is usually less severe than testicular torsion and can have a more insidious onset (as in this case). Both cause a red swollen testis but, in torsion of the hydatid, the tenderness is usually localized to the upper pole of the testes, in contrast to the extremely tender testicle, found high in the scrotum, in testicular torsion. The pain in testicular torsion is also often referred to the abdomen. Other distinguishing features of testicular torsion include nausea and vomiting. The cremasteric reflex is preserved in torsion of the hydatid, and there may be a 'blue dot' (the torted hydatid) visible on the scrotum when it is transilluminated.

Irreversible infarction of a twisted testicle occurs within 6 to 12 hours, so affected patients should be taken to theatre for surgical exploration without further investigation. (Generally, to preserve spermatogenesis, torsion should be relieved within 4 hours.) Surgical management includes untwisting of the testicle and bilateral fixation of the testes to the tunica vaginalis to prevent further torsion. Bilateral fixation is required because anatomical abnormalities of the testes that predispose to torsion usually occur on both sides.

A hydrocele presents with a swollen scrotum but is usually soft and non-tender. It is difficult to palpate the testicle as it lies within the fluid collection. Epididymitis, an inflammation of the epididymis, presents with a swollen painful testicle. There is often an associated fever as well as nausea. It can be difficult to distinguish from testicular torsion but Prehn's sign is indicative of epididymitis (tenderness relieved by elevating the scrotum). There may also be associated urinary symptoms including frequency and dysuria.

Giovanni Baptista Morgagni, Italian anatomist (1682–1771).
Hydatid, from Greek *hydatis* = drop of water.

34. SPLENOMEGALY

A – Acute lymphoblastic leukaemia

This child is most likely to have leukaemia with a combination of splenomegaly, bruises, lethargy and pallor. Acute lymphoblastic leukaemia (ALL) accounts for 80% of childhood leukaemias and is therefore the most likely answer. ALL has a peak incidence at around 5 years, which slowly decreases in adolescence. It is slightly more common in boys and a higher incidence is seen in Caucasians.

Acute myeloid leukaemia (AML) is not nearly as common in childhood, though it accounts for 80% of all acute leukaemias when including adults. There is an increased incidence of leukaemia in Down syndrome with an equal incidence of AML and ALL. Bloom syndrome (an autosomal recessive syndrome characterized by short stature, facial photosensitive rash, narrow face, subfertility and immune deficiency) and neurofibromatosis are also associated with an increased risk.

Features of leukaemia depend on the degree of infiltration into the bone marrow and other sites in the body. These range from an incidental finding on full blood count in a well child to life-threatening situations where the child is in tumour lysis syndrome. The symptoms are related first to the direct infiltration of the bone marrow by leukaemic cells (bone and muscle pain) or direct infiltration of other organs (hepatosplenomegaly or lymphadenopathy). Other symptoms are related to the decreased production of normal marrow elements including white cells, haemoglobin and platelets. Anaemia leads to pallor, lethargy, dizziness and exertional dyspnoea. The white cell count may be normal, low or high but the neutrophils are nearly always low. This leads to an increase in infections and the inability to recover from seemingly mild infections. Platelets are often low, resulting in bruising, epistaxis, bleeding gums and petechiae. Occasionally, if the leukaemia is already in the central nervous system, children may present with nausea, vomiting or even a focal neurological deficit.

Cystic fibrosis is often picked up on neonatal screening (Guthrie card) though it can present with failure to thrive and recurrent chest infections. Splenomegaly can be seen in cystic fibrosis, secondary to liver disease, but is unlikely to be a presenting sign. Neglect and physical abuse can present with failure to thrive and bruising, but in an acutely unwell child with splenomegaly this is unlikely to be the cause. Glandular fever, caused by Epstein–Barr virus, can present with lethargy and prolonged fever. However, pharyngitis is the typical presentation, not a chest infection. Splenomegaly may be present, but bruising is not a feature.

35. EPILEPSY SYNDROMES

B – Benign rolandic epilepsy

This child has a typical history of benign rolandic epilepsy, which accounts for 20% of all childhood epilepsy. Seven- to ten-year olds are most likely to be affected (but it can be seen from 3 to 13 years of age), and there is a male preponderance. Rolandic seizures are usually nocturnal involving the mouth and face. They often begin with an odd sensation at the corner of the mouth, which leads to twitching of the mouth and then the rest of the ipsilateral face. Excessive salivation, grunting and slurred speech can occur, and they can progress to generalized seizures. The EEG often shows high amplitude spikes in the left centrotemporal region. This area of the brain is near the motor strip (the Rolandic fissure, hence the name of the epilepsy). It is a benign condition, and children often grow out of it by adolescence.

Juvenile myoclonic epilepsy usually begins around puberty and can be precipitated by alcohol. There are usually severe symmetrical jerks of the arms and trunk, which can proceed to generalized fits. They often occur in the morning on waking.

Absence seizures are generalized seizures affecting consciousness that typically last a few seconds. The child stares blankly and is unresponsive. They are often noticed in school and can be confused with daydreaming. There is no involuntary movement or falling to the ground, but when children become alert after the seizure they have no recollection of the event. Absence seizures occur between the ages of 2 and 10 years, are more common in girls and children frequently grow out of them. The EEG typically shows three spike–wave complex cycles per second. There is a family history in 20% of cases.

Lennox–Gastaut type epilepsy is rare and presents between 1 and 4 years of age. Features include daily seizures, episodes of status epilepticus, slowed psychomotor development and behavioural disorders. It has a poor prognosis. The EEG shows slow spike–waves with multiple abnormalities.

Henri Gastaut, French neurologist (1915–1995).
William Gordon Lennox, American neurologist (1884–1960).
Luigi Rolando, Italian anatomist (1773–1831).

36. IMMUNIZATION

C – Meningitis C

Immunizations and the immunization schedule commonly appear in written papers. Much more commonly, though, is an objective structured clinical examination (OSCE) station in which you will need to counsel a parent about the need for immunizations. As part of this, you should have a basic understanding of which immunizations are given at certain ages.

The current immunization programme (2015) is described here:

Timing	Immunization (each injection on a separate line)
2 months old	DTaP/IPV/HiB
	PCV
	Rotavirus
3 months old	DTaP/IPV/HiB
	MenC
	Rotavirus
4 months old	DTaP/IPV/HiB
	PCV
12–13 months old	HiB/MenC
	MMR
	PCV
2, 3 and 4 years old	Children's flu vaccine
3 years and 4 months – 5 years old	DTaP/IPV booster
	MMR
Girls 12–13 years old	HPV (2 injections between 6 months to 2 years apart)
13–15 years old	MenC booster
13–18 years old	Td/IPV booster

DTaP: diphtheria, tetanus and acellular pertussis; Td: tetanus and diphtheria; IPV: inactivated poliovirus vaccine; HiB: *Haemophilus influenza* type B; PCV: pneuomococcal vaccine; MenC: meningitis C; MMR: measles, mumps and rubella; HPV: human papillomavirus vaccine.

Meningococcal B vaccine has recently been approved to be added to this schedule at 2, 4 and 12 months, though at time of writing it has not been actually implemented. An up-to-date schedule can be found at: http://www.nhs.uk/Conditions/vaccinations/Pages/vaccination-schedule-age-checklist.aspx

37. MANAGEMENT OF CARDIAC DISEASE

D – Insertion of a feeding nasogastric tube

This child has a ventricular septal defect (VSD). The history also suggests that he is developing heart failure due to the extra work of the left side of the heart supplying the systemic circulation as well as blood flowing to the right heart via the septal defect. This boy has a quiet

(Grade I) murmur. Remember that quiet murmurs often signify a large lesion as there is little turbulent flow. A small defect on the other hand usually causes a loud murmur due to the highly turbulent flow across the septum.

Heart failure can be caused by structural lesions (e.g. coarctation, VSD, atrioventricular septal defect [AVSD], large patent ductus arteriosus [PDA]) or by the failure of a structurally normal heart (e.g. supraventricular tachycardia, myocarditis, cardiomyopathy). The signs of heart failure are breathlessness, poor feeding, sweating and recurrent chest infections. On examination, you may find a child who is failing to thrive, tachypnoeic and tachycardic with a murmur, hepatomegaly or a displaced apex due to cardiomegaly.

The definition of heart failure is the inability of the heart to keep up with the metabolic requirements of the tissues of the body. The management of heart failure starts with supportive steps to maximize the provision of metabolic requirements to the body. Therefore, inserting a nasogastric tube and starting high caloric feeds will reduce the associated growth retardation. Growth retardation is caused by a failure to take adequate feeds due to breathlessness and to a high metabolic rate in the symptomatic child. Commencing oxygen therapy will also aid in the provision of oxygen to the tissues.

It is likely that this child will need pharmacological management. Diuretics (thiazide or loop) will reduce the load on the heart. ACE inhibitors are frequently used in conjunction with diuretics. There is now little evidence for the use of digoxin. Surgery is the definitive treatment and is usually delayed until the child is big enough to tolerate the procedure. Some children need to have surgical correction in the first year of life; they include babies with severe heart failure and failure to thrive or those with pulmonary hypertension with the potential to progress to pulmonary vascular disease.

38. OPHTHALMIA NEONATORUM

A – *Chlamydia trachomatis*

Ophthalmia neonatorum is the term used for conjunctivitis occurring in the first few weeks of life. A standard swab for microscopy and culture should be performed along with a conjunctival scraping. The aim of the scraping is to gain cells within which chlamydial organisms can be found.

The most common causes of ophthalmia neonatorum are:

- *Staphylococcus aureus*
- *Chlamydia trachomatis*
- *Neisseria gonorrhoeae*
- Chemical irritation (silver nitrate)

Chlamydia is now among the most common causes of neonatal conjunctivitis. *C. trachomatis* is an intracellular organism and is treated with tetracycline eye drops and oral erythromycin for 2 weeks. The other organisms here are not intracellular and therefore cannot be responsible. *C. trachomatis* can also cause pneumonia, and this should be considered if the child develops any respiratory symptoms.

It is important that the mother of this child attends a genitourinary clinic for investigation and treatment of her sexually transmitted infection. Partner tracing is imperative.

39. COUGH

E – Whooping cough

Whooping cough is caused by the bacterium *Bordetella pertussis*. It is now less common in the UK due to the introduction of the diphtheria, tetanus, pertussis (DTP) vaccine, though in recent years there has been a recent surge of cases. As of this writing, pregnant women are being offered the pertussis vaccine in the third trimester of pregnancy to help protect their newborn baby until they are old enough for the 2-month immunizations. In a child who has moved from outside the UK, you should always consider that immunizations may not have been given. Illness usually begins with coryza, and a dry cough develops after a few days. This cough becomes more pronounced and occurs in paroxysms. Repeated episodes of coughing classically end with an inspiratory 'whoop'. Another name for pertussis is the '100-day cough' as the symptoms often continue for that duration. No treatment can change the course of the illness, although erythromycin is said to reduce the period of infectivity. Complications are uncommon but include pneumonia and bronchiectasis. Immunization does not give total protection and protection is not necessarily lifelong.

Bronchiolitis classically presents in the first year of life with a high-pitched cough and wheeze. In this case, you would be right to suspect an inhaled foreign body though you would usually hear a difference in the air entry between the left and right hemithoraces. Also, this cough usually has an abrupt onset without the signs and symptoms of an upper respiratory tract infection.

Pertussis, from Latin *per* = throughout + *tussus* = cough ('intensive coughing').

40. DIAGNOSIS OF SEIZURES

B – Carboxyhaemoglobin levels

Carbon monoxide (CO) can be produced by natural gas combustion devices (especially if poorly ventilated), motor vehicle exhausts and by burning charcoal or kerosene. It is therefore more likely that you will come into contact with CO poisoning in the winter months when heating devices are used. CO has a very high affinity for binding with haemoglobin (250 times greater than oxygen), although binding is reversible. Poisoning causes acute symptoms associated with hypoxia, such as headaches, dizziness and nausea. Cyanosis does not occur, and the skin remains pink. Syncope and seizures can occur, and this may be followed by coma and death.

Blood saturations and blood gases are not useful for diagnosing CO poisoning as they will not accurately determine the degree of hypoxia. A blood gas may show metabolic acidosis, which corrects on treating the hypoxia. The diagnosis of CO poisoning is made by taking a carboxyhaemoglobin (COHb) level. Smokers will have a naturally higher COHb level (up to 9%). A COHb >5% in a non-smoker confirms CO poisoning. You will not be able to gain an accurate result if the patient has been given 100% oxygen for more than one hour.

Management is with 100% oxygen using a tight fitting mask, which speeds dissociation of CO from Hb by up to five times. Patients may need intervention for low blood pressure (fluids) and seizures (anticonvulsants). Hyperbaric oxygen is required for severe symptoms or if the COHb is >40%.

In this case, the source of the CO needs to be found and should be either removed or fixed. Regular servicing of natural gas burning devices will prevent many cases of CO poisoning. Household CO detectors are also now being incorporated into smoke alarms.

41. GENETIC INHERITANCE

E – Tuberous sclerosis

The inheritance of disorders is a relatively common exam question and needs to be memorized. Knowing the inheritance of certain disorders is important for counselling parents regarding the risk of future children being affected.

Inheritance patterns

Chromosomal abnormalities	Autosomal recessive inheritance
Trisomy 21 (Down)	Congenital adrenal hyperplasia
Trisomy 13 (Patau)	Cystic fibrosis
Trisomy 18 (Edwards)	Friedreich's ataxia
Turner (45XO)	Galactosaemia
Fragile-X syndrome	Haemochromatosis
Klinefelter syndrome (47 XXY)	Oculocutaneous albinism
	Sickle cell disease
Autosomal dominant inheritance	Tay–Sachs
Achondroplasia	Thalassaemia
Tuberous sclerosis	
Ehlers–Danlos	X-linked recessive inheritance
Familial hypercholesterolaemia	Red–green colour blindness
Huntington disease	Duchenne muscular dystrophy
Marfan syndrome	Haemophilia A & B
Neurofibromatosis	Glucose-6-phosphate dehydrogenase deficiency
Noonan syndrome	
Osteogenesis imperfecta	X-linked dominant inheritance
Polyposis coli	Vitamin D-resistant rickets
	Incontinentia pigmenti

42. MANAGEMENT OF ECZEMA

E – All of the above

Atopic eczema (atopic dermatitis) is a chronic inflammatory itchy skin condition that usually develops in early childhood and follows a remitting and relapsing course. There is often a breakdown of the skin barrier, which makes the skin susceptible to trigger factors, including irritants and allergens. Guidelines on the management of atopic eczema have been published by NICE.*

When assessing a child, identify potential trigger factors, including irritants (such as soap and detergents), skin infections, contact allergens, food allergens and inhaled allergens.

Emollients are the foundation of good eczema care. They should be:

- Used more often and in larger amounts than other treatments
- Used on the whole body even when atopic eczema is clear
- Used while using other treatments
- Used instead of soaps and detergent-based wash products
- Easily available to use at nursery, preschool or school

43. SYNCOPE

E – Reflex anoxic seizure

Whenever a child has a 'funny turn' or possible loss of consciousness it is vital to take a thorough history, preferably from the person who witnessed the event. The parents often think their child has had a fit when in fact there are many other causes for the loss of consciousness.

This girl has had a reflex anoxic seizure. These often occur after pain, discomfort or minor head injuries, with other triggers including fever, cold drinks or a fright. The child (usually an infant or toddler) becomes very pale and can fall to the ground. Episodes occur due to a reflex cardiac asystole secondary to increased vagal response. They can occasionally be associated with tonic–clonic movements, as in this case, but the child recovers rapidly and is their usual self soon after the event (unlike after an epileptic seizure).

Breath-holding attacks occur in young children, typically toddlers, and are associated with the child being upset, angry or crying. The child usually holds their breath at the end of expiration and can then occasionally go blue and apnoeic. It is usually seen while the child is screaming. Loss of consciousness can occur though it is usually only for a brief period and occurs only after breath-holding has occurred for a while. Simple vasovagal attacks occur when a child has been standing for long periods or is in a hot stuffy room. The child will often remember feeling dizzy, lightheaded, experience ringing in their ears or blurred vision before the

---

* National Collaborating Centre for Women's and Children's Health. *Atopic eczema in children: Management of atopic eczema in children from birth up to the age of 12 years.* London: RCOG Press, 2007. Available at: www.nice.org.uk/nicemedia/pdf/CG057FullGuideline.pdf

syncope. Cardiac arrhythmias can lead to syncope. These can occur with no warning and may be related to exercise. Supraventricular tachycardia can lead to syncope though the child usually experiences palpitations or dizziness prior to the syncope. A prolonged QT interval, though rare, is a cause of syncope and can be easily ruled out with an ECG.

44. INVESTIGATION OF JAUNDICE (1)

B – Split bilirubin
Any baby who is jaundiced after 14 days (21 days if premature) needs to have a split bilirubin assay performed. A split bilirubin assay measures conjugated and total bilirubin levels. If the conjugated fraction is greater than 20% (and >18 μmol/L), then the baby should be seen in a specialist paediatric liver centre. Examining the stool of a jaundiced neonate is very important as an acholic stool (pale stools due to the absence of bilirubin) suggests an obstruction in the biliary tree. Detailed investigation is warranted in children with prolonged conjugated hyperbilirubinaemia. The most important diagnosis to rule out is biliary atresia. Investigations should also be directed at ruling out infection, metabolic disorders, hypothyroidism and familial cholestatic syndromes.

The mnemonic TORCH is used to remember the main congenital infections.

T – Toxoplasmosis
O – Other (syphilis)
R – Rubella
C – Cytomegalovirus (CMV)
H – Herpes

The most common of these is CMV. Features common to all TORCH infections are jaundice, low birth weight, prematurity, microcephaly, seizures, anaemia, failure to thrive and encephalitis.

45. MANAGEMENT OF URINARY TRACT INFECTION

A – A 3-day course of oral antibiotics
Infants below 3 months of age should be referred immediately to a paediatric specialist and treated with intravenous antibiotics in line with treating any feverish illness in such a young age group.

If the infant or child is older than 3 months and has acute pyelonephritis or upper urinary tract infection an oral course of antibiotics for 7 to 10 days should be used. If oral antibiotics are not tolerated (e.g. excessive vomiting or lethargy), then intravenous antibiotics should be given initially, followed by oral antibiotics for a total of 10 days.

If the infant or child is older than 3 months and has a lower urinary tract infection then a course of oral antibiotics for 3 days is usually adequate. Local guidelines should be followed for the choice of antibiotics: trimethoprim, co-amoxiclav and cephalosporins are all suitable. Again, if the child is unable to manage oral medication then parenteral antibiotics may be used.

If the child is at a high risk of a serious illness, or looks seriously unwell, treatment with parenteral antibiotics is essential.

FURTHER READING

1. National Collaborating Centre for Women's and Children's Health (UK). *Urinary Tract Infection in Children: Diagnosis, Treatment and Long-term Management.* NICE Clinical Guideline 54. London: RCOG Press, 2007.

46. PURPURIC RASH

C – Conjunctivitis

This girl has Henoch–Schönlein purpura (HSP). HSP is an immunologically mediated diffuse vasculitis, especially of the small blood vessels, often preceded by an upper respiratory tract infection (especially β-haemolytic streptococci). It usually occurs between 3 and 10 years of age and is twice as common in boys. The characteristic finding is a palpable purpuric rash, which can occur anywhere, but is most commonly seen on the buttocks and lower extremities.

The rash in HSP normally resolves after 3 to 4 weeks, but it can come and go for up to a year after the initial presentation. Other complications of HSP are arthritis (80%), gastrointestinal involvement (abdominal pain and intussusception) and renal involvement (glomerulonephritis) leading to acute renal failure (in 1%). The prognosis in HSP is very good, and most children will have complete resolution without any serious long-term complications. It is important to check the blood pressure and dip the urine of every child presenting with HSP.

Treatment is supportive with analgesia for arthritis and abdominal pain. A short course of systemic steroids can be used in gastrointestinal disease to provide symptomatic relief of the abdominal pain.

Eduard Heinrich Henoch, German paediatrician (1820–1910).
Johann Lukas Schönlein, German paediatrician (1793–1864).

47. SKIN RASH (1)

D – Psoriasis

Guttate psoriasis occurs almost exclusively in children and young adults. The lesions found are 0.5 to 2 cm oval scaling red papules and small plaques. The lesions are numerous and distributed over the torso and proximal extremities. Guttate psoriasis is often preceded by streptococcal infections (as in this case). The possibility of a concurrent streptococcal infection should be investigated in any new cases of guttate psoriasis.

Classical psoriasis is a relatively common papulosquamous condition. It is characterized by well-demarcated, erythematous papules and plaques, which have a scaly surface. Infections, stress, trauma and certain medications may cause exacerbations.

Atopic eczema can flare up after an acute illness but does not tend to be scaly. Chronic atopic eczema can have a lichenified appearance and classically affects the limb extensors rather than the torso. Scarlet fever also presents with a rash after a group A β-haemolytic streptococcal infection. In scarlet fever, the rash occurs 12 to 24 hours after the onset of the illness and is a fine diffuse erythematous maculopapular rash that has the texture of goose flesh. Other features of scarlet fever include a strawberry tongue, desquamation of the rash after 2 to 3 days (especially of the palms and soles) and lymphadenopathy.

Guttate, from Latin *gutta* = drops.

48. APGAR SCORE

C – 8

Before assessing the Apgar score, the baby should be warmed and dried. The Apgar is usually performed at 1, 5 and 10 minutes of life. It was devised to allow a rapid and repeatable assessment of the newborn. The score has a maximum of 10, with two possible points in five areas of assessment. The need for intervention actually depends on just three of the five components: respiratory activity, heart rate and colour.

Virginia Apgar, American pediatric anesthetist (1909–1974).

The Apgar score		
	0	1	2
Heart rate	Absent	<100	>100
Respiration	Absent	Gasping or irregular	Regular
Muscle tone	Limp	Diminished	Normal
Reflex irritability	No response to stimulation	Feeble cry when stimulated	Cough or good cry
Colour	Blue	Pink with blue extremities	Pink

The criteria can be remembered using the mnemonic APGAR:

A	Appearance	→	colour
P	Pulse	→	heart rate
G	Grimace	→	irritability
A	Activity	→	muscle tone
R	Respiration	→	respiratory function

49. HEADACHE

D – Migraine

Headache can be a vague and non-specific symptom in many different diagnoses. It is therefore important to get an accurate pain history. The mnemonic SOCRATES can be used to assess any pain including headaches:

S Site
O Onset
C Character
R Radiation
A Associated features
T Timing
E Exacerbating/relieving features; ever-before?
S Severity

Red-flag symptoms include an acute onset of severe pain, pain worse on lying down, vomiting, developmental regression or personality change, unilateral pain, papilloedema, hypertension, an increase in head circumference and focal neurological signs.

Migraines can be unilateral or bilateral. They are often associated with nausea, vomiting and photophobia. Occasionally migraines are associated with an aura that can range from flashing lights or black spots to unilateral weakness or paraesthesia. However, these signs are only transient and should disappear soon after the headache is better. A family history of migraines is often seen as well as other associated factors such as the oral contraceptive pill and foods containing tyramine (e.g. cheese and red wine).

Idiopathic intracranial hypertension (previously known as benign intracranial hypertension) usually occurs in young women and is associated with obesity. There is a raised intracranial pressure (ICP) in the absence of a mass lesion. This can be idiopathic or precipitated by drugs (tetracyclines, oral contraceptive pill and steroid withdrawal). Features include headache, transient diplopia and bilateral papilloedema. A CT scan is normal and a lumbar puncture will confirm a raised cerebrospinal fluid pressure. Management options include weight loss, avoidance of precipitating drugs and repeated lumbar puncture. The aim of treatment is to prevent permanent visual loss.

Space-occupying lesions are associated with signs and symptoms of raised ICP. This includes early morning headaches, headaches that are relieved by vomiting, focal neurological deficits or blurring of vision. There may be evidence of papilloedema. Hypertension and bradycardia are seen in severe raised ICP. Tension headaches are often described as a band-like pressure that is precipitated by stress, and they are worse late in the day. Cluster headaches are sudden severe brief attacks of unilateral, periorbital pain associated with eye watering. They can occur frequently, up to eight times a day, and often at similar times of day.

50. MANAGEMENT OF CONSTIPATION

E – Movicol disimpaction regimen

This child has chronic constipation and has secondary soiling. Incontinence occurs in chronic constipation due to the leakage of liquid stool from above the impacted stool. Until full disimpaction has been achieved, the soiling is likely to remain. The objectives of treatment are to first remove faecal impaction, restore a bowel habit where soft stools are passed without discomfort and then to ensure self-toileting and passing stools in appropriate places (in younger children). It is essential to establish a good rapport with both parents and the child as there may be feelings of guilt, blame and shame that all need to be recognized and dealt with sensitively.

Disimpaction

The objective of disimpaction is to fully clear the rectum of retained faeces. The use of polyethylene glycol (Movicol) in disimpaction has been shown to be extremely effective. The disimpaction regime consists of starting with two sachets of Movicol on day 1 and then increasing the number of sachets by two every 2 days till a maximum of eight sachets a day. Treatment should be continued until impaction has resolved or for a maximum of 7 days. Suppositories and rectal enemas can also be used to disimpact, but most paediatricians try and avoid rectal routes unless oral disimpaction has failed. Very rarely, disimpaction under anaesthetic may be required.

Maintenance therapy

Osmotic laxatives have the best evidence for effectiveness, and these would include lactulose and Movicol. A randomized controlled trial showed that Movicol was more effective and had fewer side effects than lactulose. The dose should be adjusted to achieve the regular passage of soft, formed stools. The chronic use of stimulant laxatives, such as senna, is contentious although they are often used alongside osmotic laxatives. Prolonged use can cause an atonic colon and hypokalaemia. Adequate intake of fluid and fibre should always be encouraged and a dietician may be needed.

Behaviour modification

Regular toileting and unhurried time on the toilet should be encouraged. A reward system, especially one that is geared towards successful use of the toilet, as opposed to clean pants, is important.

Practice Paper 4: Questions

1. GLASGOW COMA SCALE

A 13-year-old female is admitted to the emergency department having been involved in a road traffic accident. She does not open her eyes spontaneously but does so when you say 'Jane, open your eyes'. She starts talking, but not appropriately, shouting out occasional words. She will not follow simple commands, but when you press on her fingernail bed, she uses her other arm to push you away.

What is her Glasgow Coma Score?

A. 10
B. 11
C. 12
D. 13
E. 14

2. DIAGNOSIS OF URINARY TRACT INFECTION

A 2-year-old girl presents to the general practitioner with a fever and vomiting. On examination, there is no obvious focus for infection. A urine sample is obtained and sent for urgent microscopy and culture. Before sending the sample to the laboratory, a urine dipstick analysis is performed in the clinic.

Which of the below dipstick results most likely represents a urinary tract infection?

A. Leucocytes negative, nitrites negative
B. Leucocytes negative, nitrates positive
C. Leucocytes 2+, nitrates negative
D. Leucocytes 2+, nitrites positive
E. Leucocytes 2+, nitrates positive

3. HEPATITIS

An 8-year-old boy presents to his general practitioner with jaundice. About a week earlier, he had a brief period of fever, diarrhoea and nausea. These symptoms have now resolved. His mother thought this was caused by 'food poisoning' after a scout camp.

Which of the following is the most likely cause for his jaundice?

A. Hepatitis A
B. Hepatitis B
C. Hepatitis C
D. Hepatitis D
E. Hepatitis E

4. HAEMOGLOBINOPATHIES

An 8-year-old girl is undergoing a routine tonsillectomy. At pre-assessment, she appears well but slightly pale. The remainder of the examination is unremarkable except for enlarged non-inflamed tonsils. You receive the results of her blood tests and her blood film reveals a microcytic, hypochromic anaemia. Haemoglobin electrophoresis shows increased levels of HbA_2 and HbF. No HbH is seen.

What is the most likely diagnosis?

A. α-Thalassaemia minor
B. β-Thalassaemia major
C. β-Thalassaemia trait
D. Iron deficiency anaemia
E. Sickle cell anaemia

5. MANAGEMENT OF SICKLE CELL ANAEMIA

An 8-year-old boy with known sickle cell disease arrives at hospital complaining of severe pain in the fingers of his right hand. He is generally well. He has a normal heart and respiratory rate. His temperature is 37.1°C, and there is no evidence of infection. You place him on oxygen as his oxygen saturations are 94% on air.

What is the next most important treatment to give him?

A. Hydroxycarbamide
B. Intravenous antibiotics
C. Intravenous fluids
D. Intravenous sodium bicarbonate
E. Pain relief including opioids

6. HYPERACTIVITY DISORDER

Duncan is a 6-year-old boy who has been at school for almost 2 years. The teachers are concerned that he has a lot of energy associated with difficulties in maintaining attention on tasks. They feel this is significantly impairing his academic development.

Which of the following is true regarding attention deficit hyperactivity disorder?

A. The behaviour should persist for at least 12 months.
B. The behaviour should be consistent with the child's developmental age.
C. The symptoms only occur in one setting.
D. There must be a significantly impaired social or academic development.
E. There can be another explanation for the symptoms.

7. MICROORGANISMS

A 5-month-old girl presents with fever and irritability. A 'clean catch' urine specimen is sent from the emergency department. Once on the ward, the nurse informs you she has had a phone call from the lab and that the microscopy of the urine has revealed pyuria and a Gram-negative bacillus.

Which of the following organisms is causing this girl's urinary tract infection?

A. *Campylobacter jejuni*
B. *Escherichia coli*
C. Group A streptococcus
D. *Niesseria meningitidis*
E. *Treponema pallidum*

8. ELECTROLYTE DISTURBANCE (2)

A 6-year-old girl is seen in the paediatrics follow-up clinic. She was an inpatient 5 months ago with meningococcal meningitis. Since she was discharged from hospital, she has been drinking increasingly excessively and passing large amounts of urine. Her mother reports that the child has to get up during the night to urinate. She was previously dry by day and night; however, she has now had a number of episodes of nocturnal enuresis. She passes large volumes of urine even when she is not drinking much. You insert a cannula and take blood for an analysis of urea and electrolytes.

You receive the following blood results:

Na	152 (135–145 mmol/L)
K	4.2 (3.5–5.0 mmol/L)
Urea	6.2 (1.5–4.5 mmol/L)
Creatinine	83 (40–110 µmol/L)
pH	7.37 (7.35–7.45)
Glucose	4.2 (3.4–5.5 mmol/L)

Which of the following is the most likely cause of the electrolyte disturbance?

A. Chronic renal failure
B. Primary aldosteronism
C. Diabetes insipidus
D. Diabetes mellitus
E. Syndrome of inappropriate ADH secretion

9. LUMBAR PUNCTURE

A 5-month-old boy presents to the emergency department with a short history of irritability and poor feeding. He is systemically unwell, poorly perfused and has a fever of 39.0°C. The admitting doctor performs a septic screen (including lumbar puncture) and starts empirical intravenous antibiotics. You are called by the on-call microbiologist with the following results of the lumbar puncture:

Blood sugar	4.8 mmol/L
CSF sugar	3.9 mmol/L
CSF protein	0.18 g/dL (range 0.2–0.4 g/dL)
CSF white cell count	36 lymphocytes/mm^3
CSF red cell count	50 red cells/mm^3
Microscopy	No organisms seen

Which of the following is the most likely diagnosis?

A. Bacterial meningitis
B. Intracranial haemorrhage
C. Normal result
D. TB meningitis
E. Viral meningitis

10. STRIDOR

A 2-year-old boy presents to the emergency department with a new onset of 'noisy breathing' and a cough. He has been unwell for 2 days with a runny nose and temperature of 38.0°C. When you arrive, he is sitting up and drinking from a bottle. He has a loud stridor and a harsh cough. There is moderate subcostal recession. He is mildly tachycardic. His capillary refill time is <2 seconds. His oxygen saturations are 98% on air.

Which of the following is the most likely diagnosis?

A. Epiglottitis
B. Laryngotracheobronchitis
C. Laryngomalacia
D. Pharyngitis
E. Subglottic stenosis

11. AUTISM SPECTRUM DISORDER

You see a 3-year-old boy as there is concern regarding poor language skills and delayed social development. His mother reports that he displays ritualistic behaviour and becomes very upset if these rituals are not adhered to. It is thought that he may have autism spectrum disorder.

Which of the following statements is true regarding autism spectrum disorder?

A. Aetiology is well described.
B. It affects girls more commonly than boys.
C. Language skills do not help predict long-term function.
D. It presents before the age of 3 years.
E. There is no increased risk of autistic disorder in siblings.

12. VOMITING IN A BABY

A mother brings her 6-week-old baby boy to the general practitioner as she is worried he is vomiting. He weighs 4.6 kg and is bottle-fed. He is taking 4 oz (120 mL) every 4 hours but vomits after nearly every bottle. The vomiting is occasionally 'projectile'. Her baby is not taking his feeds well and is crying excessively. Examination is unremarkable, and he displays normal growth.

What is the most likely diagnosis?

A. Colic
B. Gastro-oesophageal reflux
C. Normal variant
D. Overfeeding
E. Pyloric stenosis

13. RASH AND FEVER

A 4-year-old boy presents to the emergency department with a 36-hour history of feeling generally unwell. He has a temperature of 38.1°C, and his cheeks are bright red. He also has a maculopapular blanching rash covering his limbs. There are no lesions in his mouth.

Which of the following is the most likely diagnosis?

A. Chickenpox
B. Erythema infectiosum
C. Measles
D. Meningococcal sepsis
E. Scarlet fever

14. SKIN RASH (2)

A 15-year-old female was recently started on the oral contraceptive pill. A few weeks later, she presented with a urinary tract infection that was successfully treated with trimethoprim. Now, a month later, she has developed a series of painful lesions in her mouth that are associated with multiple skin lesions over her lower limbs. The peripheral lesions are round and deep red with a central area of pallor.

Which of the following is the most likely cause of her rash?

A. Echovirus
B. *Escherichia coli*
C. Herpes simplex
D. Oral contraceptive pill
E. Sulphonamide antibiotic

15. SYNDROME RECOGNITION (2)

You are referred a 15-year-old female from primary care as the parents are worried because she is the shortest in her class. She enjoys school and is doing well. On examination, you find her height to be below the second centile and her weight to be on the fiftieth centile. She has developed some pubic hair but still has little breast tissue and no menarche. Her mother informs you that she was herself late to develop signs of puberty. You also notice slightly low set ears and a low hairline. The remainder of her examination is normal.

What is the most likely diagnosis?

A. Congenital hypothyroidism
B. Klinefelter syndrome
C. Noonan syndrome
D. Normal child
E. Turner syndrome

16. CONTRAINDICATIONS TO IMMUNIZATION

A 4-year-old boy was born prematurely and is known to have vertically acquired HIV. He is asymptomatic, and his latest CD4 count was 1250/μL. For the last 48 hours, he has had a 'cold' but no associated fever. He had an acute exacerbation of his asthma 2 months ago, which was treated with a one-week course of prednisolone 30 mg. He is known to have an allergy to eggs but this does not cause anaphylaxis. He is due his measles, mumps and rubella (MMR) booster.

Why is the MMR vaccine contraindicated in this child?

A. Egg allergy
B. HIV infection
C. Prematurity
D. Steroid treatment for asthma
E. Upper respiratory tract infection

17. FEBRILE ILLNESS (3)

A 4-year-old girl presents to the emergency department with a 7-day history of fever associated with abdominal pain. On examination, she has a widespread rash, red conjunctiva and cervical lymphadenopathy. On examining her mouth, you notice that her lips are red and cracked.

Bearing in mind the most likely underlying cause of her symptoms, which one of her features does not fulfil the diagnostic criteria?

A. Abdominal pain
B. Cervical lymphadenopathy
C. Conjunctivitis
D. Fever of at least 5 days' duration
E. Polymorphous rash

18. DIABETIC REGIMENS

A 10-year-old boy has recently been diagnosed with type 1 (insulin-dependent) diabetes. He wants to discuss the type of treatment regimen that would best suit him. He does not particularly like giving the injections but has got used to it and would like to have as tight a control as possible. However, he is very unwilling to give himself any injections while at school as he is embarrassed in front of his friends.

What treatment regimen would be best suited?

A. Continuous subcutaneous insulin infusion (insulin pump therapy)
B. Diet control alone
C. Multiple daily injection regimen with carbohydrate counting
D. Three times daily injection insulin regimen
E. Twice times daily injection insulin regimen

19. SHORTNESS OF BREATH

A 9-month-old girl presents with shortness of breath. She started having a 'runny nose' 24 hours ago, and her mother says she felt hot to touch. She now has a high-pitched cough. Examination reveals bilateral fine crepitations and an intermittent wheeze.

Which of the following organisms is most likely to be responsible?

A. Adenovirus
B. Influenza virus
C. Mycoplasma
D. Parainfluenza virus
E. Respiratory syncitial virus

20. DIAGNOSIS OF NEPHROTIC SYNDROME

A 5-year-old boy presents to the emergency department as his mum has noticed he is 'puffy around his eyes and ankles'. He is normally fit and well but has been lethargic over the last few days and has vomited on a few occasions.

Urine dipstick reveals:

Protein	3+
Leucocytes	Negative
Nitrites	Negative

A preliminary diagnosis of nephrotic syndrome is made.

Which of the following results would establish this as the correct diagnosis?

A. Blood albumin concentration 20 g/L (normal = 35–50 g/L)
B. Blood pressure 150/80
C. Blood urea concentration 9.0 mmol/L (normal = 3–7 mmol/L)
D. Microscopic haematuria
E. Weight gain >10%

21. INVESTIGATION OF DEVELOPMENTAL DELAY

A mother brings her 2-year-old son to the development clinic as he is not walking yet and does not use many words. He only says 'mama' and 'dada'. He is able to sit unsupported and commando-crawls but cannot stand or walk. He feeds himself with a spoon and fork and is able to build a tower of three bricks. On examination, he does not appear dysmorphic but has enlarged calf muscles. Chromosomal analysis is normal.

Which investigation is most likely to reveal the diagnosis?

A. Brain MRI scan
B. Creatine kinase
C. Electroencephalogram
D. Genetic testing
E. Metabolic screen

22. PAINFUL RASH

A 7-year-old boy presents with tonsillitis associated with a painful rash. He has multiple lesions over his shins. They are 1 to 5 cm in size, raised, tender and are hot to touch. He has recently been started on antibiotics for his tonsillitis.

Which of the following is the cause of the rash?

A. Epstein–Barr virus
B. Group A streptococcus
C. Reaction to erythromycin
D. Systemic lupus erythematosus
E. Tuberculosis

23. INVESTIGATION OF CHRONIC COUGH (2)

An 18-month-old girl presents with a recurrent cough, which is occasionally productive. She is small for her age. Mum reports multiple episodes of wheeze.

Which of the following is the gold standard investigation to confirm her diagnosis?

A. Chest X-ray
B. Genetic mutation analysis
C. Immune-reactive trypsin
D. Nasal potential difference
E. Sweat test

24. ANAEMIA

A 2-year-old girl is found to be anaemic. She has been growing well and drinks plenty of milk and fruit juices. Her mother feels she is well apart from looking 'slightly pale'. Examination is unremarkable.

Her full blood count reveals the following:

Hb	82 g/dL (range 95–140 g/dL)
MCV	70 fL (range 85–105 fL)
MCH	19 pg/cell (range 23–31 pg/cell)

What is the most likely cause for her anaemia?

A. β-Thalassaemia trait
B. Folate deficiency
C. Haemolytic anaemia
D. Iron deficiency
E. Lead poisoning

25. COMPLICATIONS OF UNDESCENDED TESTES

A 5-year-old boy is seen in clinic and is found to have an undescended testis on the right side. You are unable to palpate a testis either in the scrotum or the inguinal canal. An abdominal ultrasound is performed and shows a right-sided intra-abdominal testicle.

Which of the following is a reason to perform an orchidopexy?

A. Decrease the risk of direct hernias in later life
B. Decrease the risk of epididymitis
C. Decrease the risk of malignancy back to that of the normal population
D. Psychological benefit
E. Significant improvement in fertility

26. INVESTIGATION OF JAUNDICE (2)

A 6-hour-old baby is jaundiced. His mother is blood group O, rhesus D negative and her waters broke 48 hours before she delivered. The baby is breastfeeding well. On examination, the baby is clinically well.

Which of the following would you perform?

A. Bilirubin level
B. Blood culture
C. Direct antibody test
D. Full blood count
E. All of the above

27. MANAGEMENT OF ANAEMIA

An 8-year-old girl with arthritis has some routine blood tests taken by the general practitioner. She is currently on methotrexate for her arthritis. Her mother is worried she is a fussy eater and does not enjoy eating meat. On examination, she has some ulceration at the corners of her mouth.

Her full blood count reveals:

Hb	8.9 g/dL (range 9.5–14.0)
MCV	109 fL (range 85–105)

What is the best treatment for her?

A. Intramuscular vitamin B_{12}
B. Oral ferrous sulphate
C. Oral folic acid
D. Oral vitamin B_{12}
E. Multivitamin tablet

28. INVESTIGATION OF SEIZURES

A 10-year-old girl presents to the emergency department with a seizure that lasted 2 minutes before resolving on its own. Her mother described her as suddenly collapsing to the ground, going stiff and then shaking all four limbs. She was 'drowsy' for 15 to 20 minutes after the seizure. The girl has no recollection of the event. Her temperature is 36.2°C, and she was well before the event. Examination, including a full neurological assessment, is normal. Blood sugar level was 4.5 mmol/l. Electrolytes were normal.

Which investigation should next be performed?

A. 12-lead ECG
B. Electroencephalogram
C. Head MRI
D. Serum prolactin
E. None of the above

29. MANAGEMENT OF EPILEPSY

A 7-year-old girl has absence seizures requiring treatment with an anti-epileptic medication (AEM). Her mother has noticed that she has put on weight recently and wondered if this was a side effect of her epilepsy medication. She also tells you that when her daughter started her medication she started to lose some of her hair, though this has now resolved.

What medication is she on?

A. Carbamazepine
B. Gabapentin
C. Lamotrigine
D. Phenytoin
E. Sodium valproate

30. THE ACUTELY PAINFUL JOINT

A 4-year-old girl presents to the emergency department unable to weight-bear and with a 'swollen right knee'. She has a temperature of 38.3°C. On examination, she looks unwell and cannot move her right leg. Her knee is hot, red, swollen and tender. Blood tests show a raised C-reactive protein and high white cell count.

What is the advised treatment for this condition?

A. Immediate IV antibiotics, followed by joint aspiration the following day
B. Immediate IV antibiotics, continuing for 4 to 6 weeks, with no need for aspiration
C. Joint aspiration followed by IV antibiotics, continuing for 10 days
D. Joint aspiration followed by IV antibiotics, continuing for 4 to 6 weeks
E. Joint aspiration followed by high-dose oral antibiotics for 3 months

31. SURFACTANT DEFICIENCY

A 36-weeks' gestation, male infant is born by elective caesarean section because of intrauterine growth restriction. After birth, he is found to have septicaemia and respiratory distress. He requires intubation and ventilation. A chest X-ray reveals a 'ground glass appearance'. His respiratory distress is therefore attributed to surfactant deficiency.

Which of the following is *not* a risk factor for surfactant deficiency?

A. Elective caesarean section
B. Intrauterine growth restriction
C. Male gender
D. Prematurity
E. Sepsis

32. INVESTIGATION OF HAEMATURIA

A 9-year-old girl presents to the general practitioner with 'red urine'. She is complaining of some abdominal pain but is otherwise well. She has a history of recurrent urinary tract infections, and she recently had a throat infection that was treated for 3 days with oral penicillin. Examination is unremarkable.

A urine dipstick reveals:

Blood	3+
Leucocytes	Negative
Nitrites	Negative

What investigation would best reveal the cause of her haematuria?

A. Abdominal X-ray
B. Abdominal ultrasound
C. Antistreptolysin-O titre/throat swab
D. Full blood count
E. Urine for microscopy and culture

33. CAUSES OF SPEECH DELAY

A mother brings her 2½-year-old daughter to a drop-in speech and language service. Mum is concerned that her daughter only uses a handful of words. Her mother understands what her daughter is saying but other people do not. She is a bright girl who has good understanding and enjoys playing with other children. Her mother has no concerns about her hearing. On assessment, she has normal development in all the other areas and a normal examination.

What is the likely cause for her speech delay?

A. Autism
B. Expressive language disorder
C. Global developmental delay
D. Hearing loss
E. Neglect

34. FEEDING

A 6-week-old boy presents with vomiting. He is described as a hungry baby and will take 210 mL (7 oz) feeds every 4 hours. He weighs 5 kg and is gaining weight along his centile (fiftieth). After many feeds, he will effortlessly vomit into his mouth and down his clothes. He is otherwise clinically well. Examination is unremarkable.

Which of the following is the most likely cause of this baby's vomiting?

A. Abdominal colic
B. Gastro-oesophageal reflux
C. Malrotation of the gut
D. Overfeeding
E. Pyloric stenosis

35. INVESTIGATION FOLLOWING URINARY TRACT INFECTIONS

A 10-month-old baby boy presents for the second time to hospital with a urinary tract infection. He recovers quickly with a course of antibiotics. Your consultant asks you to organize follow-up for him.

What investigations does this boy need?

A. Inpatient renal ultrasound scan (USS)
B. Renal USS in 1 week
C. USS and dimercaptosuccinic acid (DMSA) as outpatient
D. USS and micturating urogram (MCUG) as outpatient
E. USS, MCUG and DMSA as outpatient

36. MANAGEMENT OF CHRONIC ASTHMA

A 7-year-old boy has a chronic cough and wheeze. He had a good response to a β-agonist, demonstrated by his peak expiratory flow rate (PEFR). He was initially managed with a short-acting β-agonist, but his symptoms persisted and a regular inhaled steroid was added (400 µg/day).

If no improvement is seen, which of the following would be the next step in the management?

A. Add an inhaled long-acting β-agonist
B. Add an oral leukotriene receptor antagonist
C. Increase the inhaled steroid dose
D. Increase the short-acting β-agonist dose
E. Start daily oral steroids

37. NEURAL TUBE DEFECTS

You review a 2-year-old boy in clinic. He had a neural tube defect when he was born, which was operated on soon after birth. His mother describes it as a sac of jelly at the base of his spine. On examination today, he has a full range of movement of both his arms and legs and his power, tone and reflexes appear normal. He is still in nappies, but his mother is beginning to toilet train.

What was the neural tube lesion likely to be?

A. Anencephaly
B. Encephalocele
C. Meningocele
D. Myelomeningocele
E. Spinal bifida occulta

38. RISK FACTORS FOR HIP DISEASE

A 7-year-old boy with a history of hypothyroidism presents with a limp. Mum has noticed the limp over the last few weeks, and it seems to come and go. He is also complaining of pain in his left leg. On examination, he has limited range of movement of the left hip. His height and weight are both on the seventy-fifth centile.

This boy is more likely to have Perthes disease rather than a slipped capital femoral epiphysis because:

A. He is a boy
B. He has hypothyroidism
C. He is obese
D. He is tall
E. He is 7 years old

39. CAUSES OF CEREBRAL PALSY

A 2-year-old boy is known to have quadriplegic cerebral palsy. He was born at 36 weeks' gestation and required five inflation breaths at birth as he was not breathing. He was briefly admitted to the special care baby unit to establish his feeds, and he required a day of phototherapy for jaundice but was discharged at 7 days of life. At 9 months of age, he suffered from meningitis and was admitted to the paediatric intensive care (PICU) and ventilated for 4 days. The only other history of note was that he fell off his parent's bed at the age of 4 months and was observed in hospital for a few hours.

What is the most likely cause of his cerebral palsy?

A. Head injury
B. Hypoxic insult
C. Kernicterus
D. Meningitis
E. Prematurity

40. INVESTIGATION OF CONSTIPATION

A 3-year-old boy presents with a history of constipation since the age of 6 months. His general practitioner is worried he has Hirschsprung disease and refers him to you. His mother describes his stools as being normal until she started weaning him at the age of 6 months. Since then he has never passed a proper stool and appears in pain and strains. He passes small amounts of 'rabbit poo droppings' and is still in nappies as he soils continually. On examination, he has no palpable abdominal masses and his lower limb reflexes are normal. Inspection of his anus is normal.

Which of the following investigations is required?

A. Abdominal X-ray
B. Examination under anaesthesia
C. Thyroid function tests
D. Rectal biopsy
E. No investigation required

41. HIP PAIN

A mother brings her 5-year-old son to the emergency department as he is refusing to walk and is complaining his right hip hurts. There is no history of trauma; the child is fit and well except for a mild cold he had a week ago. On examination, he appears well with a temperature of 36.8°C. He has limited movement of his left leg and appears in pain on passive movement.

Which one investigation will confirm the most likely diagnosis?

A. Full blood count
B. Hip MRI
C. Hip ultrasound
D. Hip X-ray
E. None of the above

42. INVESTIGATION OF ENURESIS

An 8-year-old girl presents to the general practitioner with a history of bedwetting. She is wetting the bed nearly every night, and there has never been a period when she has been dry at night. She does not wet during the day, and there is no history of constipation. On examination, you find no anomalies.

Which investigation needs to be performed before starting treatment?

A. 24-hour blood pressure monitoring
B. Renal ultrasound
C. Urea and electrolytes
D. Urinalysis
E. None of the above

43. MANAGEMENT OF DIARRHOEA

A 10-month-old boy presents with a 4-day history of watery, sweet-smelling diarrhoea. He had been vomiting but this had now settled, though he is still not eating anything. His mother is worried he is dehydrated and, on assessment, you find him to have a normal capillary refill time but moderate dehydration.

What is the best treatment for this child?

A. Intravenous bolus of saline, followed by oral rehydration therapy
B. Rehydration with half-strength formula milk
C. Rehydration with intravenous dextrose 5% and saline 0.45%
D. Rehydration with oral rehydration therapy alone
E. Rehydration with oral rehydration therapy and erythromycin

44. ABDOMINAL PAIN IN A CHILD (2)

An 8-year-old boy presents with abdominal pain in the 'lower right part of his tummy'. He has had a cold for the last 3 days. On examination, he is slightly tender in his right iliac fossa but he has no guarding or signs of peritonism. His temperature is 37.9°C. A urine dipstick reveals: leucocytes 1+, nitrites negative, blood negative.

What is the most likely cause of his abdominal pain?

A. Appendicitis
B. Constipation
C. Mesenteric adenitis
D. Pneumonia
E. Urinary tract infection

45. CYANOSIS

You are called to see a 12-hour-old baby. On examination, the baby is jittery, lethargic and has very blue peripheries. You are concerned about sepsis and so perform a blood culture. Blood tests show haemoglobin 17 g/dL, haematocrit 0.69 and C-reactive protein <5 mg/L. A chest X-ray is normal, as is a nitrogen washout test.

What is the most likely cause of this baby's clinical features?

A. Congenital pneumonia
B. Polycythaemia
C. Sepsis
D. Tetralogy of Fallot
E. Transposition of the great vessels

46. MANAGEMENT OF DEHYDRATION

A 7-year-old boy presents to your acute unit. He is known to have insulin-dependent diabetes. He is acutely unwell with polyuria, abdominal pain, vomiting and confusion. He is clinically dehydrated and has lost more than 5% of his body weight.

How quickly would you correct his dehydration?

A. 8 hours
B. 12 hours
C. 24 hours
D. 36 hours
E. 48 hours

47. THE VOMITING INFANT (2)

A 1-year-old girl presents with fevers and vomiting for 2 days. She has also passed two loose stools today. She is more lethargic than normal and has not been feeding well. On examination, she is well perfused and alert. You are unable to find any focus of her fever on examination, although there appears to be some discomfort when you palpate her lower abdomen.

Urine dipstick reveals:

Leucocytes	1+
Nitrites	Positive
Ketones	Negative

What is the most likely cause for this child's vomiting?

A. Diabetic ketoacidosis
B. Gastroenteritis
C. Meningitis
D. Tonsillitis
E. Urinary tract infection

48. ARTERIAL BLOOD GASES (2)

You see a 6-week-old boy with a short history of projectile vomiting and hunger. The junior paediatric doctor takes a venous blood sample while inserting a cannula. A venous blood gas revealed the following:

pH	7.48
PaCO$_2$	5.8 kPa
Base excess	+5
PaO$_2$	3.8 kPa

Normal reference ranges for arterial blood gases are:

pH	7.36–7.44
PaCO$_2$	4.7–6.0 kPa, 35–45 mmHg
Base excess	±2
PaO$_2$	>10.6 kPa, >80 mmHg (in air)

Which of the following is your interpretation of this blood gas?

A. Hypoxia
B. Metabolic alkalosis (uncompensated)
C. Metabolic alkalosis with partial respiratory compensation
D. Respiratory alkalosis (uncompensated)
E. Respiratory alkalosis with partial metabolic compensation

49. INVESTIGATION OF THE UNWELL NEONATE

You are urgently paged to the postnatal ward. A newborn baby has just stopped breathing for a minute and 'had a fit' from which he has now recovered. He is 12 hours old and is being breastfed.

Which of the following is the most important investigation to perform at this point?

A. Blood culture
B. Blood gas
C. Blood sugar level
D. C-reactive protein
E. Lumbar puncture

50. DEVELOPMENTAL MILESTONES (2)

You see a boy in clinic and are asked to perform a developmental assessment. He can walk well and even runs but is not able to kick a ball. He can create a tower of three blocks and scribbles, though he cannot copy a straight line. He uses nearly 10 words but is not putting them together. He is able to feed himself with a spoon but is not able to use a fork. His mother tells you he is always copying her when she does the housework.

What is his developmental age?

A. 12 months
B. 15 months
C. 18 months
D. 2 years
E. 2½ years

Practice Paper 4: Answers

1. GLASGOW COMA SCALE

B – 11

The Glasgow Coma Scale (GCS) is a useful tool for objectively recording the conscious state of a patient, both as an initial and continuing assessment. The maximum score is 15, which implies full consciousness, and the minimum score is 3, which implies deep unconsciousness. The scale comprises three tests: eye, verbal and motor (EVM) responses. It is the best response to each of these categories that is used in the score.

In this case, the patient scores 3 for eyes as she opens them to speech; 3 for verbal as she is only using inappropriate words and 5 for motor as she localizes to pain.

The AVPU (alert, voice, pain, unresponsive) scale is often used in children to assess consciousness quickly. This reports the best level of consciousness of the child.

	Glasgow Coma Scale		
	Eyes	**Verbal**	**Motor**
1	Does not open eyes	Makes no sounds	Makes no movements
2	Opens eyes to pain	Makes incomprehensible sounds	Extensor (decerebrate) posturing to pain
3	Opens eyes to speech	Says inappropriate words	Flexor (decorticate) posturing to pain
4	Opens eyes spontaneously	Converses but is disoriented	Withdrawal movement to pain
5	×	Oriented, converses normally	Localizing movement to pain
6	×	×	Follows commands

The Paediatric Glasgow Coma Scale is a modified version of the GCS used in infants.

	Paediatric Glasgow Coma Scale		
	Eyes	**Verbal**	**Motor**
1	Does not open eyes	Makes no sounds	Makes no movements
2	Opens eyes to pain	Infant moans to pain	Extensor (decerebrate) posturing to pain

Continued

Paediatric Glasgow Coma Scale			
	Eyes	**Verbal**	**Motor**
3	Opens eyes to speech	Infant cries to pain	Flexor (decorticate) posturing to pain
4	Opens eyes spontaneously	Infant is irritable and continually cries	Infant withdraws from pain
5	×	Infant coos or babbles	Infant withdraws from touch
6	×	×	Infant moves spontaneously or purposely

2. DIAGNOSIS OF URINARY TRACT INFECTION

D – Leucocytes 2+, nitrites positive

All children with a non-specific fever should have a urine sample taken. The aim of urine collection is to obtain a good quality sample from which the diagnosis of urinary tract infection (UTI) can be confidently confirmed or excluded. A clean catch is the best method and is usually always possible but requires patience on the parents' behalf. Non-invasive collection methods include a collection bag that goes over the penis or vulval area. However, these are associated with a significant risk of contamination leading to a misleading diagnosis and/or inappropriate treatment. Cotton wool balls, gauze and sanitary towels should not be used to obtain urine samples. Where none of these are possible, a suprapubic aspiration can be performed.

Where possible, an urgent microscopy and culture should be performed and, depending on the result, action can be taken as appropriate. All children less than 3 years of age should have a microscopy and culture performed. Pyuria is the production of urine that contains white cells; these are visible on microscopy.

Microscopy results	Pyuria positive	Pyuria negative
Bacteriuria positive	The infant or child should be regarded as having UTI	The infant or child should be regarded as having UTI
Bacteriuria negative	Antibiotic treatment should be started *only if clinically diagnosed as having UTI*	The infant or child should be regarded as *not* having UTI

If urgent microscopy is not available, dipstick testing can be used to make a provisional diagnosis while awaiting formal culture. Urine dipsticks measure pH, specific gravity, glucose, ketones, blood, leucocytes and nitrites. Nitrites (not nitrates) are produced by many bacteria and indicate a urine infection. Leucocytes (suggesting pyuria) are also indicative of infection. Following is a table of how to interpret the leucocyte and nitrite results.

Leucocytes and nitrite both positive	The child should be regarded as having UTI and antibiotic treatment should be started. A sample should be sent for culture.
Leucocytes negative and nitrite positive	This child is likely to have a UTI and antibiotic treatment should be started if the urine test was carried out on a fresh sample of urine. A sample should be sent for culture for confirmation.
Leucocytes positive and nitrite negative	Antibiotic treatment for UTI should not be started, unless obvious urinary symptoms. A sample should be sent for microscopy and culture. Leucocytes can be indicative of an infection outside the urinary tract.
Leucocytes and nitrite are negative	The child should not be regarded as having UTI and antibiotic treatment should not be started.

If a child is seriously unwell, treatment should not be delayed while waiting for a sample or for a result.

FURTHER READING

1. National Collaborating Centre for Women's and Children's Health. *Urinary Tract Infection in Children*. NICE Clinical Guideline 54. London: NICE, 2007. Available at: www.nice.org.uk:80/nicemedia/pdf/CG54NICEguideline.pdf

3. HEPATITIS

A – Hepatitis A

Hepatitis A accounts for more than half of all cases of viral hepatitis in children. It is transmitted via the faecal–oral route and often presents as a bout of gastroenteritis. Hepatitis E is also transmitted via the faecal–oral route but is endemic only in certain areas.

Viral hepatitis presents as follows: there is a preicteric phase, characterized by headache, anorexia, malaise, abdominal discomfort, nausea and vomiting; this is followed by an icteric phase (jaundice and tender hepatomegaly).

The treatment of hepatitis A is supportive, with rest and hydration. Hospitalization may be required if there is severe vomiting and dehydration. Deranged liver function (abnormal clotting) and hepatic encephalopathy would also be an indication for admission.

Viral hepatitis summary*

	Hepatitis A virus	Hepatitis B virus	Hepatitis C virus	Hepatitis D virus	Hepatitis E virus
Virus	RNA	DNA	RNA	RNA	RNA
Transmission	Faecal–oral	Contact with infectious blood, semen and other body fluids	Contact with blood of an infected person	Transfusion, sexual, inoculation, perinatal	Faecal–oral

Continued

	Hepatitis A virus	Hepatitis B virus	Hepatitis C virus	Hepatitis D virus	Hepatitis E virus
Incubation period	15–30 days (average 28)	60–180 days (average 120)	30–60 days (average 45)	Co-infection with hepatitis B	35–60 days
Fulminant liver failure	Rarely	<1% unless hepatitis D	Uncommon	2%–20%	20%
Increased risk of hepatocellular carcinoma?	No	Yes	Yes	No	No
Prevention	Good hygiene	Transfusion safety, safe sex education, needle exchange	Transfusion safety, needle exchange	Transfusion safety, safe sex education, needle exchange	Good hygiene

*Adapted from *Nelson Essentials of Paediatrics*. Oxford: Elsevier, 2006.

FURTHER READING

1. Centers for Disease Control and Prevention. ABCs of hepatitis. Available at: http://www.cdc.gov/hepatitis/Resources/Professionals/PDFs/ABCTable.pdf

4. HAEMOGLOBINOPATHIES

C – β-Thalassaemia trait

Microcytic, hypochromic anaemia is seen in both thalassaemias and iron deficiency anaemia. 'Haemoglobinopathies' is the collective name for a group of blood disorders where there is an abnormality in haemoglobin synthesis. It includes the thalassaemias as well as sickle cell anaemia. The haemoglobinopathies range from asymptomatic disease to severe and even fatal forms. To understand thalassaemia, it is useful to know the normal structure of haemoglobin.

Normal haemoglobin is composed of a tetramer of globin chains (two α-globin and two non-α-globin chains, HbA – $\alpha^2\beta^2$). In the fetus, the two α chains pair up with two γ chains to produce fetal haemoglobin (HbF). In adults, the majority of the haemoglobin is HbA (two α chains and two β chains). About 2% of adult haemoglobin is HbA_2 (two α chains and two δ chains). About 1% of adult haemoglobin is in the fetal form (HbF).

β-Thalassaemia major is an autosomal recessive disorder in which there is a complete lack of production of the β-globin chain. It occurs mainly in Mediterranean and Middle Eastern families and is due to a point mutation on chromosome 11. Because patients with β-thalassaemia major have mutations on both alleles and cannot synthesize any β-globin, they cannot produce functioning adult haemoglobin (HbA – $\alpha^2\beta^2$). This condition typically presents within the first year of life when the production of fetal haemoglobin (HbF – $\alpha^2\gamma^2$) begins to fall. Affected children become generally unwell and fail to thrive secondary to a severe microcytic anaemia.

Ferritin levels are normal because there is no iron deficiency. A compensatory increase in the synthesis of HbF and haemoglobin A_2 (HbA$_2$ – $\alpha^2\delta^2$) occurs, which can be detected on serum electrophoresis. Clinical features include failure to thrive, lethargy, pallor and jaundice. On examination, there is often hepatosplenomegaly (secondary to extramedullary haematopoiesis) with bossing of the skull and long bone deformity (due to excessive intramedullary haematopoiesis). The treatment of β-thalassaemia major is with regular blood transfusions, aiming to maintain haemoglobin levels high enough to reduce extramedullary production. Regular iron chelation therapy (with desferrioxamine) is required to prevent iron overload and deposition in vital organs such as the heart, liver and endocrine glands. If untreated, death is inevitable in the first years of life. Allogenic bone marrow transplant is a treatment option but carries a high risk.

β-Thalassaemia minor (also known as β-thalassaemia trait) describes people who are heterozygous for the β-chain chromosomal mutation. Affected persons have only a mild hypochromic, microcytic anaemia and are usually asymptomatic. Again iron and ferritin levels are normal, and Hb electrophoresis shows an elevated HbA$_2$ and HbF, as in this case.

α-Thalassaemia is common in Southeast Asia. There are four α genes and therefore four variants of α-thalassaemia.

- α-Thalassaemia minima (one gene corruption): asymptomatic, haemoglobin electrophoresis pattern is normal.
- α-Thalassaemia minor (two corruptions): this resembles mild β-thalassemia trait. Mild hypochromic anaemia is present. Feritin and iron are normal. Haemoglobin electrophoresis pattern is normal. In contrast to patients with β-thalassemia, elevation of HbA$_2$ is not seen in the α-thalassemias; slight elevations of HbF have been reported.
- Haemoglobin H (HbH) disease (three corruptions): HbH is a β-chain tetramer that is functionally useless. Haemoglobin electrophoresis pattern shows 5% to 30% HbH. Treatment options are as for β-thalassaemia.
- α-Thalassaemia major (four corruptions): leading to tetramers of fetal γ-chains (Hb Barts), which cannot carry oxygen and results in stillbirth as it is incompatible with life.

Thalassaemia, from Greek *thalassa* = sea + *haima* = blood. It is so-called as the disease is especially prevalent in 'countries by the sea' (i.e. the Mediterranean).

5. MANAGEMENT OF SICKLE CELL ANAEMIA

E – Pain relief including opioids

This boy is presenting with a painful sickle cell crisis and requires analgesia immediately. Sickle cell disease is a homozygous inheritance of faulty β-globin genes most commonly found in African, Mediterranean and Middle Eastern communities. A single amino acid substitution (glutamine → valine) results in abnormal haemoglobin (HbS). When exposed to low oxygen tensions or acidaemia, highly structured polymers become brittle and distorted, leading to sickling (crescentic shape) of the red cells. This results in red cells that are prematurely destroyed in the spleen (the mean lifespan of the red cell is reduced from 120 to 10–12 days). Sickled cells can also become trapped in the microcirculation, leading to thrombosis and ischaemia. HbS can be detected on haemoglobin electrophoresis.

Children develop a progressive anaemia from about 3 months of age. Splenic infarction can lead to asplenia and an increased risk of infections. Frontal bossing (prominent forehead and supraorbital ridges) may be seen secondary to excess erythropoiesis in the marrow of atypical sites. Most affected children experience 'crises' throughout their life varying in frequency and severity.

Types of sickle crisis include:

- Vaso-occlusive (swelling/pain in fingers or toes due to vaso-occlusion – 'dactylitis')
- Bone crisis (acute pain in long bones)
- Splenic sequestration (acute painful enlargement of the spleen)
- Chest (respiratory symptoms with chest X-ray changes)
- Haemolytic (accelerated anaemia due to increased haemolysis)
- Aplastic (worsening of anaemia due to reduced erythropoiesis, triggered by parvovirus B19 infection)

These crises are usually precipitated by infection, acidosis, dehydration, alcohol/drugs, hypothermia, hypoxia, pregnancy or stress.

Symptomatic management during a crisis includes removing the precipitate stress, i.e. treat hypothermia, hypoxia (with oxygen) or infection. Adequate analgesia is essential; a combination of non-opioids and opioids is often needed. Analgesia should be started within 30 minutes of arrival in hospital, and the pain should be controlled within 60 minutes of starting analgesia.

Maintaining hydration is important. A fluid balance chart should be started in all these patients, and they should be encouraged to take fluids orally. If the patient is unable to drink sufficient amounts or is vomiting, then intravenous or nasogastric fluids are necessary. Nasogastric fluids can be helpful as they avoid intravenous cannulation, which can pose a risk of venous thrombosis and ulceration. If infection is a possibility, broad-spectrum antibiotics are started.

Blood transfusions are given when the haemoglobin is low (usually not until <6.0 g/dL as affected children have usually accommodated to relatively low haemoglobin levels). There is a high risk of iron overload in children who are given frequent blood transfusions, and exchange transfusion may be required to remove the sickled red cells. Children presenting with acute chest syndrome (sickle cell crisis in the lung) need to be treated with adequate ventilation, antibiotics and blood transfusions depending on the severity. Acute chest syndrome presents with fever, cough, sputum, dyspnoea and hypoxia, and new infiltrates are seen on chest X-ray.

There are a number of preventative measures used in children with sickle cell disease. These include adequate nutrition and fluid intake, avoidance of the cold and prompt treatment of infections. Prophylactic penicillin and extra immunizations, including influenza and an extra pneumococcal vaccine, are given to all children with sickle cell disease. Hydroxycarbamide (previously known as hydroxyurea) is used to reduce the frequency of crises. Guidelines for the management of sickle cell crises have been published by the British Society of Haematologists (www.bcshguidelines.com).*

6. HYPERACTIVITY DISORDER

D – There must be a significantly impaired social or academic development

Attention deficit hyperactivity disorder (ADHD) usually presents before the age of 7 and is present in approximately 1% of school-aged children. Regarding the options given: the behaviour must be present for at least 6 months, the behaviour is inconsistent with the child's developmental age, the symptoms must occur in more than one setting (i.e. pervasive) and there can be no other explanation for the symptoms. Therefore, the right option here is that there is a significant impairment of social and/or academic skills.

Boys are far more likely to be affected by ADHD. The symptoms have a significant impact on a child's development, including social, emotional and cognitive functioning. These symptoms cause significant morbidity and dysfunction for the child, their family and their peer group.

The three core symptoms of ADHD comprise developmentally inappropriate levels of:

- Inattention (difficulty in concentrating)
- Hyperactivity (disorganized, excessive levels of activity)
- Impulsive behaviour

It is possible to have just one of these features without the others (e.g. marked hyperactivity without inattention or impulsive behaviour).

In addition to the above core symptoms, the following criteria should be fulfilled:

- The behaviour should have persisted for at least 6 months
- The behaviour should be inconsistent with the child's developmental age
- There must be clinically significant impairment in social or academic development
- The symptoms should occur in more than one setting
- There should be no other explanation for the symptoms (e.g. psychiatric illness)

---

* Rees D. Guidelines for the management of the acute painful crisis in sickle cell disease. *Br J Haematol* 2003;120:744–752.

The diagnosis is difficult and requires gathering information from all those involved in the child's life.

Treatment packages are tailored to the child's needs. These include psychosocial intervention (e.g. family-based psychosocial intervention of a behavioural type for the treatment of co-morbid behavioural problems), educational support and social services support. If pharmacological intervention is required to manage behavioural symptoms, psychostimulants (e.g. methylphenidate) are the first-line treatment, followed by tricyclic antidepressants.

7. MICROORGANISMS

B – *Escherichia coli*

The presence of organisms on microscopy confirms a urinary tract infection. Medically important bacteria can be classified depending on their morphology and staining reactions. In clinical life, a microbiologist will usually be at hand to type organisms; however, organism classification comes up in exams. There is no easy way to overcome this; you just have to learn them. For more information, see *Lecture Notes on Medical Microbiology.**

Gram-positive cocci

| Staphylococcus | → | *S. aureus, S. epidermidis* |
| Streptococcus | → | *S. pneumoniae, S. pyogenes* |

Gram-positive bacilli

Bacillus	→	*B. anthracis, B. cereus*
Clostridium	→	*C. difficile, C. tetani, C. perfringens*
Corynebacterium	→	*C. diphtheriae*
Listeria	→	*L. monocytogenes*

Gram-negative dipplococci

| Niesseria | → | *N. meningitidis, N. gonorrhoeae* |

Gram-negative bacilli

Escherichia	→	*E. coli*
Klebsiella	→	*K. pneumoniae*
Proteus	→	*P. mirabilis*
Salmonella	→	*S. typhi*
Shigella	→	*S. sonnei*
Yersinia	→	*Y. enterocolitica, Y. pestis*
Pseudomonas	→	*P. aeruginosa*
Bordatella	→	*B. pertussis*
Haemophilus	→	*H. influenzae*
Legionella	→	*L. pneumophila*

---

* Elliott TS, Hastings M, Desselberger O. *Lecture Notes on Medical Microbiology*. 3rd ed. Oxford: Wiley-Blackwell, 2007.

Gram-negative comma-shaped/curved bacteria

Vibrio	→	*V. cholerae*
Campylobacter	→	*C. jejuni*
Helicobacter	→	*H. pylori*

Spiral-shaped bacteria

Treponema	→	*T. pallidum*
Borrelia	→	*B. burgdorferi*

Acid-fast bacteria

Mycobacterium	→	*M. tuberculosis*

Cell-wall-deficient bacteria

Mycoplasma	→	*M. pneumoniae*

8. ELECTROLYTE DISTURBANCE (2)

C – Diabetes insipidus

This girl most likely has central diabetes insipidus (DI) secondary to her recent episode of meningitis. Conn syndrome is primary aldosteronism caused by an adrenal aldosteronoma (aldosterone-secreting benign adrenal neoplasm). There are other causes of primary hyperaldosteronism than Conn. Her potassium and pH are normal, making this less likely. In primary hyperaldosteronism, there would be hypokalaemia and a metabolic alkalosis. Chronic renal failure is possible following an episode of meningococcal septicaemia (not meningitis) due to an insult to the kidneys. If this were the case, the serum creatinine levels would be raised. Diabetes mellitus would cause a high blood sugar level. Syndrome of inappropriate ADH secretion (SIADH) can occur during acute meningitis and is characterized by reduced urine output and hyponatraemia (low sodium).

The differential diagnosis of polyuria and polydipsia includes diabetes mellitus, chronic renal failure, DI (central or nephrogenic) and psychogenic polydipsia.

DI is characterized by the excretion of excessive quantities of dilute urine with thirst and is related to the dysfunction of antidiuretic hormone (ADH). ADH is secreted by the posterior pituitary gland and increases water reabsorption in the kidney. There are two types of DI: cranial DI (which is due to a lack of ADH secretion from the pituitary) and nephrogenic DI (which results from a lack of response of the kidneys to circulating ADH). Causes of cranial DI include infections (this case), head injury, surgery, sarcoidosis and the DIDMOAD syndrome (characterized by Diabetes Insipidus, Diabetes Mellitus, Optic Atrophy and Deafness). Nephrogenic DI can be due to metabolic abnormalities (hypokalaemia, hypercalcaemia), drugs (lithium, demeclocycline), genetic defects and heavy metal poisoning.

Patients with DI may pass up to 20 L of water in a day. In this case, the diagnosis is clinically likely. The diagnosis is confirmed using the water deprivation test. The patient is deprived of water, and the urine and plasma osmolalities are measured every 2 hours. If there is a raised plasma osmolality (>300 mOsm/kg) in the presence of urine that is not maximally concentrated (i.e. <660 mOsm/kg), then the patient has DI. At this point in the test, the patient is given an intramuscular dose of desmopressin (a synthetic analogue of ADH). If the patient now starts concentrating their urine, then they have cranial DI. If the urine osmolality remains <660 mOsm/kg, then nephrogenic DI is confirmed. The treatment of cranial DI is with desmopressin. Nephrogenic DI is improved by thiazide diuretics.

Diabetes insipidus, from Greek *diabainein* = to siphon + Latin *in* = not + *sapere* = to taste; in other words, to pass tasteless urine.

9. LUMBAR PUNCTURE

E – Viral meningitis

Cause	Appearance of fluid	White cell count/mm³	Protein	Glucose
Normal	Clear	0–5	0.2–0.4 g/dL	>50% of blood sugar
Bacterial	Turbid	>5 (neutrophils)	Raised	<50% of blood sugar
Viral	Clear	>5 (lymphocytes)	Low	Normal
TB meningitis	Clear/viscous	Very high number of lymphocytes	Very high	Very low

In this case, the emergency doctor was right to perform a septic screen and start antibiotics. The lumbar puncture (LP) result is suggestive of viral meningitis. However, the microscopy only gives a diagnostic prediction, and antibiotics should continue until the blood culture and cerebrospinal fluid (CSF) culture return as negative. Early bacterial meningitis can present initially with lymphocytes in the CSF; however, neutrophils are more common.

There are several contraindications to performing an LP. Antibiotics should never be delayed while waiting to perform an LP as the CSF result can still be interpreted after antibiotics have been commenced.

Contraindications to LP include:

- Airway compromise
- Respiratory instability
- Cardiovascular instability
- Coagulopathy (clinically evident with non-blanching rashes or bleeding)

- Clinical signs of raised intracranial pressure (high blood pressure, bradycardia)
- Focal neurological signs
- Soft tissue infection at intended puncture site

10. STRIDOR

B – Laryngotracheobronchitis

Infectious croup (also known as laryngotracheobronchitis) now accounts for the vast majority of laryngotracheal infections. Parainfluenza virus is the most common causative organism. It occurs most commonly between 6 and 36 months of age. Croup presents over a period of days with coryzal symptoms followed by a severe cough and stridor. Affected children are unwell and usually have a low-grade fever. The stridor is harsh, and it is unusual for children with croup to drool or not be able to drink (unlike epiglottitis).

Epiglottitis is now rare due to the introduction of the HiB (*Haemophilus influenza* type B) vaccine; however, you should always be aware of it. Never examine the tonsils of a child who has a stridor as it could potentially exacerbate airway obstruction. Epiglottitis has an acute onset with no preceding coryza. The child looks septic and has a high-grade fever (>38.5°C). Children with epiglottitis have a very quiet cough and quiet stridor. They often drool excessively due to the pain of swallowing (odynophagia). Laryngomalacia, where the cartilage of the upper larynx is too soft and collapses during inspiration causing partial airway obstruction, is a common cause of stridor that may appear at birth but most commonly appears at 2 to 4 weeks of life. Symptoms are often worse when the child is supine or agitated. The stridor usually resolves in the first year of life without intervention. Children with an upper respiratory tract infection (URTI) such as pharyngitis present with cough, coryza and fever. It should not independently cause a stridor or respiratory distress. Subglottic stenosis can be congenital or acquired and presents with a stridor in an otherwise well infant.

The Westley croup score is the most widely acknowledged system for assessing the severity of laryngotracheobronchitis (croup) and the effectiveness of therapy:

- **Inspiratory stridor**
  - None   0 points
  - Upon agitation   1 point
  - At rest   2 points
- **Recession (sternal, subcostal, intercostal)**
  - Mild   1 point
  - Moderate   2 points
  - Severe   3 points

- **Air entry**
  - Normal   0 points
  - Mild decrease   1 point
  - Marked decrease 2 points
- **Cyanosis**
  - None   0 points
  - Upon agitation 4 points
  - At rest   5 points
- **Level of consciousness**
  - Normal   0 points
  - Depressed   5 points

Score

Mild disease	<3
Moderate disease	3–6
Severe disease	>6

11. AUTISM SPECTRUM DISORDER

D – Presents before the age of 3 years

Clinical manifestations of autism spectrum disorder (ASD) should be present by 3 years of age. If the delays occur later than this, then a different developmental disorder should be considered.

The following are true regarding ASD:

- It affects boys more commonly than girls.
- There is an increased risk of ASD in siblings.
- The aetiology is unknown.
- Language skills and IQ are the best predictors of long-term function.

The criteria for the diagnosis of ASD are based on a triad of impairments:

1. Social
   - Impaired, deviant and delayed or atypical social development, especially interpersonal development
2. Language and communication
   - Impaired and deviant language and communication, verbal and nonverbal
   - Impairment in pragmatic aspects of language
3. Thought and behaviour
   - Rigidity of thought and behaviour and impoverished social imagination
   - Ritualistic behaviour, reliance on routines, impairment of imaginative play

Management is tailored to each child. Preschool intervention within the home environment/nursery is possible if the diagnosis is made early. Schooling varies; many will attend mainstream school with support and others require support through a special unit. Schooling often requires a highly structured environment to minimize disruption. Speech and language therapy (SALT) assessment and input is also required to aid communication skills. ASD not only affects the child but all members of the family, so adequate social support including respite care is important.

12. VOMITING IN A BABY

B – Gastro-oesophageal reflux

Gastro-oesophageal reflux (GOR) is extremely common in infants, partly as their lower oesophageal sphincter is not competent. Infants with reflux often present with difficulty feeding. They can appear to be in pain (arching their back and crying) during or soon after a feed. While parents may describe the vomiting in GOR as 'projectile', it is technically regurgitation as the stomach contents are emptied effortlessly. An exact description from parents or observation of the vomiting is helpful in the diagnosis. More severe symptoms of GOR include apnoeic episodes, aspiration, failure to thrive and a chronic cough or wheeze.

GOR is a clinical diagnosis, and it is rare that investigations are required. In severe cases, a pH study may be performed – measuring the lower oesophageal pH over a 24-hour period. A pH <4 for more than 4 hours is indicative of reflux. If the history is strongly suggestive of reflux, a trial of treatment is undertaken without any investigation. GOR often resolves spontaneously without therapy, especially within the first year of life as the infant's sphincter matures and the infant spends more time upright. Simple measures such as positioning the baby upright after feeding and thickening feeds are the first interventions.

There is still not a strong consensus on whether medical treatments actually benefit infants with GOR. Medical options in GOR include:

- Antacids (e.g. Gaviscon)
- H$_2$-receptor antagonists (e.g. ranitidine)
- Protein pump inhibitors (e.g. omeprazole)
- Gastric motility agents (e.g. erythromycin or domperidone)

In severe cases, a Nissen fundoplication is performed (where the fundus of stomach is wrapped around the lower oesophagus).

Infants should receive, on average, 150 to 180 mL/kg/day of milk. Infants who are fed considerably more than this (overfeeding) can often vomit after feeds. Babies with pyloric stenosis will vomit after every feed but are usually good feeders (unlike in this case) and want more milk once they have vomited. Colic is not a diagnosis but rather a description of a fussy baby. It is defined as >3 hours total crying, for >3 days in any week for >3 weeks. The crying usually occurs in the evenings, without any identifiable cause. During these episodes, an otherwise healthy infant aged 2 weeks to 4 months is difficult to console, stiffens, draws up their legs and passes flatus. Colic is not usually associated with vomiting. It is important to understand that medical causes (e.g. GOR or cow's milk protein allergy) should be ruled out before describing a baby as 'colicky'.

Rudolf Nissen, German surgeon (1896–1981).

13. RASH AND FEVER

B – *Erythema infectiosum*

Erythema infectiosum (also known as Fifth disease or slapped cheek syndrome):

- *Organism:* erythrovirus (parvovirus B19)
- Incubation period: 6 to 14 days
- *Main features:* initially presents with appearance of slapped cheeks followed by maculopapular rash on limbs, malaise and fever
- *Complications:* arthralgia, aplastic anaemia
- *Investigation findings:* full blood count to rule out aplastic crisis if clinically anaemic

Varicella (also known as chickenpox):

- *Organism:* varicella zoster
- *Incubation period:* 10 to 21 days (average 14–16 days)
- *Main features:* rash on trunk and scalp made up of vesicles and pustules. The onset of fever coincides with the pustular phase of the rash.
- *Complications:* encephalitis (presenting as ataxia), pneumonitis and conjunctival lesions. If infection occurs with damaged skin (e.g. eczema), then the risk of serious illness is much higher.

Measles

- *Organism:* measles virus
- Incubation period: 1 to 12 days
- *Main features:* miserable child, fever, coryza, cough, conjunctivitis, macular or maculopapular rash starting on the face working down to the trunk. Koplik's spots (white pin heads) are found in the mouth. The fever and coryza precede the rash by approximately 4 days.
- *Complications:* pneumonia, otitis media and encephalitis

Meningococcal sepsis

- *Meningococcal disease:* 25% septicaemia alone, 60% septicaemia + meningitis, 15% meningitis alone
- Organism: *Neisseria meningitidis* (Gram-negative diplococcus)
- Incubation period: 2 to 10 days
- *Main features:* mild non-specific symptoms followed by shock, fever and a widespread macular rash that becomes purpuric (non-blanching)
- *Complications:* brain damage, loss of digits and limbs, deafness, blindness and death

- *Investigation findings:* N. meningitidis can be grown from pharyngeal swabs, blood cultures, aspirate of skin lesions or cerebrospinal fluid. Diagnosis is increasingly relying on polymerase chain reaction (PCR).

Scarlet fever

- *Organism:* group A β-haemolytic streptococcus (e.g. *Streptococcus pyogenes*)
- Incubation period: 1 to 7 days
- *Main features:* tonsillitis, erythematous rash predominantly on the trunk and a sore coated tongue (strawberry tongue), desquamation (peeling) of skin of palms and soles (towards end of the illness)
- *Complications:* otitis media, rheumatic fever, acute nephritis
- *Investigation findings:* raised antistreptolysin-O titres, group A streptococcus on throat swab

Fifth disease is so-called because it is the fifth of the classical childhood exanthema (rashes):

- First disease: measles
- Second disease: scarlet fever
- Third disease: rubella
- Fourth disease: no longer accepted as a medical disorder
- Fifth disease: erythema infectiousum
- Sixth disease: roseola infantum (human herpes virus 6 and 7)

14. SKIN RASH (2)

C – Herpes simplex

This female has erythema multiforme (EM) most likely caused by herpes simplex (herpes labialis or cold sore). All of the listed options are causes of EM except the oral contraceptive pill, which causes erythema nodosum. Trimethoprim is commonly used to treat urinary tract infections. It is also commonly used in conjunction with sulphonamides in the form of co-trimoxazole. EM presents with characteristic target lesions (1–3 cm oval or round, deep red, well-demarcated, flat macules), though it may also present with macules, papules, wheals, vesicles and bullae. Infections account for 90% of cases of EM with herpes being the most common cause.
Causes of EM include:

- Infections: herpes simplex (majority of cases), mycoplasma, coxsackievirus, echovirus, parapoxvirus, varicella zoster, adenovirus, EBV, CMV, viral hepatitis, erythrovirus, HIV, salmonella, tuberculosis, typhoid, dermatophytes
- Drugs: non-steroidal anti-inflammatories (NSAIDs), antiepileptics, sulphonamides, penicillins, barbiturates
- Pregnancy
- Idiopathic

Stevens–Johnson syndrome is a severe form of EM with mucosal bullae of the mouth, conjunctiva and anogenital region. Treatment is based on identifying and treating the underlying cause and providing symptomatic support. Antihistamines can help in reducing symptoms of itching. Steroids are given in severe cases. Most cases (80%) in children are caused by the herpes simplex virus.

15. SYNDROME RECOGNITION (2)

E – Turner syndrome

This female has Turner syndrome, one of the most common chromosomal disorders, which was first described in 1938. It is due to the absence of an X chromosome (45XO) or the presence of an abnormal X chromosome.

Features of Turner syndrome include:

- Webbing of the neck
- A low hairline
- Shield-shaped chest
- Widely spaced nipples
- Wide carrying angle (arms turn out at the elbow)
- Low set ears (80%)
- Lymphoedema of hands and feet in the neonatal period
- Normal intelligence, though often have problems with spatial/temporal processing

As with most syndromes, features are variable and not all the features are always present. However, nearly all females with Turner syndrome have slow growth and early ovarian failure. Kidney abnormalities, coarctation of the aorta, dissection of the aorta, bicuspid aortic valve, otitis media and autoimmune thyroiditis are all seen in increased frequency in females with Turner syndrome.

Turner syndrome is often not diagnosed until adolescence when the female fails to go through puberty. Premature ovarian failure occurs, and there are usually characteristic 'streak' gonads instead of functioning ovaries. Adrenarche, the beginning of pubic and axilla hair growth, usually occurs at a normal age as this is not under the influence of oestrogen. Breast development and menstruation do not occur except in a small minority. Infertility is almost universal. The structure of the uterus, vagina and external genitalia is normal, and pregnancy with a donor egg is possible.

Noonan syndrome (autosomal dominant) is often confused with Turner syndrome as the patients often have a webbed neck and low hairline, short stature and a wide carrying angle. However, Noonan syndrome can affect males and females and is associated with mental retardation and pulmonary valve stenosis. Those with Noonan syndrome have characteristic dysmorphic facies (widely spaced eyes, epicanthic folds and low set ears).

Klinefelter syndrome only affects males and is caused by an extra X chromosome (47 XXY). Affected males are often tall and do not go through puberty. It is associated with a slightly lower IQ than would be expected.

Harry Fitch Klinefelter, American endocrinologist (1912–1990).
Jacqueline Noonan, American pediatric cardiologist (1921b).
Henry Turner, American endocrinologist (1892–1970).

16. CONTRAINDICATIONS TO IMMUNIZATION

D – Steroid treatment for asthma

Public Health England states that 'Almost all individuals can be safely vaccinated with all vaccines. In very few individuals, vaccination is contraindicated or should be deferred. Where there is doubt, rather than withholding vaccine, advice should be sought from an appropriate consultant paediatrician or physician, the immunization co-ordinator or consultant in health protection.'[*]

All vaccines are contraindicated in those who have had a confirmed anaphylactic reaction to a previous dose of a vaccine containing the same antigens or a confirmed anaphylactic reaction to another component contained in the relevant vaccine.

Live vaccines can cause severe, or fatal, infections in severely immunocompromised children. This is due to extensive replication of the vaccine strain. Children treated with high-dose oral or rectal steroids are immunocompromised for up to 3 months after the course has finished. A week-long course of prednisolone is significant (particularly if greater than 2 mg/kg). Not only does this child need to have his MMR delayed but he most likely needs to see a respiratory paediatrician regarding his asthma management as he is very young to require such a prolonged course of oral steroids.

In general, vaccination should be postponed if the child is suffering from a significant acute illness. However, minor illnesses without fever or systemic upset are not contraindications.

Hypersensitivity to egg is a contraindication to the influenza vaccine, yellow fever vaccine and tick-borne encephalitis vaccine. The MMR vaccine can be safely given to most children with a history of egg allergy. For children who have had a confirmed anaphylactic reaction to egg, specialist advice should be sought with a view to immunization under controlled conditions.

Children with HIV are at risk from live vaccines. They can, however, receive the live vaccines for MMR and varicella unless they are severely immunocompromised (CD4 count <500/μL, or <200/μL in children more than 6 years of age). HIV-positive individuals should never receive BCG or yellow fever vaccines.

---

[*] The Green Book. Information for public health professionals on immunisation. *Public Health England* 2013.

17. FEBRILE ILLNESS (3)

A – Abdominal pain

This girl has Kawasaki disease. Kawasaki disease is a vasculitis that occurs during childhood. Most children (85%) are under the age of 5 years, and it is most common in Japanese boys. The exact cause is still unknown; however, a peak during winter and spring months has led to the theory of an infective origin. The diagnostic criteria for complete Kawasaki syndrome are as follows: Fever of at least 5 days' duration *plus* four out of the following five criteria (plus the lack of another known disease process that could explain the illness):

- Bilateral conjunctival injection without exudates
- Oral mucosal erythema: red, fissured lips, strawberry red tongue
- Polymorphous rash
- Extremity changes: peripheral oedema/erythema and periungual desquamation
- Cervical lymphadenopathy

Kawasaki disease causes coronary aneurysms, myocardial infarction, myocarditis and pericarditis. It is the leading cause of acquired paediatric heart disease. The mainstay of treatment is intravenous immunoglobulins, which have been shown to reduce the length of symptoms and also significantly reduce the rate of cardiac complications.

Tomisaku Kawasaki, Japanese paediatrician (1925b).

18. DIABETIC REGIMENS

D – Three times daily injection insulin regimen

There are various insulin regimens, and different children are suited to different forms. The traditional two-injection regimen is still used especially in young children. Its advantage is the need for only two injections per day, but it is often hard to achieve tight control without experiencing hypoglycaemic events. It is also not as useful when children or young adults are not eating at regular times of the day or are exercising.

In this case, a three-injection regimen would be most suited. This is when long-acting insulin is given at night, followed by mixed insulin (short- and long-acting) given in the morning and rapid-acting insulin given at teatime to cover the evening meal. This regimen allows for tighter control than a two-injection regimen and allows the child not to have any injections at school. However, with different insulin preparations being given at different times, confusion can occur and the flexibility that comes with a multiple-injection regimen is not present.

The multiple-injection regimen ('basal-bolus') is now the most commonly used regimen but requires good understanding and co-operation on behalf of the patient. It consists of an injection of long-acting insulin (e.g. glargine) in the evening, which gives a background level over 20 to 24 hours. Short-acting insulin (e.g. novarapid) is then given with meals and snacks during the day. Approximately 30% to 50% of the child's calculated insulin requirement is given as the long-acting form. Carbohydrate counting is used to determine how much short-acting insulin is needed with each meal. The advantage of this regimen is that when compliance is good, the glycaemic control can be a lot tighter and they are less likely to have episodes of hypoglycaemia compared with the two- or three-injection regimen. It also allows the child to eat at anytime and makes glycaemic control easier during an intercurrent illness. The disadvantages include having to inject more frequently, as well as injecting when they are at school.

Insulin pumps achieve optimal control. A subcutaneous device is kept *in situ* for up to 72 hours, and a basal rate of insulin (short-acting) is given continuously. The basal rate can vary during different times of the day as required. The child can then administer boluses of insulin when eating without having to repeat injections. The pump does not measure the blood glucose level, and so the child still needs to do this peripherally. Insulin pumps require commitment and competence to use the therapy effectively. This boy has only just been diagnosed with diabetes; therefore, it is too early to start on a pump. Patients and families must learn how to administer subcutaneous insulin safely and effectively in case of pump failure. The advantages of pump therapy are excellent control with fewer episodes of hypoglycaemia. Patients also appreciate the need for fewer injections. However, the pump needs to be on at all times and, if it gets disconnected by mistake for any period of time, diabetic ketoacidosis can rapidly ensue due to the lack of background long-acting insulin.

19. SHORTNESS OF BREATH

E – Respiratory syncitial virus

Extra respiratory noises include wheeze (an expiratory noise caused by lower airway obstruction/narrowing) and stridor (inspiratory noise caused by upper airway narrowing).

This child has bronchiolitis, which is most commonly caused by the respiratory syncitial virus (RSV). The other organisms given here do cause bronchiolitis but far less commonly. Diagnosis is confirmed by a nasopharyngeal aspirate (NPA). Bronchiolitis is very common, especially during the autumn and winter months. These children present with respiratory distress, coryza, fever, hyperinflation, widespread crackles and a wheeze. Management is supportive with adequate oxygen and hydration. Rarely, some children will need intensive management with ventilatory support. Antibiotics, steroids and bronchodilators are not effective.

Children at high risk of severe bronchiolitis include those with:

- Prematurity (<37 weeks)
- Age less than 12 weeks
- Chronic pulmonary disease, especially chronic lung disease
- Congenital heart disease
- Congenital and anatomic defects of the airways
- Immunodeficiency

20. DIAGNOSIS OF NEPHROTIC SYNDROME

A – Blood albumin concentration 20g/L

Nephrotic syndrome is not a single disease entity as such but rather a kidney disorder. It is characterized by a triad of:

- Proteinuria (>0.05 g/kg/day)
- Hypoalbuminaemia (<30 g/L)
- Oedema

Hyperlipidaemia is also often present but is not required to confirm the diagnosis.

Oedema is characteristically around the eyes (periorbital) but can occur throughout the body and is usually more pronounced in the morning. Children can develop ascites (transudate) and are at risk of spontaneous pneumococcal peritonitis. They are at risk of infection from encapsulated organisms (e.g. *Pneumococcus*) due to the renal loss of IgG proteins. Other symptoms include abdominal pain, diarrhoea, vomiting and lethargy. Renal function is usually normal but renal failure can develop in a few cases. Blood pressure must be monitored as it can be raised (such as in this case). Haematuria is occasionally seen in nephrotic syndrome but is not a diagnostic requirement. Affected children are often hypovolaemic despite being oedematous. Diuretics and intravenous albumin may be necessary if fluid retention is severe. Patients are also placed on prophylactic penicillin due to the susceptibility to infection. Nephrotic syndrome in children often responds well to steroids especially if it is a minimal change disease.

Causes of nephrotic syndrome include glomerulonephritis, congenital nephrotic syndrome, systemic lupus erythematosus, Henoch–Schönlein purpura and certain drugs such as penicillamine, non-steroidal anti-inflammatory drugs (NSAIDs) and paracetamol. The majority of children with nephrotic syndrome (90%) have minimal change glomerulonephritis.

Remember the rule of thirds for prognosis regarding minimal change glomerulonephritis:

- One-third have only a single episode
- One-third develop occasional relapses
- One-third have frequent relapses, which stop before adulthood

21. INVESTIGATION OF DEVELOPMENTAL DELAY

B – Creatine kinase

Global developmental delay is defined as significant delay in two or more developmental domains. First-line investigations include chromosomal analysis, fragile-X testing, creatine kinase (CK), urea and electrolytes (U&Es), lead level, urate, full blood count (FBC), ferritin, thyroid function tests and biotinidase levels.

Most cases of developmental delay never have a cause found. Chromosomal analysis brings the highest yield of abnormal results. Syndromes such as Down, DiGeorge and Williams all can present with developmental delay. The DNA-based test for the fragile-X gene should also be routinely performed as this inherited cause of learning difficulties has subtle dysmorphia and is difficult to diagnose clinically. Biotinidase should be tested early as biotinidase deficiency is treatable and may present with global developmental delay without other symptoms. Iron deficiency should be tested for, as it can be associated with developmental delay and is easily treated. Thyroid function tests are performed as congenital hypothyroidism needs to be treated promptly and certain syndromes are associated with hypothyroidism.

When investigating developmental delay, neuroimaging is often performed as a second-line investigation. Detailed genetic testing should not be performed unless there are other indications such as odd behaviour, dysmorphia or a family history. An EEG is not recommended unless there are associated seizures or speech regression (Landau–Kleffner syndrome = sudden or gradual aphasia + abnormal EEG). A full metabolic screen is only initially performed if there is a history of consanguinity, organomegaly or regression.

This boy is likely to have Duchenne muscular dystrophy (DMD). All boys presenting with developmental delay, especially gross motor delay, should have CK levels measured to rule out DMD. DMD is an X-linked recessive disorder resulting in a lack of dystrophin production in the muscles. This leads to progressive muscle weakness, wasting and eventually death. Children present in the first 5 years of life with delayed walking, frequent falling, difficulty climbing stairs and pseudohypertrophy of the calves. Gowers' sign (where the child uses their hands to 'climb up' their legs when rising from the ground) is usually positive. Some boys also have delayed speech or global developmental delay. CK is raised, often 100 times above normal, and a muscle biopsy (revealing reduced dystrophin) establishes the diagnosis.

Guillaume Benjamin Amand Duchenne, French neurologist (1806–1875).

FURTHER READING

1. McDonald L, Rennie A, Tolmie J, Galloway P, McWilliam R. Investigation of global developmental delay. *Arch Dis Child* 2006;91:701–705.

22. PAINFUL RASH

B – Group A streptococcus

The rash described here is erythema nodosum (EN); in this case, it is caused by group A streptococcal tonsillitis. EN presents with red nodules or plaques that are symmetrical, tender and hot to touch. They are most commonly found on the shins but may also be found on the thighs, ankles, knees, arms, face and neck. Frequently, no cause is found. Treatment is based on identifying and treating the underlying cause.

Causes of EN include:

- Infection
  - Group A streptococcus
  - Tuberculosis
  - Invasive fungal infections
- Drugs
  - Sulphonamides
  - Oral contraceptive
  - Barbiturates
- Inflammatory bowel disease
- Systemic lupus erythematosus
- Sarcoidosis
- Idiopathic

23. INVESTIGATION OF CHRONIC COUGH (2)

E – Sweat test

Cystic fibrosis (CF) is the most common lethal autosomal recessive disease of Caucasians. In the UK, there is a carrier rate of 1 in 25 leading to the disease affecting approximately 1 in 2500. CF is caused by an abnormal gene coding for the cystic fibrosis transmembrane regulator protein (CFTR), located on chromosome 7. This protein functions as a channel across the membrane. The channel transports negatively charged chloride ions into and out of cells. Cells that produce mucus, sweat, saliva, tears and digestive enzymes are all affected. The most common mutation in CF is the ΔF508 mutation, although well over a thousand different mutations have been identified. The poor transport of chloride ions and water across epithelial cells of the respiratory and pancreas exocrine glands in CF results in an increased viscosity of secretions. The range of presentations is varied, including recurrent chest infections, failure to thrive from malabsorption and liver disease. In the neonatal period, infants may present with prolonged neonatal jaundice, bowel obstruction (meconium ileus) or rectal prolapse.

The gold standard investigation for CF is the sweat test. The abnormal function of sweat glands results in the excess concentration of sodium chloride (NaCl) in sweat. Sweat is stimulated by pilocarpine iontophoresis, collected on filter paper and analyzed.

Normal sweat NaCl concentration = 10–14 mmol/L
Sweat NaCl concentration in CF = 80–125 mmol/L

At least two sweat tests should be performed as diagnostic errors and false positives are common.

Chest X-rays are frequently required in CF to monitor disease progress or during an acute infective episode but would not be diagnostic. Immune-reactive trypsin (IRT) is now used as a national screening tool on the neonatal Guthrie card. A raised IRT is strongly suggestive of CF, but the diagnosis still needs to be confirmed with either genetic mutation analysis or a sweat test. Genetic mutation analyses can be used for the pre- or postnatal diagnosis of CF; however, not all mutations have been identified. Nasal potential difference is used to measure the voltage across nasal epithelium, which correlates with the transport of sodium and chloride across cell membranes.

24. ANAEMIA

D – Iron deficiency

This child is likely to have iron deficiency as she has a microcytic, hypochromic anaemia. Iron deficiency is the most common form of anaemia in children – as much as 50% in certain populations. It is often due to poor intake of iron-rich foods. Children who drink a large amount of cow's milk are particularly vulnerable as only 10% of iron is absorbed from the milk compared with 50% in breast milk. All formula milk and most breakfast cereals are fortified with iron.

Anaemias are often categorized according to the morphology of the red cells. The three different classifications for the size of the red cell are: microcytic (small), normocytic and macrocytic (large).

- Microcytic anaemia: there is a failure or insufficiency in haemoglobin synthesis. The red blood cells are smaller than normal, i.e. mean cell volume (MCV) <85 fL. The red cells are often hypochromic (pale in colour). This is quantified by a low mean-corpuscular haemoglobin (MCH). A good way of remembering the causes of microcytic anaemia is by using the acronym 'TAILS' (thalassaemias, anaemia of chronic disease, iron deficiency anaemia, lead poisoning and sideroblastic anaemia). Sideroblastic anaemia is the inability to completely form haem molecules. Lead poisoning is now uncommon in the UK. It presents with irritability, failure to thrive, abdominal pain, pica (eating non-nutritious substances) as well as microcytic anaemia.
- Normocytic anaemia: occurs when the overall haemoglobin levels are decreased but the red blood cells are of normal size (MCV 85–105 fL). Causes include acute blood loss, anaemia of chronic disease, aplastic anaemia (bone marrow failure) and haemolytic anaemias. Remember that chronic disease can also cause a microcytic anaemia.
- Macrocytic anaemia: usually, this is due to a failure of DNA synthesis. The red blood cells are larger than normal (MCV >105 fL). The most

common cause is megaloblastic anaemia that is due to either a deficiency in vitamin B_{12} or in folic acid. Other causes of macrocytic anaemia include liver disease and hypothyroidism.

25. COMPLICATIONS OF UNDESCENDED TESTES

D – Psychological benefit

Cryptorchidism is defined as the failure of the testis to descend from its intra-abdominal location into the scrotum. The testes develop in the abdomen of the fetus. They remain high in the abdomen until the seventh month of gestation, when they move from the abdomen through the inguinal canal into the scrotum, guided by the gubernaculum (a fold of peritoneum). This process is influenced by anti-Mullerian hormone (AMH) and testosterone. Maldevelopment of the gubernaculum, or deficiency or insensitivity to either AMH or testosterone, can prevent the testes from descending into the scrotum.

Cryptorchidism can lead to complications, including psychological distress, decreased fertility and an increased risk of torsion, indirect hernias and malignancies. There is a huge psychological benefit in bringing a testicle down into the scrotum, and this should not be underestimated as one of the reasons for performing an orchidopexy. During orchidopexy, the inguinal canal is closed once the testicle has been brought down, thus decreasing the risk of indirect (rather than direct) hernias.

Infertility is observed in 10% of patients with unilateral and 40% of patients with bilateral cryptorchidism. At least one contributing mechanism for reduced spermatogenesis in cryptorchid testes is temperature. The temperature of testes in the scrotum is at least a couple of degrees cooler than in the abdomen, and it is postulated that an increased temperature could damage fertility. Subtle or transient hormone deficiencies that lead to the lack of descent into the scrotum can also impair the development of spermatogenic tissue as well as the high rate of epididymal abnormalities in boys with cryptorchidism. Even after an orchidopexy, fertility does not improve significantly especially if the orchidopexy is performed after the age of 2.

One of the strongest arguments for early orchidopexy is prevention and early treatment of testicular cancer. There is a 4- to 40-fold increased risk in men born with undescended testes, with the most common tumour being a seminoma. Even after orchidopexy, there is an increased risk of malignancy; this is probably due to an inherent abnormality in the undescended testicle. However, with orchidopexy and testicular self-examination, men are able to detect the malignancy much earlier than if the testis had been left in the abdomen.

Cryptorchidism, from the Greek *crypto* = hidden + *orchid* = testicle.
Johannes Peter Müller, German physiologist (1801–1858).

26. INVESTIGATION OF JAUNDICE (2)

E – All of the above

As many as half of newborn babies will be clinically jaundiced in the first week of life. Bilirubin is produced by the breakdown of fetal haemoglobin (HbF), which is replaced with adult haemoglobin (HbA).

Investigation is not required as long as the following criteria are fulfilled:

- Jaundice is not apparent in the first 24 hours of life.
- The infant remains clinically well.
- The serum bilirubin is below treatment level.
- The jaundice resolves by 14 days.

In this case, the most important single test at this point would be a bilirubin level. This is because high levels of unconjugated bilirubin can cross the blood–brain barrier and cause permanent neuronal damage (kernicterus). Jaundice can be treated with phototherapy, which converts unconjugated bilirubin into non-toxic isomers, which are then excreted.

This baby has several risk factors for 'pathological' jaundice:

- Jaundice before 24 hours of life.
- Rhesus D negative mother – and so this could be rhesus haemolytic disease of the newborn (red cell alloimmunization). A direct antibody test (Coombs' test) would reveal any active haemolysis present. A full blood count is required to see if the infant is anaemic due to possible haemolysis. The incidence of rhesus disease of the newborn has fallen dramatically due to the use of anti-D immunoglobulin in rhesus D negative mothers.
- Prolonged rupture of membranes, which would put the infant at risk of sepsis. Sepsis can cause jaundice in the first 24 hours of life. Therefore, a blood culture and C-reactive protein (CRP) should be performed and the baby started on empirical antibiotics, such as amoxicillin and gentamicin, until the blood culture returns negative.

Kernicterus, from Greek *kern* = nucleus + *icterus* = yellow ('yellow brain').

27. MANAGEMENT OF ANAEMIA

C – Oral folic acid

This girl has macrocytic anaemia, which is most likely due to folate deficiency. Children who are on anticonvulsants (e.g. phenytoin), methotrexate, antimalarials (e.g. pyrimethamine) or high-dose trimethoprim can display folate deficiency as a side effect. Clinical features of folate deficiency include glossitis (a smooth, beefy red tongue), angular stomatitis (fissuring at the corners of the lips), nausea and vomiting, abdominal pain and anorexia. Folate deficiency is easily treated with oral folate supplementation in the form of folic acid. A 4-month course is generally sufficient to replenish body stores. Folate deficiency is also seen during periods of rapid growth such as in infancy, and in malabsorption due to coeliac or inflammatory bowel disease.

Another cause of macrocytic anaemia is vitamin B_{12} deficiency. Clinical features of vitamin B_{12} deficiency are very similar to folate deficiency with the addition of peripheral neuropathy, depression and dementia. Macrocytic anaemia is also seen in malabsorption as well as in certain worm infestations (the fish tapeworm competes for vitamin B_{12} and in chronic cases can lead to deficiencies). A rare cause of vitamin B_{12} deficiency is pernicious anaemia. Parietal cells produce intrinsic factor, which is essential for the uptake of vitamin B_{12} in the terminal ileum. Pernicious anaemia describes the autoimmune loss of parietal cells and/or intrinsic factor, thus preventing the absorption of vitamin B_{12}. It is most common in women more than 60 years of age. Around 90% of patients demonstrate antiparietal antibodies (but some normal women also have it), and 60% are found to have anti-intrinsic factor antibody (which is a more specific marker). Vitamin B_{12} deficiency is treated with intramuscular injections of hydroxocobalamin (a natural analogue of vitamin B_{12}) rather than oral forms.

Pernicious, from Latin *perniciosus* = ruinous.

28. INVESTIGATION OF SEIZURES

A – 12-lead ECG

This girl has experienced her first non-febrile seizure. Many people believe that all children who have had a seizure or fit of any kind need an EEG; however, this is not the case. An EEG should be performed to *support* a diagnosis of epilepsy and not be used in isolation; they are not done until after a second seizure. Remember that EEGs produce both false positives and false negatives. EEGs can be useful in determining seizure type and epilepsy syndromes and thus enable children to be given accurate prognoses.

Neuroimaging is warranted in certain circumstances, and magnetic resonance imaging (MRI) would be the modality of choice. However, neuroimaging is not required in most cases. Indications for MRI include any suggestion of a focal seizure – if the child is under the age of 2, or if the seizures are continuing despite medication. In this case, the girl has experienced only one generalized seizure and MRI is not necessary.

All children who have had a 'convulsive seizure' (such as in this case) should have an ECG. The ECG may reveal a cardiac cause for the fit and, in particular, a prolonged QTc interval needs to be excluded. The girl in this case collapsed suddenly before fitting, so an ECG is warranted to exclude a cardiac cause.

Serum prolactin, which is thought to rise after epileptic seizures, is no longer recommended as an investigation due to its lack of both sensitivity and specificity.

FURTHER READING

1. National Collaborating Centre for Primary Care. *The Epilepsies*. Clinical Guideline 20. London: NICE, 2004. Available at: www.nice.org.uk:80/nicemedia/pdf/CG020NICEguideline.pdf
2. Scottish Intercollegiate Guidelines Network. *Diagnosis and Management of Epilepsies in Children and Young People*. Edinburgh: SIGN, 2005. Available at: www.sign.ac.uk/pdf/qrg81.pdf

29. MANAGEMENT OF EPILEPSY

E – Sodium valproate

For children with absence seizures, the first-line drugs are sodium valproate and lamotrigine.* Recognized side effects of sodium valproate include transient hair loss, weight gain, liver damage and blood dyscrasias. Sodium valproate is also associated with a higher risk of fetal malformations if taken in pregnancy, particularly neural tube defects. Lamotrigine side effects include skin rash, drowsiness, insomnia and agitation.

Carbamazepine and gabapentin should not be used in absence seizures as they can worsen the symptoms.

Carbamazepine is often used in tonic–clonic seizures as well as focal seizures. Common side effects include allergic skin reactions, blurred vision, ataxia and nausea. Carbamazepine is also a hepatic enzyme-inducing drug and therefore can cause problems if the child is taking other medications. For example, it increases the metabolism, and thus removal, of oestrogen and progesterone from the blood stream. Adolescents who are using the oral contraceptive pill and who are on carbamazepine should take extra protection to prevent pregnancy. Gabapentin may cause fatigue and emotional lability.

Phenytoin is no longer used as a first-line drug. It can be used in focal or tonic–clonic seizures. Phenytoin side effects include gum hyperplasia, hirsutism, coarsening of facial features, ataxia and slurred speech.

30. THE ACUTELY PAINFUL JOINT

D – Joint aspiration followed by IV antibiotics, continuing for 4 to 6 weeks

This girl has septic arthritis; an infection within a joint. This is a medical emergency. It can rapidly irreversibly destroy a joint and is also life-threatening. Septic arthritis presents with an unwell child with a fever and a short history of a hot swollen joint. There is restricted movement in the joint with pain on passive movement. The hip joint is most commonly

---

* Stokes T, Shaw EJ, Juarez-Garcia A, Camosso-Stefinovic J, Baker R. *The Epilepsies: The Diagnosis and Management of the Epilepsies in Adults and Children in Primary and Secondary Care*. London: Royal College of General Practitioners, 2004. Available at: www.nice.org.uk:80/nicemedia/pdf/CG020fullguideline.pdf

affected in children, although any joint may be involved. In 5% of cases, the child will have two or more joints involved.

Investigations in a suspected case should include blood cultures, full blood count and erythrocyte sedimentation rate (ESR) or C-reactive protein (CRP). Ultrasound can be useful in demonstrating an effusion in a deeply placed joint such as the hip and can also be used to guide aspiration. Joint aspiration is vital and yields yellowish pus, which should be sent for an urgent Gram staining, microscopy, culture and sensitivity. Joint aspiration should be performed before starting antibiotics so that the culture and sensitivity are more accurate. However, if aspiration is to be delayed, then antibiotics should be started. High blood white cell counts and a raised CRP are consistent with septic arthritis though these are also seen in transient synovitis. Patients who have a negative microscopy and culture, but who are still likely to have septic arthritis, must be treated as such.

Management of septic arthritis is by empirical intravenous antibiotics, which should aim to cover the most likely organisms (*Staphylococcus aureus, Streptococcus* sp. and *Haemophilus influenzae* type B in unimmunized children).

Exact antibiotics will be guided by local policies, but a broad-spectrum antibiotic, such as a third-generation cephalosporin, is often used until the organism has been cultured and sensitivities determined. Total duration of treatment needs to be for 4 to 6 weeks. Intravenous antibiotics may be converted to a high-dose oral version after 2 weeks if the infection is under control, but close monitoring of compliance and clinical progress is required. In addition, septic joints need to be drained. This can be done via repeated joint aspirations, but surgical drainage may be required.

31. SURFACTANT DEFICIENCY

B – Intrauterine growth restriction

A preterm baby is defined as a baby born prior to 37 completed weeks' gestation. Intrauterine growth restriction describes a baby that is small for its corrected gestation. Preterm babies develop respiratory disease because of a deficiency of surfactant production by the type II pneumocytes in the lung. Surfactant is required to reduce the surface tension within the lungs (i.e. making them less stiff).

The outcome of premature babies has been significantly improved by the production of exogenous surfactant, which can be administered directly into the lungs via an endotracheal tube.

Causes of increased incidence of surfactant deficiency are:

- Prematurity
- Male gender
- Sepsis
- Maternal diabetes

- Second twin
- Elective caesarean section

  A reduced incidence of surfactant deficiency is associated with:

- Female gender
- Prolonged rupture of membranes
- Maternal opiate use
- Intrauterine growth restriction
- Antenatal steroids

If a pregnant woman is between 24 and 32 weeks' gestation and there is a strong likelihood of her delivering prematurely, then there is good evidence that giving the mother two doses of glucocorticoid prior to delivery will significantly improve the outcome for the baby. This evidence was from the first Cochrane Review ever produced.

32. INVESTIGATION OF HAEMATURIA

C – Antistreptolysin-O titre/throat swab

There are many causes of haematuria, and it is important to establish whether there is frank blood (macroscopic) or just blood indicated on dipstick testing (microscopic). Bright red macroscopic haematuria suggests lower urinary tract pathology. Brown (cola)-coloured urine suggests a renal origin. Both beetroot and rifampicin can also cause the urine to turn red.

Fever, dysuria, frequency and urgency would indicate infection as the cause, and a clean catch urine specimen for urinalysis, microscopy and culture should be sent. Children, particularly infants, may have no other signs of infection, so all children presenting with haematuria should have a urine sample sent. Once a urine infection has been ruled out, further investigation is necessary.

Acute glomerulonephritis can cause haematuria. This is caused by damage to the glomerulus secondary to an immune-mediated process. It is relatively rare in the UK, but the most common form occurs after streptococcal infection (typically 2 weeks after a throat or skin infection). An antistreptolysin-O titre and throat swab are useful to establish if there has been a recent streptococcal infection and, in this case, it is the most likely cause for the haematuria (post-streptococcal glomerulonephritis). Complement levels are sometimes low, particularly in nephrotic syndrome, but this is not a reliable diagnostic test. The urine can look smoky, and there may be red cell casts visible on urine microscopy.

Pain, particularly severe colicky pain, may signal renal stones, and an abdominal X-ray with or without an ultrasound scan may reveal them. Henoch–Schönlein purpura (HSP) can cause haematuria and/or proteinuria. There is no definite investigation for the diagnosis of HSP, but a history of a purpuric rash with or without joint pain would make it more likely.

33. CAUSES OF SPEECH DELAY

B – Expressive language disorder

By 2½ years of age, children should use at least 50 words (some will use >400 words) and be able to use simple word combinations, understand two-stage commands and be able to ask for food, drink, toys and so on. Speech and language need to be separated. Speech is the act of communication through the articulation of verbal expression and is a motor act. Language is the knowledge of a system of symbols (words, gestures, images) that enables communication. It is the ability to understand (receptive) and express (expressive) speech and is associated with meaning rather than sounds.

Speech delay in this age group can be due to numerous causes. This little girl is likely to have an expressive language disorder. These children have normal intelligence and understanding but have a problem 'translating' their ideas into speech. They often do well with intervention from the speech therapists. Children with maturation delay or 'late bloomers' tend to improve without the need for intervention.

If a child has hearing loss, speech often does not develop normally. All children with significant speech delay should have a hearing test, even if their parents are not concerned with their hearing. This child should therefore have an audiology assessment. Speech delay can be part of a general developmental delay, and an underlying chromosomal or neurological abnormality may be detected. It is also often seen in children with cerebral palsy. Children who have autism spectrum disorder (ASD) can present with speech delay. Autism is characterized by delayed and deviant language development, failure to develop the ability to relate to others and by ritualistic and compulsive behaviours.

Neglect and social deprivation can lead to speech delay due to poor stimulation. Speech development can be slower in twins, younger siblings, children in lower socioeconomic classes and children exposed to more than one language. Structural abnormalities can also cause problems with speech. This may include a missed cleft palate or malocclusion of the jaw.

34. FEEDING

D – Overfeeding

A 6-week-old infant should be taking approximately 150 to 180 mL/kg/day. Many parents will describe fluid volumes in ounces, so it is well worth remembering that there are approximately 30 mL in one ounce. The vomiting baby is a very common problem. If a baby takes, or is given, too much milk, the stomach cannot hold the volume and the child will effortlessly vomit the milk back. Advice should be given that the volume of feeds needs to be reduced, even with the description of a 'hungry baby'.

Effortless vomiting also occurs in gastro-oesophageal reflux, although you would need to know if the symptoms continue on a normal feed volume before making the diagnosis. Reflux leads to vomiting, oesophagitis, recurrent apnoea, recurrent pulmonary aspiration and failure to thrive.

In pyloric stenosis, the vomit is forcefully ejected and is described as being projectile. (Once seen, it is never forgotten as it will travel the length of a room!) Examination will reveal a smooth mass just below the right costal margin, which is the hypertrophied pylorus. These infants are often dehydrated on presentation due to recurrent vomiting and the inability of milk to get beyond the pylorus. In this case, the child is thriving and the vomiting is not projectile.

35. INVESTIGATION FOLLOWING URINARY TRACT INFECTIONS

C – USS and dimercaptosuccinic acid (DMSA) as outpatient

Investigations for children with urinary tract infections (UTIs) have been rationalized in the last few years. Useful investigations after a UTI are USS of the urinary tract, DMSA scan and MCUG, but these are not required in all patients:

- A USS of the urinary tract is performed to check for structural abnormalities such as obstruction.
- DMSA is a radiolabelled compound that becomes fixed in functioning proximal renal tubular cells. DMSA is not taken up by scarred, nonfunctioning areas of the kidney and can therefore detect defects in the renal parenchyma. The DMSA scan is performed 4 to 6 months after the most recent infection.
- An MCUG is performed to demonstrate the presence of vesico-ureteric reflux. Contrast is injected via a catheter into the bladder, and X-rays are taken of the bladder and kidney while it empties. It is important to establish the diagnosis of vesicoureteric reflux and the severity so that corrective surgery can be performed early to prevent kidney damage.

Recommended imaging schedule for infants younger
than 6 months

All infants with UTIs (<6 months) need to have a renal USS. If they have had a simple UTI which responds to antibiotics, this can be performed as an outpatient in 6 weeks and no further imaging is required. If this is abnormal, however, an MCUG is recommended. If they have an atypical UTI or recurrent UTI, a USS should be performed as an inpatient along with a DMSA and MCUG as an outpatient.

Recommended imaging schedule for infants and children
6 months or older but younger than 3 years

None is required unless UTI is atypical or recurrent (such as this case); then, a USS followed by a DMSA scan should be performed as an outpatient. An MCUG should not be routinely performed unless any of the following features are present: dilation on ultrasound, poor urine flow, non-*E. coli* infection or a family history of vesicoureteric reflux.

Recommended imaging schedule for children 3 years or older

No imaging is required if they have a simple UTI that responds well to antibiotics. Children with atypical UTIs should have a USS as an inpatient, and those with recurrent UTIs should have a USS as an outpatient followed by a DMSA in 4 to 6 months.

These recommendations are taken from the NICE guidelines for UTIs in children.*

36. MANAGEMENT OF CHRONIC ASTHMA

A – Add an inhaled long-acting β-agonist

The management of asthma is done in a structured step-wise manner. This is to ensure consistency of care.

There are five steps for children between 5 and 12 years:

- Step 1 – Inhaled short-acting β-agonist
- Step 2 – Add inhaled steroid 200 to 400 mg/day
- Step 3 – Add inhaled long-acting β-agonist (LABA)
  - 3a – Good response – continue LABA
  - 3b – Benefit from LABA but not full control – increase inhaled steroid dose
  - 3c – No response to LABA – stop LABA, increase inhaled steroid dose and/or trial of other therapies (e.g. leukotriene receptor antagonist or slow-release theophylline)
- Step 4 – Increase inhaled steroid dose to 800 mg/day
- Step 5 – Use daily steroid tablet

Pharmacological management can significantly improve symptoms, but it is important to consider lifestyle changes. These include allergen avoidance, house dust mite control and smoking cessation (advise parents regarding the effect on children).

37. NEURAL TUBE DEFECTS

C – Meningocele

Since the introduction of folic acid supplementation in pregnancy, the incidence of neural tube defects has decreased by 75%. It is now seen in 0.3 in 1000 births. Such defects result from failure of the neural tube to close normally during early pregnancy.

This patient is likely to have had a meningocele – an exposed sac of meninges. With a meningocele, the spinal cord remains intact and

---

* National Collaborating Centre for Women's and Children's Health. *Urinary Tract Infection in Children.* NICE Clinical Guideline 54. London: NICE, 2007. Available at: www.nice.org.uk:80/nicemedia/pdf/CG54NICEguideline.pdf

functions normally and thus the child's neurology is normal, such as in this case. The sac can rupture, and there is an increased risk of developing meningitis and hydrocephalus. Surgical correction is always necessary, and long-term follow-up is needed as neurological problems may develop as the child grows.

In a myelomeningocele, a meningeal sac herniates through a defect in the lower vertebrae and contains elements of the spinal cord and lumbo-sacral roots. The majority (80%) are seen in the lumbrosacral region. Neurological deficits range from minimal bladder dysfunction, mobility and intellectual problems in small defects to loss of lower limb function, anaesthesia and urine and faecal incontinence in more severe defects.

In spina bifida occulta, the vertebral bodies fail to fuse posteriorly. Tethering of the cord can occur with growth and is associated with neurological dysfunction. There can be weakness of the legs with spasticity and abnormal gait. Sensory abnormalities include paraesthesia. The loss of bladder and bowel control, leading to incontinence or constipation, can be of sudden or gradual onset and decreases in anal sphincter tone may be seen. There is no sac present in the lumbosacral area, but there may be cutaneous markers over the area including tufts of hair, a sinus or port wine stain. Diagnosis can be made on ultrasound scan (below the age of 2) or, ideally, magnetic resonance imaging. Bony anomalies may also be seen radiologically.

An encephalocele is a cranium bifida (i.e. a protrusion of the meninges and brain through a fault in the skull). Anencephaly is the most severe form of a neural tube defect. There is absence of the skull vault, the skin and significant parts of the brain. Affected babies do not survive long and many are stillborn.

Meninges, from Greek *meninx* = membrane.

38. RISK FACTORS FOR HIP DISEASE

E – He is 7 years old
Perthes disease (or Legg–Clavé–Perthes disease) describes idiopathic avascular necrosis of the femoral head, which is followed by revascularization and re-ossification over a period of 2 to 3 years.

Risk factors for Perthes disease:

- Age 3 to 12 years, with peak incidence at 5 to 7 years of age
- Male–female ratio is 4:1
- African races are rarely affected
- Underlying condition (e.g. renal failure, glucocorticoid use, systemic lupus erythematosus, HIV)

In 10% of patients, the condition is bilateral. Presentation is insidious with hip pain (which may be referred to the groin or knee) and a limp. Examination may reveal a reduced range of movements in all directions of the hip joint, secondary to irritation of the capsule, though internal rotation and abduction are usually more affected. There may be a fixed flexion deformity of the opposite leg (to compensate for shortening of the affected leg), and there may be some muscle wasting on the affected side. X-ray will show a collapsed, irregular, sclerotic femoral head (secondary to osteopaenia of surrounding bone), with an increased joint space. Magnetic resonance imaging may be more sensitive in detecting changes early. Treatment depends upon the extent of disease and the amount of femoral head that is involved. Mild disease may be treated conservatively with bed rest, analgesia and repeat imaging to monitor progress. More severe disease may be treated by abduction bracing/splinting or by femoral osteotomy. The prognosis is worse in older children, in girls and if more than half the femoral head is affected. Complications include early osteoarthritis and coxa magna (overgrowth of the femoral head).

Slipped capital femoral epiphysis (SCFE) describes posterolateral displacement of the femoral head. Slippage occurs through the femoral head growth plate.

Risk factors for SCFE:

- Age 10 to 15 years (mean age 12 years in girls and 13.5 years in boys)
- Male–female ratio is 3:2
- Obesity
- Microgenitalia
- Hypothyroidism
- Tall stature

Twenty to forty percent of cases are bilateral. SCFE presents with a limp and with hip pain referred to the knee. It may follow minor trauma. There may be restriction in abduction and internal rotation of the hip. The affected leg is often shortened and externally rotated. The diagnosis is confirmed on a lateral view X-ray of the affected hip. Management is by surgical pinning of the epiphysis. Complications of a SCFE include premature epiphyseal fusion and avascular necrosis.

Georg Clemens Perthes, German surgeon (1869–1927).

39. CAUSES OF CEREBRAL PALSY

D – Meningitis

There are numerous causes of cerebral palsy, and it is a misconception that the majority of cases of cerebral palsy are due to birth asphyxia.

Premature babies are at a higher risk of cerebral palsy because myelination of the motor pathways occurs between 5 and 8 months postconception. In this case, the baby is already 36 weeks postconception making an association between his spasticity and prematurity unlikely. Hypoglycaemia can also lead to cerebral palsy. While hypoxic events at birth can lead to cerebral palsy, only about 6% of cases are due to avoidable factors during labour. The child needs to be moderately asphyxiated for damage to occur. Trauma, both at birth and postnatally, can also lead to cerebral palsy, but a head injury needs to be significant and in this case it is unlikely to be the cause.

Prenatal insults are probably the most common cause of cerebral palsy, and up to 60% are probably due to an early prenatal abnormality. Impairment of placental function can damage the motor pathways and lead to cerebral dysgenesis and cerebral malformation. Congenital infections and cerebral malformations are other prenatal causes.

Infections such as meningitis and encephalitis that affect the child before their second birthday can lead to cerebral palsy and in this patient is the most likely cause as he was significantly unwell requiring PICU admission. Kernicterus (brain damage secondary to high levels of unconjugated bilirubin) used to be a relatively common cause for cerebral palsy but, due to treatment of rhesus disease and the use of phototherapy, kernicterus is now rarely seen in developed countries. In this boy, the levels of bilirubin are unlikely to have been high enough to cause kernicterus. Strokes, though rare in children, do occur and typically cause a hemiplegia.

40. INVESTIGATION OF CONSTIPATION

E – No investigation required

This boy is likely to have simple constipation and no further investigation is necessary at this stage. Constipation is the passage of stool, which is difficult or painful and is often associated with soiling. Fewer than three stools per week are considered abnormal.

In simple or idiopathic constipation, the rectum becomes distended with the chronic loading of hard stool. The stretched rectum becomes desensitized and does not convey a feeling of fullness and thus the urge to defecate, which in turn leads to further distension with stool. Often loose stool, from the proximal colon, passes around the impacted stool and, due to the absence of sensation, leaks out unnoticed, causing soiling. An inadequate intake of food or fluid leads to constipation in children, and it must be remembered that large amounts of milk lead to hard stools.

No investigations are needed when simple or idiopathic constipation is thought to be the diagnosis. An abdominal X-ray can reveal faecal loading, but this is an unnecessary investigation unless bowel obstruction is thought to be the cause. An anal fissure can lead to constipation due to the pain caused on defecation, and this is usually associated with fresh blood when passing a stool. It can be secondary to passing a large hard stool but is also seen in Crohn disease; examination under anaesthesia is sometimes needed in small children to assess the anal area. Constipation can occur in hypothyroidism. However, one would only test for thyroid disease if there was clinical evidence on examination, if the constipation was intractable to treatment or if there was evidence of growth faltering.

Hirschsprung disease is a congenital disorder with aganglionic stretches of the bowel causing the area to be tonically contracted, resulting in obstruction. This starts from the anus and progresses up the colon to differing levels. Colon dilation is seen secondary to bowel obstruction. Diagnosis is made on rectal biopsy and around 95% present in the first year of life. There is delay in passing meconium in the first 24 hours of life followed by intermittent bowel obstruction or chronic constipation. Very occasionally it can present later in life, but a normal bowel habit in the early months, as in this case, makes it a very unlikely diagnosis.

Harald Hirschsprung, Danish paediatrician (1830–1916).

41. HIP PAIN

E – None of the above

This boy has an irritable hip. Irritable hip (or transient synovitis) is common in children and presents with a painful limp that gradually resolves. The cause is uncertain, and the diagnosis is one of exclusion. Therefore, the list of tests here will not confirm the diagnosis (transient synovitis) but rather rule out other causes of the symptoms.

In transient synovitis, infection and trauma are thought to be precipitating factors. However, research has found that infection, usually of the upper respiratory tract, is present in only 30% of cases and significant trauma in only 5% of cases. It is most commonly seen in boys between the ages of 2 and 12 years. There is a history of acute-onset hip pain and a limp. Often knee pain and the inability to bear weight follow. This is usually unilateral but rarely can be seen bilaterally. On examination, there is restricted movement in the affected limb, especially of extension and adduction.

Investigations in irritable hip are performed not only to confirm the diagnosis but to exclude other problems such as septic arthritis, osteomyelitis and Perthes disease. Blood tests including full blood count (FBC), white cell count (WCC) and C-reactive protein (CRP) are usually normal, whereas in septic arthritis or osteomyelitis they are deranged. X-rays are poor at demonstrating effusions; therefore, the imaging of choice is ultrasound, which picks up 95% of effusions where one is present. To definitely exclude septic arthritis, the effusion needs to be aspirated and cultured.

Symptoms usually persist for 1 to 2 weeks, then resolve spontaneously. If symptoms continue, consider other diagnoses such as Perthes disease, slipped upper femoral epiphysis or malignancy.

42. INVESTIGATION OF ENURESIS

E – None of the above

Enuresis refers to the involuntary passing of urine. It can be nocturnal or diurnal (during the day) or both. It is common in school-aged children, particularly boys; affecting 15% of 5-year olds and 5% of 10-year olds.

In this case, the child has primary nocturnal enuresis (i.e. has never been dry). If a child has been dry and then starts to wet again, this is known as secondary enuresis. Secondary enuresis needs much more careful assessment and relevant investigation.

History taking should seek to exclude urinary symptoms, a family history and psychosocial problems. Clinical examination should include growth parameters and examining the abdomen and genitalia. Neurological problems, such as spina bifida and cerebral palsy, are rare causes of nocturnal enuresis but need to be ruled out by a lower limb neurological and spinal examination.

Blood pressure should be performed, which, if elevated, could indicate renal disease. This only needs to be a spot check rather than 24-hour monitoring. Previously, all children would require urinalysis. Urinalysis could help identify diabetes mellitus or a urinary tract infection (UTI). A urinalysis is now only performed if clinically indicated: secondary enuresis, daytime symptoms, signs of ill health and/or a history of either UTI or diabetes are indications. This child therefore does not require any investigation prior to treatment.

There are a number of strategies for tackling nocturnal enuresis. First, contributory factors (constipation, stress, urinary tract infection, diabetes mellitus) need to be considered and addressed. Non-pharmacological measures include reward systems such as star charts, encouraging adequate drinking and voiding during the day as well as ease of access to the bathroom. Alarms that wake the child up if they wet the bed can be used. Medical options include desmopressin (an antidiuretic hormone analogue that causes a reduction in the nocturnal production of urine) and oxybutynin (an anticholinergic that dampens bladder contractions) if there are elements of bladder instability.

After the age of 4 years, enuresis resolves spontaneously in 5% of affected children each year.

Enuresis, from Greek *en* = in + *ourein* = to urinate.

43. MANAGEMENT OF DIARRHOEA

D – Rehydration with oral rehydration therapy alone

Acute diarrhoea is most commonly caused by infection. The most common infections in children are viral, as in this case, with rotavirus and adenovirus being the main offenders. Patients with diarrhoea and vomiting are at risk of becoming dehydrated and developing electrolyte imbalance (e.g. hypernatraemia, hypokalaemia). The initial management of patients without severe dehydration or electrolyte disturbance is with oral fluids, ideally in the form of oral rehydration solutions (ORS), which replace lost water and electrolytes. Intravenous rehydration is only necessary if oral rehydration is not tolerated or is unsuccessful. Half-strength formula milk should not be used; once the child has recovered, they can go straight back onto their normal milk. If ORS is not tolerated orally, then it can be given via a nasogastric tube rather than progressing immediately to intravenous therapy.

Bacteria such as *Escherichia coli, Salmonella* and *Shigella* also cause diarrhoea. Bacterial gastroenteritis may result in diarrhoea that is more frequent but lower in volume than viral causes, and blood and mucus are often apparent in the stool. Again rehydration is the initial management. Antimicrobials are only used in certain infections. Antimotility agents are not indicated for infectious diarrhoea.

Other causes of acute diarrhoea include appendicitis, intussusception, overflow from constipation and colitis due to inflammatory bowel disease. Chronic diarrhoea can be found in inflammatory bowel disease, malabsorption (e.g. cystic fibrosis, coeliac disease) and parasitic infestations. Toddler's diarrhoea is a normal variant whereby thriving toddlers present with chronic non-specific loose stools, often with bits of undigested food. Diagnosis is one of exclusion, and no treatment is required.

44. ABDOMINAL PAIN IN A CHILD (2)

C – Mesenteric adenitis

Mesenteric adenitis describes inflammation of the intra-abdominal lymph nodes. It is usually associated with, or follows, an upper respiratory tract infection or gastroenteritis. Mesenteric adenitis often mimics appendicitis and commonly presents with right iliac fossa pain. Features that may be helpful in distinguishing the two are a high-grade fever (>38.5°C), shifting tenderness, lack of rebound tenderness and absence of anorexia in mesenteric adenitis. There is no specific investigation, and it is a diagnosis of exclusion. Mesenteric adenitis is a self-limiting condition and treatment is conservative (analgesia and antipyretics).

Urinary tract infections can also present with abdominal pain, but in this case the urine dipstick does not support the diagnosis. Remember that in children pain can be poorly localized and that lower lobe pneumonia can present with abdominal pain. Constipation often causes abdominal pain, which can present acutely. Children with constipation can present with overflow diarrhoea, so they may open their bowels daily but no formed or substantial amount of stool is passed. Hard, impacted faeces can often be felt when performing an abdominal examination. Other medical causes of abdominal pain include gastroenteritis, diabetic ketoacidosis and Henoch–Schönlein purpura, due to widespread vasculitis.

45. CYANOSIS

B – Polycythaemia

Cyanosis is detected clinically when there is >5 g/dL of deoxygenated haemoglobin. Polycythaemia is defined as a central venous haematocrit of >0.65. Haematocrit is a measure of blood viscosity and is also known as the packed cell volume (PCV). Hyperviscosity can present with jitteriness, lethargy, hypotonia, hyperbilirubinaemia, hypoglycaemia, seizures, stroke, renal vein thrombosis and necrotizing enterocolitis. Because the haemoglobin level is so high in polycythaemia (17 g/dL in this case), it is very easy for these infants to achieve >5 g/dL deoxygenated haemoglobin and therefore appear cyanosed.

Transposition of the great vessels and tetralogy of Fallot are both cyanotic congenital heart defects. The nitrogen washout test (also known as the hyperoxia test) involves taking a preductal arterial blood gas and then repeating the blood gas after applying 100% oxygen for 10 to 15 minutes (i.e. washing out the nitrogen). A low PaO_2 (<20 kPa) after 10 to 15 minutes of 100% oxygen suggests a fixed right-to-left shunt (e.g. tetralogy of Fallot).

With these features, you would be right to be concerned about congenital sepsis. The C-reactive protein (CRP) of <5 mg/L is very reassuring, though you would want to start empirical antibiotics until the blood culture returns negative. The key result described here is the haematocrit of 0.69, which is diagnostic of polycythaemia. Management would initially involve intravenous fluids to 'dilute' the blood. Exchange transfusion could also be considered.

46. MANAGEMENT OF DEHYDRATION

E – 48 hours

This boy likely has diabetic ketoacidosis (DKA). However, to make a diagnosis of DKA the patient must have ketones in the urine or blood and have a pH <7.3 with hyperglycaemia. The clinical history may include polyuria, polydipsia, weight loss, abdominal pain, weakness, vomiting or confusion. This patient is dehydrated and will require slow rehydration over 48 hours, initially with normal saline. Rapid correction of dehydration and a rapid drop in the blood glucose can cause cerebral oedema and therefore should be avoided. Meticulous attention to electrolytes, glucose levels and fluid balance is required to avoid complications.

During a period of hyperglycaemia, the intracellular osmolality in the brain rises slowly with the increasing glucose. If the blood glucose is dropped too quickly, an osmotic shift of fluid into the brain tissues can occur. Signs of neurological deterioration include headache, irritability, slowing heart rate, raised blood pressure and a reduced conscious level. The first step with these signs would be to rule out hypoglycaemia. If raised intracranial pressure is suspected, it needs to be treated aggressively with fluid restriction (two-thirds of the normal intake), intravenous mannitol and ITU admission for ventilation.

The gold standard algorithm for managing DKA has been produced by the British Society of Paediatric Endocrinology and Diabetes (BSPED).*

---

* BSPED recommended DKA guidelines, 2009. Available at www.bsped.org.uk/clinical/docs/ DKAGuideline.pdf

47. THE VOMITING INFANT (2)

E – Urinary tract infection

Vomiting in children is a very non-specific symptom. The most likely cause of vomiting in infants and young children is infection, but it is important to rule out surgical causes. A surgical cause is often associated with a tender or distended abdomen, no bowel movements and the cardinal sign of bilious vomiting, which must always be taken seriously. Bilious vomit in the newborn is green.

Gastroenteritis is a common cause of vomiting, though other infections such as tonsillitis and otitis media often only present with vomiting and fever. More serious infections, such as meningitis and pneumonia, are also associated with vomiting, as is diabetic ketoacidosis. More obscure causes such as intracranial pathology, drugs, poisons and metabolic diseases should also be considered.

This child is most likely to have a urinary tract infection (UTI) as the urine is both leucocyte and nitrite positive. UTIs in children often present with fever and vomiting alone. Otitis media and tonsillitis are ruled out by examination. Meningitis is unlikely in a relatively well child with a positive urine dipstick.

48. ARTERIAL BLOOD GASES (2)

B – Metabolic alkalosis (uncompensated)

The history and results are strongly suggestive of pyloric stenosis. The classical blood gas findings are that of a hypokalaemic, hypochloraemic metabolic alkalosis, due to the loss of acid and the renal excretion of K^+ ions in return for H^+ (in an effort to compensate for the alkalosis). The hypertrophied pylorus is often palpable in the abdomen when giving the baby a feed (known as the test feed). Definitive management is by surgical incision through the longitudinal and circular muscle of the pylorus (pyloromyotomy or Ramstedt's procedure). On this blood gas, the blood oxygen level appears low, but this is to be expected as the sample was venous (deoxygenated) blood. An arterial sample would give a more accurate representation of respiratory function but is painful and difficult in this age group.

Although named for Conrad Ramstedt, a German surgeon (1867–1963), who first performed the procedure in 1911, the first pyloromyotomy was actually performed in 1910 by Harold Stiles, a British surgeon (1863–1946).

49. INVESTIGATION OF THE UNWELL NEONATE

C – Blood sugar level

If you had arrived while this newborn was apnoeic (not breathing), the priority would have been to manage the airway and provide respiratory breaths with a bag and mask. Use the mnemonic ABC-DEFG (airway, breathing, circulation, don't ever forget glucose) in any resuscitation situation involving children. This is particularly important if there has been a seizure-like episode. In this case, the blood sugar was 0.9 mmol/L. A bolus of 10% dextrose (5 mL/kg) was given with success.

A newborn that has an apnoea and is hypoglycaemic could also easily have a serious infection and you should therefore perform a full blood count, C-reactive protein and blood culture. Empirical antibiotics (e.g. gentamicin and amoxicillin) should be commenced until infection has been ruled out. A blood gas would also be useful as metabolic disease can also cause hypoglycaemia and the apnoea may be due to respiratory compromise.

50. DEVELOPMENTAL MILESTONES (2)

C – 18 months

It is important to know the developmental milestones, but it is also equally important to know at what age to worry if a milestone has not been reached.

There are four areas of development:

- Gross motor
- Fine motor and vision
- Hearing and language
- Social

It is useful when assessing the child to look at the areas individually as some children may be delayed in only one aspect of their development. Every book gives slightly different milestones for different ages, so it is therefore useful to learn ranges rather than exact ages.

Practice Paper 5: Questions

1. ALCOHOL USE (1)

A 29-year-old man admits to drinking three pints of normal strength beer every lunchtime, two 175 mL glasses of red wine and four single (25 mL) measures of vodka each evening.

How many units of alcohol does he consume each day?

A. 10 units
B. 11.5 units
C. 12 units
D. 13 units
E. 17 units

2. BIPOLAR DISORDER (1)

A 46-year-old woman is brought into hospital by the police. She had been found 'behaving inappropriately' in the town centre, walking around in her underwear and declaring she was spending all her lottery winnings. On examination, her speech is pressured and she is overly amorous towards the doctor assessing her.

Which of the following symptoms is *not* consistent with mania?

A. Grandiose delusions
B. Flight of ideas
C. Increased need for sleep
D. Reckless spending
E. Reduced social inhibitions

3. CAUSES OF WEIGHT LOSS (1)

A 32-year-old woman presents to the general practitioner complaining that her periods have stopped. She has lost 20 kg from her normal healthy weight over the past few months and is now 38 kg. She admits to strict dieting and exercising excessively in an attempt to reduce her weight. Her motivation is to change the way she looks; she says she is embarrassed by her obesity.

Which of the following is the most likely cause for her weight loss?

A. Anorexia nervosa
B. Bulimia nervosa
C. Hyperthyroidism
D. Mania
E. Obsessive–compulsive disorder

4. THE MENTAL HEALTH ACT (1)

A 21-year-old man is found wandering the streets by a police officer. He appears distressed, disorientated and is muttering to himself. He becomes instantly aggressive and states the police cannot touch him as he is the son of God.

Under which Section of the Mental Health Act 1983 can the police officer take the man from a public place to a place of safety?

A. Section 2
B. Section 3
C. Section 5(2)
D. Section 135
E. Section 136

5. COGNITIVE IMPAIRMENT

A 76-year-old man is seen on the ward round by the house officer a day after his elective left knee replacement. She is surprised that the patient cannot remember that he has had an operation.

Which of the following is suggestive of a diagnosis of dementia rather than delirium?

A. A score of 27 on the mini mental state examination
B. Abrupt onset
C. Clouding of consciousness
D. Concurrent infection
E. Insidious onset

6. PSYCHIATRY OF SEXUALITY (1)

A 54-year-old man sees his general practitioner complaining of gradually worsening impotence over the last year. He is in debt and had found out 2 months ago that his wife was having an affair. He admitted to drinking up to 40 units of alcohol per week. His past medical history includes hypertension, for which he takes atenolol.

What is the most appropriate initial management plan?

A. Psychosexual counselling
B. Self-help exercises
C. Sildenafil
D. Stop atenolol and reduce alcohol consumption
E. Use of a vacuum constriction device

7. ALCOHOL USE (2)

The recommended weekly consumption of alcohol for men should not exceed:

A. 7 units
B. 14 units
C. 21 units
D. 28 units
E. 30 units

8. DIAGNOSIS OF DEMENTIA (1)

A 68-year-old woman presents with sudden-onset loss of concentration and worsening confusion. This has become progressively more severe on many discrete occasions without recovery in between.

What is the most likely cause of her confusion?

A. Lewy body dementia
B. Normal pressure hydrocephalus
C. Parkinson disease
D. Pick disease
E. Vascular dementia

9. DIAGNOSIS OF SCHIZOPHRENIA

A 20-year-old woman presents with evidence of delusions of a religious nature, persecutory auditory hallucinations and thought broadcasting. According to her mother, these symptoms have been present for the last 2 weeks.

According to ICD-10 criteria, how long should symptoms be present before a probable diagnosis of schizophrenia can be made?

A. Greater than or equal to 2 weeks
B. Greater than or equal to 1 month
C. Greater than or equal to 2 months
D. Greater than or equal to 6 months
E. Unspecified duration

10. SUBSTANCE USE (1)

A 63-year-old man is admitted to hospital with an exacerbation of chronic obstructive pulmonary disease (COPD). On the third day, he complains of sweating and tremor. On examination, he is confused, anxious, tachycardic and appears to be responding to visual hallucinations. He says he can see thousands of miniature soldiers marching on the floor.

Which of the following is the most likely cause?

A. Alcohol use
B. Alcohol withdrawal
C. Amphetamine withdrawal
D. Sedative use
E. Sedative withdrawal

11. ELECTROCONVULSIVE THERAPY (1)

A 42-year-old woman is about to undergo electroconvulsive therapy. Her family asks you about the possible side effects.

Which of the following is recognized as a late side effect of this therapy?

A. Death
B. Hallucinations
C. Headaches
D. Memory loss
E. Muscle aches

12. SIDE EFFECTS OF PSYCHIATRIC MEDICATION (1)

A 62-year-old man has been taking haloperidol for schizophrenia since his initial diagnosis 20 years ago. On examination, he displays continual facial movements, which look as though he is chewing his own mouth. These movements have been present for some time.

From which one of the following side effects is he suffering?

A. Acute dystonia
B. Akathisia
C. Parkinsonism
D. Serotonin syndrome
E. Tardive dyskinesia

13. DEMENTIA

An 81-year-old man has a 10-month history of worsening forgetfulness. He has, however, had frequent episodes of relative lucidity during this period. He occasionally sees dogs running around his house, although he does not own any, and his walking has slowed markedly. His sleeping pattern is now irregular.

Which of the following descriptions suggests a clinical diagnosis of Lewy body dementia?

A. Bradykinesia, limb rigidity, repeated falls
B. Fluctuating cognition, recurrent auditory hallucinations
C. Motor features of Parkinsonism, fluctuating cognition
D. Recurrent visual hallucinations, syncope
E. Transient loss of continence, visual hallucinations

14. PERSONALITY DISORDERS (1)

A 35-year-old man attends the general practice because he is concerned about his partner. He has become very suspicious of her and feels he cannot trust her. Although he does not know why he feels like this, he has various possible conspiratorial explanations.

Which of the following personality disorders is most appropriate?

A. Dissocial
B. Emotionally unstable – impulsive type
C. Paranoid
D. Schizoid
E. Schizotypal

15. FEATURES OF DEPRESSION (1)

A 78-year-old woman is assessed in the emergency department following a deliberate overdose of 70 paracetamol tablets. She mentions that she has been feeling very under the weather this week and she had no one to talk to.

Which of the following features would suggest a better prognosis of her mood in this case?

A. Acute onset
B. Associated personality disorder
C. Insidious onset
D. Lack of social support network
E. Older age group

16. FEATURES OF SCHIZOPHRENIA (1)

An 18-year-old male with a previous diagnosis of schizophrenia complains of hearing voices and difficulty in concentration, and he has become socially withdrawn. He is rather quiet at interview and does not respond to questions apart from one-word answers.

Which one of the following positive symptoms of schizophrenia does he have?

A. Anhedonia
B. Blunted affect
C. Hallucinations
D. Poverty of speech
E. Poverty of thought

17. PSYCHIATRY OF SEXUALITY (2)

A 32-year-old man has begun to gain sexual excitement from soft materials such as wool and cotton. He is now relying on it in order to become aroused.

Which of the following words best describes his behaviour?

A. Exhibitionism
B. Fetishism
C. Sadomasochism
D. Transvestism
E. Voyeurism

18. FIRST-RANK SYMPTOMS

A 29-year-old man complains to his general practitioner that a colleague at work has been deleting the ideas from his head before he has had time to say them or to write them down. He is referred to the psychiatrist with a presumptive diagnosis of schizophrenia.

Which one of the following is *also* a first-rank symptom of schizophrenia?

A. Grandiose delusions
B. Nihilistic delusions
C. Second person auditory hallucinations
D. Thought broadcasting
E. Visual hallucinations

19. MANAGEMENT OF PSYCHOSIS

A 38-year-old man attends the general practice for monitoring his anti-psychotic medication. The 'traffic light' notification system is used for the monitoring of which antipsychotic drug?

A. Chlorpromazine
B. Clozapine
C. Olanzapine
D. Quetiapine
E. Risperidone

20. MINI MENTAL STATE EXAMINATION

A 72-year-old man is being assessed by a psychiatrist for memory impairment. He scores 20 on the mini mental state examination.

Which of the following scores is suggestive of cognitive impairment?

A. Less than 30
B. Less than 28
C. Less than 25
D. Less than 20
E. Less than 15

21. SLEEP DISORDERS (1)

A 22-year-old woman complains of problems staying awake during the day. She often falls asleep at inappropriate moments and has occasionally collapsed when she has fallen asleep in a standing position. The periods of sleep are of a sudden onset but last only a few minutes.

Which of the following terms best describes this sleep disorder?

A. Hypersomnia
B. Insomnia
C. Narcolepsy
D. Sleep apnoea
E. Somnambulism

22. MOVEMENT DISORDERS

A 34-year-old woman with severe mania was found in her hospital bedroom sitting on the floor. She was staring towards one of the walls with an elated look on her face but did not respond to the commands of the nursing staff.

Which of the following terms best describes her behaviour?

A. Echopraxia
B. Hyperkinesis
C. Motor tic
D. Negativism
E. Stupor

23. TRANSCULTRAL PSYCHIATRIC DISORDERS (1)

A 33-year-old man living in Malaysia had a gun, which used to belong to his father, in his house. One day, he grabbed it, shot his family and ran outside shooting passers-by before finally taking his own life. He had no previous psychiatric history, and there was no obvious motive.

Which of the following terms describes this condition?

A. Amok
B. Dhat
C. Koro
D. Latah
E. Susto

24. BIPOLAR DISORDER (2)

A 21-year-old man is found breakdancing in a fast food restaurant. He says that he is the best breakdancer in the world and that he felt it was only right that everyone should be able to witness his talents. He has been awake for the last 60 hours practising at home. This is his second such episode in a month.

Which of the following is the first-line drug for stabilizing his mood?

A. Fluoxetine
B. Haloperidol
C. Lithium
D. Clozapine
E. Lamotrigine

25. NEUROLEPTIC MALIGNANT SYNDROME

A 32-year-old man with schizophrenia has recently had an increase in his dose of clozapine. He presented to the emergency department unconscious with muscle rigidity. Initial blood tests revealed a raised white cell count and a creatine kinase of 5000 IU/L.

Which of the following is not a common feature of neuroleptic malignant syndrome?

A. Altered consciousness
B. Hypothermia
C. Increased creatine kinase
D. Muscle rigidity
E. Tachycardia

26. THE MENTAL HEALTH ACT (2)

A 35-year-old woman is admitted to a psychiatric unit with a probable diagnosis of postpartum psychosis. She is very distressed, states she is not ill and threatens to leave the ward.

Under which Section of the Mental Health Act 1983 may a doctor prevent her from leaving hospital?

A. Section 2
B. Section 4
C. Section 5(2)
D. Section 5(4)
E. Section 136

27. SYNDROMES IN PSYCHIATRY (1)

A 32-year-old woman attends the general practitioner in tears. She is upset because she thinks that the man at home with her is not her husband but someone disguised as her husband. Her sister, who is with her, tells the doctor that this is not true.

From which of the following conditions is she suffering?

A. Capgras syndrome
B. Couvade syndrome
C. de Clérambault syndrome
D. Folie à deux
E. Fregoli syndrome

28. NEUROTIC DISORDERS (1)

A 30-year-old soldier returns from 6 months' duty in Afghanistan, during which time he witnessed the death of a close friend from a land-mine explosion. He now describes poor sleep, 'flashbacks' of the event and irritability.

Which of the following is a risk factor for developing this condition?

A. Caucasian ethnicity
B. Low self-esteem
C. Higher social class
D. Male sex
E. Psychopathic traits

29. PERSONALITY DISORDERS (2)

A 23-year-old woman has had a string of intense and unstable relationships. She is often unpredictable. She also has a history of deliberate self-harm.

From which of the following types of personality disorders is she most likely suffering?

A. Anankastic
B. Avoidant
C. Emotionally unstable, borderline
D. Emotionally unstable, impulsive
E. Histrionic

30. ELECTROCONVULSIVE THERAPY (2)

A 56-year-old man has been referred by his psychiatrist for electroconvulsive therapy.

Which of the following is *not* an indication for such intervention?

A. Catatonia
B. Neuroleptic malignant syndrome
C. Prolonged manic episode
D. Severe depression
E. Treatment-resistant dementia

31. CAUSES OF WEIGHT LOSS (2)

A 62-year-old man with a history of persistent low mood presents to his general practitioner with weight loss and lethargy. He has lost 10 kg in the last month, but he denies having had any desire to do so. He says that he has had increasing difficulty swallowing solid foods and a has had reduced appetite.

Which of the following is the most likely cause of his weight loss?

A. Anorexia nervosa
B. Bulimia nervosa
C. Depression
D. Hyperthyroidism
E. Malignancy

32. PSYCHIATRIC DISORDERS RELATING TO WOMEN'S HEALTH (1)

A 30-year-old woman gave birth to her first child 3 days ago. It was a planned pregnancy, and there were no physical problems with the delivery or the baby. She has no past psychiatric history but has become inconsolably tearful, anxious and low in mood today.

Which of the following is the most likely diagnosis?

A. Maternity blues
B. Postnatal depression
C. Premenstrual syndrome
D. Pseudocyesis
E. Puerperal psychosis

33. DIAGNOSIS OF DEMENTIA (2)

A 37-year-old man is brought to the general practitioner by his wife because he is becoming less socially responsive and motivated. She feels he has declined gradually over the last year but has become much worse in the last few days. When asked his name, he stares blankly at the floor and says 'I don't know'. Similar responses are given for other simple questions, and the man claims it is because he has lost his memory. He has previously been fit and well and has no other symptoms.

What is the most likely cause of his symptoms?

A. Creutzfeldt–Jakob disease
B. HIV dementia
C. Huntington disease
D. Pseudodementia
E. Vascular dementia

34. PSYCHIATRIC SIGNS OF PHYSICAL ILLNESS

A 34-year-old woman presents to her general practitioner complaining of feeling sad all the time, difficulty sleeping and of weight gain. She has a history of severe asthma and is taking medication regularly for frequent exacerbations.

Which of the following conditions is most likely to be causing her mood problems?

A. Cushing syndrome
B. Delirium
C. Hypothyroidism
D. Neurosyphilis
E. Space-occupying lesion

35. NEUROTIC DISORDERS (2)

A 32-year-old man is brought to the general practitioner by his wife because he is always distressed. He worries excessively over trivial issues at work and home, and his muscles always feel tense. His mother died last year after a long illness, but there has been no recent change in his circumstances.

From which of the following conditions is he most likely suffering?

A. Acute stress reaction
B. Generalized anxiety disorder
C. Panic disorder
D. Social phobia
E. Undifferentiated somatoform disorder

36. FEATURES OF SCHIZOPHRENIA (2)

According to ICD-10 criteria, which of the following options describe the key features of hebephrenic schizophrenia?

A. Delusions and hallucinations
B. Disorganized speech and behaviour and flat affect
C. Meets the criteria for schizophrenia, but no specific symptom subtype predominates
D. Previous positive symptoms, now less marked, with prominent negative symptoms
E. Psychomotor disturbance

37. PERSONALITY DISORDERS (3)

A 42-year-old woman is described by her husband as being increasingly preoccupied with order and control. She is often doubtful, indecisive, cautious and pedantic.

From which of the following type of personality disorder is she most likely suffering?

A. Anankastic
B. Anxious (avoidant)
C. Antisocial
D. Paranoid
E. Schizoid

38. THOUGHT DISORDERS

A 20-year-old woman says that her mind is racing – so much so that she can barely speak fast enough to express all her thoughts. She speaks rapidly, frequently changing the subject without explaining her meaning.

Which of the following terms best describes this thought disorder?

A. Delusion
B. Flight of ideas
C. Obsession
D. Overvalued idea
E. Monomania

39. PSYCHIATRIC DISORDERS RELATING TO WOMEN'S HEALTH (2)

A 32-year-old woman is in her first pregnancy. She has been spotted in public talking to her unborn baby while doing the shopping. Her behaviour has been concerning some passers-by. She has no previous psychiatric history.

What is the most likely diagnosis?

A. Couvade syndrome
B. Cyclic psychosis
C. Normal behaviour
D. Pseudocyesis
E. Puerperal psychosis

40. FEATURES OF DEPRESSION (2)

Which of the following is not a key symptom of depression?

A. Anhedonia
B. Delusions of poverty
C. Disturbed sleep
D. Low energy
E. Reduced appetite

41. PSYCHIATRY OF SEXUALITY (3)

A 27-year-old woman describes a preference for sexual activity that involves bondage or inflicting pain on her partner.

Which of the following words best describes this definition?

A. Exhibitionism
B. Fetishism
C. Masochism
D. Sadism
E. Voyeurism

42. SIDE EFFECTS OF PSYCHIATRIC MEDICATION (2)

A 42-year-old woman presents to the emergency department with sweating, fever, agitation and confusion. On examination, she is shocked and has overactive reflexes. Routine observations reveal a heart rate of 118/min and a blood pressure of 186/106 mmHg. She denies illicit drug use but has recently been prescribed tramadol for chronic back pain. Her repeat prescription includes paracetamol, fluoxetine, a salbutamol inhaler and aspirin.

From which of the following conditions is she suffering?

A. Acute dystonia
B. Hyperthyroidism
C. Neuroleptic malignant syndrome
D. Opioid toxicity
E. Serotonin syndrome

43. SLEEP DISORDERS (2)

A 5-year-old girl wakes suddenly during the night, screaming. She seems very distressed. She is unable to explain why she is upset and returns to sleep after 10 minutes. The next morning the girl cannot remember the previous night's events.

Which of the following terms best describes this scenario?

A. Night terrors
B. Nightmares
C. Non-organic disorder of the sleep–wake cycle
D. Psychiatric disorder causing sleep disturbance
E. Somnambulism

44. SPEECH DISORDERS

A 32-year-old man being investigated for confusion asks, 'Please may I use the Internet... net... net... net'?

Which of the following terms best describes this speech?

A. Dysarthria
B. Expressive aphasia
C. Logorrhoea
D. Neologism
E. Perseveration

45. SUBSTANCE USE (2)

A 91-year-old man is an inpatient on an orthopaedic ward following an elective knee replacement. The nursing staff said he vomited earlier and has been poorly responsive since his operation 12 hours ago. On examination, you noticed his pupils are 2 mm and reactive and he has a respiratory rate of eight breaths per minute.

Which of the following is the most likely cause?

A. Alcohol withdrawal
B. Opiate use
C. Opiate withdrawal
D. Sedative use
E. Sedative withdrawal

46. PSYCHIATRY OF SEXUALITY (4)

An 18-year-old boy feels that he is a woman trapped in a man's body. He has changed his name to Sarah (from Sean), often goes out wearing women's clothes and is trying to get a sex change.

Which of the following words best describes his behaviour?

A. Homosexuality
B. Sadism
C. Transvestic fetishism
D. Transsexualism
E. Voyeurism

47. SYNDROMES IN PSYCHIATRY (2)

A 34-year-old man is being assessed by a psychiatrist for severe depression. The patient tells the psychiatrist that he is dead, that his arms and legs are rotting away. Further questioning elicits that he firmly believes this.

From which of the following conditions is he suffering?

A. Cotard syndrome
B. Ekbom syndrome
C. Ganser syndrome
D. Othello syndrome
E. Rett syndrome

48. SELF-HARM

A 30-year-old woman is admitted to hospital after taking an overdose of paracetamol. This is her first such episode.

What is her risk of completed suicide over the next year?

A. 0.1%
B. 1%
C. 5%
D. 10%
E. 40%

49. THE MENTAL HEALTH ACT (3)

A 22-year-old man is brought to the emergency department by his approved mental health practitioner on a Saturday night, behaving strangely. His only speech is an impersonation of a rap artist, which he does while breakdancing. He has a history of bipolar affective disorder. His social worker says that the man has stopped sleeping, and he thinks this is a manic episode. No one is available to admit the patient under Section 2 or 3.

For how long can the emergency department doctor admit the patient?

A. 6 hours
B. 24 hours
C. 48 hours
D. 72 hours
E. 7 days

50. TRANSCULTURAL PSYCHIATRIC DISORDERS (2)

A 28-year-old woman living in the Arctic Circle has a sudden-onset episode of bizarre behaviour. Her friends say that she began crying and shouting hysterically, took off her clothes and started throwing large objects. She had to be physically restrained. Later, she had no recollection of the episode.

Which of the following terms describes this behaviour?

A. Generalized anxiety disorder
B. Latah
C. Piblokto
D. Susto
E. Windigo

Practice Paper 5: Answers

1. ALCOHOL USE (1)

D – 13 units

A unit of alcohol is defined as 10 mL of ethanol (around 8 g). It is the equivalent to the amount an adult can metabolize in one hour. The number of units per given volume of drink is calculated using the percentage of alcohol by volume (usually labelled 'ABV' on the container) as follows:

$$\text{Number of units in given drink} = \frac{\text{volume of drink (mL)} \times \%\text{ABV}}{1000}$$

The average number of units in common drinks is:

- 1 pint of beer   →   2 units
- 1 small (175 mL) glass of wine   →   1.5 units
- 1 measure (25 mL) of spirit   →   1 unit

So in this scenario, this man drinks 6 units in beer, 3 units in wine and 4 units in vodka each day, totalling 13 units.

2. BIPOLAR DISORDER (1)

C – Increased need for sleep

Manic episodes present with elevated mood in 70% of cases and an irritable mood in 80% of cases. Biological symptoms of mania are decreased need for sleep, increased energy and psychomotor agitation. Cognitive symptoms include decreased concentration, flight of ideas and lack of insight. Manic patients sometimes display thought disorders, such as circumstantiality (where the speaker eventually gets to the point in a very roundabout manner) and tangential speech (where the speaker digresses further and further away from the initial topic via a series of loose associations). Psychotic features include grandiose or persecutory delusions, hyperacusis and hyperaesthesia. First-rank symptoms occur in 20% of cases. In extreme cases, there is manic stupor, in which the patient is unresponsive, akinetic, mute and fully conscious, with elated facies.

3. CAUSES OF WEIGHT LOSS (1)

A – Anorexia nervosa

A diagnosis of anorexia nervosa requires all four of the following:

- Body weight 15% below expected or body mass index (BMI) <17.5
- Self-induced weight loss (by dieting, exercising, vomiting, etc.)
- Morbid fear of being fat (an overvalued idea rather than a delusion)
- Endocrine disturbance (e.g. amenorrhoea, pubertal delay, lanugo hair)

The incidence of anorexia is 4 per 100,000 with a peak age of 18 years. Around 10% of cases of anorexia occur in males. Risk factors include being Caucasian, high social class, academic prowess and interests such as ballet or modelling. Other common features are anaemia, expressing a high interest in preparing or buying food, feeling tired and cold, bradycardia and hypotension. Treatment options include cognitive behavioural therapy (CBT)/supportive therapy and raising calorie intake. Hospitalization is indicated if there is weight loss of more than 35%. Around 50% of people with anorexia nervosa eventually recover completely. Mortality is 5%, usually from starvation or suicide. Anorexia can have two subtypes: (i) restrictive and (ii) binge eating/purging.

A diagnosis of bulimia nervosa requires all three of the following:

- Binge eating
- Methods to prevent gaining weight (e.g. vomiting, purging, laxatives, etc.)
- Morbid dread of fatness (overvalued idea, not a delusion)

The incidence of bulimia is 12 per 100,000 with females being affected 10 times more commonly than males. Individuals tend to be of a normal or above-normal weight. Complications are caused by starvation and vomiting and include hypokalaemia, dehydration, enlargement of the parotid glands, dental caries, Mallory–Weiss tear, osteoporosis and Russell's sign (thick skin on the dorsum of the hands due to repeated induced vomiting by stimulating the gag reflex with the fingers). Treatment is similar to that of anorexia but selective serotonin reuptake inhibitors may improve bingeing behaviour. Seventy percent of cases recover within 5 years, and there is no increase in mortality.

Anorexia, from Greek *an* = without + *orexe* = appetite.
Bulimia, from Greek *bous* = ox + *limos* = hunger.

4. THE MENTAL HEALTH ACT (1)

E – Section 136

These are all sections from Part II of the Mental Health Act for England and Wales 1983. They relate to compulsory detainment in hospital of patients with a psychiatric disorder that requires treatment. Around 90% of psychiatric admissions to hospital are on a voluntary (informal) basis.

Patients and their nearest relatives have the right to appeal against their detainment. This may go to Mental Health Act managers or to a mental health review tribunal, which has the authority to discharge patients. The nearest relative can also apply to discharge the patient from hospital.

The Mental Health Act was updated in 2007, specifying one small alteration to this section: '… it will not be possible for patients to be compulsorily detained or their detention continued unless medical treatment which is appropriate to the patient's mental disorder and all other circumstances of the case *is available* to that patient …'.

Section 136 is power given to the police when they perceive that the patient is at risk to themselves or to others in a public place. It allows them to remove the person to a 'place of safety'. This may be a police cell, A&E or one of the specialist 136 custody suites available in many mental health units. The limitations of Section 136 are that it may only be used in a public place and that it does not apply to private property. As a result, if a person is inside their home and is perceived to be at risk to themselves, at risk of neglect or a risk to others, a magistrate's warrant will need to be sought. These powers are under Section 135 and allow the police to break into the person's property. The warrant can only be used once and has to be used in the presence of a registered medical officer.

5. COGNITIVE IMPAIRMENT

E – Insidious onset

Dementia (meaning 'deprived of mind') can be described as a non-specific syndrome caused by several illnesses. Affected areas of cognition can be memory, attention, language and problem solving. Symptoms are usually required to be present for at least 6 months.

Delirium is characterized by fluctuating impairment of consciousness, mood changes and abnormal perceptions. It affects 10% to 25% of people over 65 years on medical wards. The patient may be obviously confused, with disruptive behaviour and expressing bizarre ideas, but it is important to recognize that delirium can also cause a decreased level of activity and speech. It develops over a short period of time and is caused by an underlying physical condition. Common causes are infection, hypoxia, electrolyte disturbances, constipation, drugs and central nervous system disease. The main principle of management is to investigate and treat the cause but to concurrently help relieve distress to the patient by optimizing their ability to orientate themselves. There should be a calm environment with adequate lighting, even at night. Patients should be wearing their glasses and hearing aids (if applicable), have continuity of staff contact where possible and ideally have family members or familiar belongings around them. In some circumstances, oral or intramuscular haloperidol or benzodiazepines can be used to relieve severe agitation, but they should be avoided where possible. The average duration of delirium is 7 days. Around 40% of patients with delirium die of the underlying condition and 5% go on to develop dementia.

6. PSYCHIATRY OF SEXUALITY (1)

D – Stop atenolol and reduce alcohol consumption

Psychosexual disorders are non-organic problems preventing an individual from participating in a satisfactory sexual relationship. However, there is frequently a combination of physical and psychological factors contributing to an impairment of function. In this scenario, these include marital difficulties, financial strain, excessive alcohol use and prescription drugs (atenolol). Other drugs that can cause erectile dysfunction include tricyclic antidepressants, benzodiazepines, antihistamines, oestrogens, statins and anti-Parkinsonism medication.

Stopping atenolol and reducing alcohol consumption are sensible initial measures in this case. Appropriate investigation will depend on the history. Biological causes should be ruled out (e.g. neuropathy, ischaemic vascular dysfunction, hypertension), and specialist referral may be needed. However, if psychological factors are involved, referral to a sexual and relationship clinic may be helpful. In cases of erectile failure (e.g. diabetic neuropathy), intracavernosal injection of papaverine or prostaglandin E1 can be used. Other physical treatments include vacuum device, nitrate creams and rod insertion.

7. ALCOHOL USE (2)

C – 21 units

In the UK, the recommended maximum weekly alcohol consumption is 21 units in men and 14 units in women. Obviously, these are general guidelines and certain people should limit their intake or abstain from alcohol altogether. Examples include people with chronic liver disease, low body weight or poor nourishment, those at the extremes of age and those on certain medications (some antibiotics, e.g. metronidazole, monoamine oxidase inhibitors, antihistamines, benzodiazepines and opioids).

8. DIAGNOSIS OF DEMENTIA (1)

E – Vascular dementia

Vascular dementia is an ischaemic disorder characterized by multiple small cerebral infarcts in the cortex and white matter. When >100 mL of infarcts have occurred, dementia is more likely to become clinically apparent, although this is not a hard and fast rule. Vascular dementia begins in the 60s with a step-wise deterioration of cognitive function. Other features include focal neurology, fits and nocturnal confusion. Risk factors for vascular dementia are similar to use of any atherosclerotic disease (male sex, smoking, hypertension, diabetes hypercholesterolaemia). Death in vascular dementia often occurs within 5 years, due to ischaemic heart disease or stroke.

Normal pressure hydrocephalus is characterized by the triad of dementia (mainly memory problems), gait disturbance and urinary incontinence. It is caused by an increased volume of cerebrospinal fluid (CSF) but with only a slightly raised pressure (as the ventricles dilate to compensate). There is an underlying obstruction in the subarachnoid space that prevents CSF from being reabsorbed but allows it to flow from the ventricular system into the subarachnoid space. Diagnosis is by lumbar puncture (to demonstrate a normal CSF opening pressure) followed by head CT/MRI (showing enlarged ventricles). Treatment is with ventriculoperitoneal shunting.

Pick disease is a form of frontotemporal dementia (it can only be differentiated from other forms at autopsy, so 'frontotemporal dementia' is the preferred term). Clinical features include disinhibition, inattention, antisocial behaviour and personality changes. Later on, apathy, akinesia and withdrawal may predominate. Memory loss and disorientation only occur late. Autopsy shows atrophy of the frontal and temporal lobes (knife blade atrophy) and Pick's bodies (cytoplasmic inclusion bodies of tau protein) in the substantia nigra. In advanced cases, the atrophy may be seen on MRI.

Arnold Pick, Czechoslovakian neurologist and psychiatrist (1852–1924).

9. DIAGNOSIS OF SCHIZOPHRENIA

B – Greater than or equal to 1 month

Psychosis should only lead to the diagnosis of schizophrenia if symptoms have been present for 1 month, and there is the absence of significant mood disorder, overt brain disease and drug intoxication/withdrawal. Important differential diagnoses are organic psychotic disorder, substance-induced psychotic disorder, delusional disorder, schizoaffective disorder and schizotypal disorder. The most appropriate diagnosis in this instance would be an acute and transient psychotic disorder, with the subtype 'acute schizophrenia-like psychotic disorder', as listed in ICD-10 (Code F 23.2).

10. SUBSTANCE USE (1)

B – Alcohol withdrawal

Alcohol withdrawal usually occurs if blood alcohol concentration falls in someone with alcohol dependence. Symptoms usually start approximately 12 hours after the last intake and include anxiety, insomnia, sweating, tachycardia and tremor. Seizures may occur after 48 hours. Treatment is supportive with a reducing dose of regular benzodiazepines (e.g. chlordiazepoxide) and vitamin B supplements (intravenous or oral). Mortality is approximately 5%.

Delirium tremens may also be a feature of alcohol withdrawal and occurs after 48 hours, lasting for 5 days. There is tremor, restlessness and increased autonomic activity, fluctuating consciousness with disorientation, a fearful affect and hallucinations. Hallucinations may be auditory, tactile or visual and delusions may also be present. Lilliputian hallucinations (seeing little people) are characteristic (named after the island of Lilliput in Jonathan Swift's novel *Gulliver's Travels*, where the inhabitants were 'not six inches high'). Delirium tremens is caused by damage to the mammillary bodies (part of the limbic system and located near the hypothalamus). Early diagnosis and treatment on a medical ward are essential as mortality rates can be high.

11. ELECTROCONVULSIVE THERAPY (1)

D – Memory loss

Electroconvulsive therapy (ECT) is the administration of an electric shock to the head (under general anaesthesia) in order to induce a seizure. The indications are severe depressive illness, especially if there is life-threatening behaviour, puerperal depressive illness, mania and catatonic schizophrenia. The absolute contraindication is raised intracranial pressure. Relative contraindications include high anaesthetic risk and known cerebral aneurysm. Long-term side effects of ECT are largely unknown, but some patients have complained of long-term memory loss. Short-term side effects are headaches, temporary confusion, muscle aches and some short-term memory loss.

12. SIDE EFFECTS OF PSYCHIATRIC MEDICATION (1)

E – Tardive dyskinesia

Typical antipsychotics block dopamine D2 receptors in the central nervous system in various pathways. This accounts for both their therapeutic results and side effects. The effect on the mesolimbic pathway improves psychotic symptoms, but action on the mesocortical pathway worsens negative symptoms. The effect on the tuberoinfundibular pathway causes the side effect of hyperprolactinaemia (→ gynaecomastia, galactorrhoea, amenorrhoea and reduced libido). Action on the chemoreceptor trigger zone has an antiemetic property.

The consequences of nigrostriatal pathway blockade are the extrapyramidal side effects. These include Parkinsonism (rigidity, bradykinesia and tremor, which can begin within 1 month and are treated with anticholinergics, e.g. procyclidine); acute dystonias (occur within 72 hours of treatment and include trismus, tongue protrusion, spasmodic torticollis, opisthotonus, oculogyric crisis and grimacing); akathisia (occurs within 60 days and features a subjective feeling of inner tension and restless leg syndrome but can be treated with β-blockers and benzodiazepines) and tardive dyskinesia (affects 20% in the long term and presents with chewing, grimacing, sucking and a darting tongue). Tardive dyskinesia is hypothesized to be caused by dopamine receptor hypersensitivity.

Other side effects of typical antipsychotics are anticholinergic effects, which cause an increased QT interval, arrhythmias and cardiac arrest; α-adrenoreceptor blocking action causes postural hypotension, and antihistamine activity causes sedation and weight gain. Chlorpromazine specifically causes greying of the skin in response to sunlight, and a reduced seizure threshold.

13. DEMENTIA

C – Motor features of Parkinsonism, fluctuating cognition

Lewy body dementia is the second most common dementia after Alzheimer. (In reality, dementia with a vascular component is probably more common than Lewy body dementia, but pure vascular dementia is less frequent.) Characteristic features of Lewy body dementia include day-to-day fluctuating levels of cognitive functioning, recurrent visual hallucinations (commonly involving people or animals), sleep disturbance, transient loss of consciousness, recurrent falls and Parkinsonian features (tremor, shuffling gait, hypokinesia, rigidity and postural instability). Although people with Lewy body dementia are prone to hallucination, antipsychotics should be avoided as they precipitate severe Parkinsonism in 60%. A Lewy body is an abnormality of the cytoplasm found within a neuron, containing clumps of α-synuclein and ubiquitin protein. They are found postmortem in the cerebral cortex in patients with Lewy body dementia, and they are also found in patients with Parkinson disease.

Frederick Lewy, German neurologist (1885–1950).

14. PERSONALITY DISORDERS (1)

C – Paranoid

The ICD-10 definition of a personality disorder is 'a severe disturbance in the characterological constitution and behavioural tendencies of the individual, usually involving several areas of the personality, and nearly always associated with considerable personal and social disruption'. They often become apparent during childhood or adolescence, and continue into adulthood. The prevalence of personality disorders is probably under-reported. It is likely to affect around 10% of the population but is higher in psychiatric settings. There are several theories regarding personality and personality disorders; the dimensional approach suggests that people with personality disorders exhibit traits that feature as a spectrum in the population but to an exaggerated degree.

There are six personality disorder types (DSM-V):

- Borderline personality disorder
- Obsessive–compulsive personality disorder

- Avoidant personality disorder
- Schizotypal personality disorder
- Antisocial personality disorder
- Narcissistic personality disorder

The key features of a borderline personality disorder are impairments in personality functioning (e.g. unstable self-image, excessive self-criticism, instability in goals/aspirations) and impairments in interpersonal functioning (compromised ability of empathy and difficulty with intimacy). It is associated with emotional liability, anxiousness, separation insecurity, impulsivity and hostility.

People with an avoidant personality disorder characteristically display social withdrawal, avoidance of intimate relationships and anhedonia (deficiency in the capacity to feel pleasure or take an interest in things). There are often intense feelings of anxiety and nervousness.

An obsessive–compulsive personality disorder is associated with rigid perfectionism and perseveration (persistence at tasks long after the behaviour has ceased to be functional); there may also be difficulties with intimacy and empathy.

The pathological personality traits in schizotypal personality disorder are eccentricity (odd, unusual or bizarre behaviour/appearance), unusual thought processes and beliefs, restricted affectivity (dampened emotional reactions), suspiciousness and a preference for being alone (withdrawal).

Characteristically, in antisocial personality disorder, there is manipulativeness, callousness and hostility. There are also traits of disinhibition, as evidenced by excessive irresponsibility, impulsivity and risk-taking. Pathological personality traits in narcissistic personality disorder include grandiosity (feelings of entitlement and self-centeredness) and excessive attention-seeking.

Narcissism comes from the name of the Greek mythological figure, Narcissus, who was cursed into falling in love with his own reflection after breaking the heart of the shy nymph, Echo. (Incidentally, Echo loved the sound of her voice so much, she was herself cursed into only being able to repeat what others said.)

15. FEATURES OF DEPRESSION (1)

A – Acute onset

The lifetime risk of depression is 10% to 25% in females and 5% to 12% in males. Marital status affects the risk of depression: the highest risk group is those who are divorced, followed by people who are separated, then single, and then married. Other risk factors are having three or more children below the age of 14, unemployment, maternal death below the age of 11 and a lack of confiding relationships. An adverse life event in the previous 6 months, chronic illness, personality disorders and a family history of bipolar disorder predispose to depression. Examples of medications that increase the risk of depression include β-blockers, steroids, anticonvulsants, benzodiazepines, antipsychotics, opiates and non-steroidal anti-inflammatory drugs.

Prognostic factors associated with a better outcome in depression include acute onset and an earlier age of onset. Prognostic factors associated with a poorer outcome include insidious onset, neurotic depression, being elderly, low self-confidence, co-morbidity (physical or psychological) and a lack of social support.

16. FEATURES OF SCHIZOPHRENIA (1)

C – Hallucinations

Schizophrenia is characterized by distortions in thought and perception, with a blunted and inappropriate affect. Intellect and clear consciousness are usually maintained, although there can be cognitive decline in people who suffer from a chronic course. The most important features are first-rank symptoms, thought disorder and negative symptoms.

Positive symptoms of schizophrenia include:

- Hallucinations
- Delusions
- Thought withdrawal, insertion and broadcasting

Negative symptoms include:

- Loss of interest in others or initiative
- Anhedonia
- Blunted affect
- Reduced speech

There is a lifetime risk of 1% with a peak onset age of 26 years in females and 23 years in males. There is a slightly higher incidence in males. Risk factors include low socioeconomic class and exposure to a high level of expressed emotion (>35 hours/week). There is also a higher incidence in those with a family history, winter/spring birthdays, maternal flu infection during the second trimester of pregnancy, decreased brain volume and increased ventricle size, adverse life events and lack of social interactions. The dopamine hypothesis is a theory regarding the mechanism of schizophrenia. Briefly, it says that the symptoms are caused in part by central dopaminergic hyperactivity in the mesolimbic–mesocortical system.

Schizophrenia, from Greek *schitz* = split/shattered + *phrenes* = mind/heart.

17. PSYCHIATRY OF SEXUALITY (2)

B – Fetishism

Paraphilias are defined as disorders of sexual preference. Fetishism focuses on inanimate objects not normally viewed as being of a sexual nature that become a source of sexual stimulation (e.g. shoes, leather, etc.). Transvestic fetishism is the use of cross-dressing in order to gain sexual excitement. Exhibitionism is the tendency to expose genitalia to strangers in public places with subsequent gratification, particularly if there are reactions of shock or horror. Type 1 exhibitionism (80% cases) occurs often in young men, showing a flaccid penis. There is often remorse afterwards. Type 2 exhibitionism is the exposure of an erect penis. This is more common in people with dissocial personality types, and there is often a lack of remorse. Voyeurism is the tendency to watch other people engaging in sexual activity.

18. FIRST-RANK SYMPTOMS

D – Thought broadcasting

Kurt Schneider listed symptoms that he felt distinguished schizophrenia from other types of psychosis. He describes these 'first-rank symptoms' as being highly suggestive of schizophrenia in the absence of organic brain disease. However, they are absent in 20% of people with schizophrenia and can be present in other psychiatric disorders, such as in depression or mania. The presence of first-rank symptoms in schizophrenia is not an indicator of prognosis.

First-rank symptoms can be categorized as follows:

- Auditory hallucinations → third person, running commentary, repeating thought
- Thought alienation → thought insertion/withdrawal/broadcast
- Influences on the body → made feelings/actions/impulses
- Other → somatic passivity and delusional perception

In third-person auditory hallucinations, the patient hears the voices of more than one person discussing matters among themselves. A running commentary is one voice describing the patient's every action. Finally, the patient can experience thought sonorization (hearing their thoughts out aloud). These 'audible thoughts' can occur either at the same time of the real thoughts (gedankenlaut-werden) or just afterwards (écho de la pensée).

In thought insertion, the patient believes that thoughts are being put into their mind by an outside agency. In thought withdrawal, they feel as if their thoughts are being removed. Thought broadcasting is where the patient feels their thoughts are being made accessible to others (i.e. others can hear them).

Made feelings, actions or impulses describe when the patient feels their feelings/actions/impulses are under control of a third party and that their free will is being taken away. In delusional perception, a real perceived event leads to a different idea or incorrect conclusion without logical reasoning. Somatic passivity is where the patient feels they are receiving bodily sensations from an outside agency (e.g. an alien is twisting their intestines).

Kurt Schneider, German psychiatrist (1887–1967)

19. MANAGEMENT OF PSYCHOSIS

B – Clozapine

Clozapine is an atypical antipsychotic. NICE guidelines* recommend that clozapine should be used in treatment-resistant schizophrenia after sequential use of at least two antipsychotics for 6 to 8 weeks, at least one of which should be an 'atypical' antipsychotic. Patients on clozapine must be registered with a central monitoring agency and have regular full blood counts – the drug must be stopped if there is evidence of neutropenia, as episodes of fatal agranulocytosis have previously been reported. All patents must be registered with the Clozaril Patient Monitoring Service (CPMS), and a normal leucocyte count must be confirmed before treatment can be started. Each time a blood sample is sent to the CPMS, the results will be telephoned through, if urgent, or posted, if not. A traffic light system is sometimes used:

- Green light   Normal, clozapine can be given
- Amber light   Caution, further sampling advised
- Red light   Stop clozapine immediately, then take daily blood samples

20. MINI MENTAL STATE EXAMINATION

C – Less than 25

The mini mental state examination (or Folstein test) permits a standardized assessment of orientation (maximum 10 points), registration/concentration/recall (maximum 11 points) and concentration and language/drawing (maximum 9 points). It is scored out of a total of 30 points. A score of >27 is normal. A score of <25 suggests cognitive impairment, graded as mild (21–24), moderate (10–20) or severe (<10). It is worth noting that although the sensitivity is high, the specificity is poor and other tests may be required to confirm the diagnosis. The mini mental state examination is not very good at detecting frontal lobe abnormalities and is not a valid test for non-English speaking patients.

21. SLEEP DISORDERS (1)

C – Narcolepsy

Narcolepsy affects <0.1% of the population. It is a neurological condition caused by a loss of inhibition of rapid eye movement (REM). It has four main features: irresistible attacks of sleep at inappropriate times, cataplexy (sudden loss of muscle tone when intense emotion occurs, leading to

---

* National Collaborating Centre for Mental Health. *Schizophrenia: Care Interventions in the Treatment and Management of Schizophrenia in Primary and Secondary Care* (update). National Clinical Practice Guideline 82. London: NICE, 2009. Available at: www.nice.org.UK/nicemedia/pdf/CG82fullGuideline.pdf

collapse), hypnogogic/hypnopompic hallucinations (hallucinations that occur on falling asleep and waking, respectively) and sleep paralysis. Not all cases of narcolepsy have all four features. When forming the diagnosis, factors that point to hypersomnia are sleeps that have a gradual onset, are worse in the mornings and that rarely occur in unusual places. Factors that suggest narcolepsy are a short duration of sleep (10–20 minutes), the inability to control sleep attacks and interrupted night-time sleep, as well as the four main features. Management falls under the remit of neurologists.

Insomnia is a condition describing a reduced quantity or quality of sleep for a prolonged period. This may involve difficulty getting to sleep/staying asleep and early morning wakening. If there is an underlying cause, this should be treated. Drug treatments are limited and include short-acting benzodiazepines such as temazepam (which have less of a hangover effect compared with longer-acting ones like diazepam) or zopiclone (which is similar). However, these drugs should be used for a limited duration as use for longer than 2 weeks increases the risk of addiction. Insomnia is more common in the elderly.

Hypersomnia is defined as either excessive daytime sleepiness with sleep attacks or an abnormal length of time taken to reach full arousal after sleeping (in the absence of an organic disorder). It affects between 0.3% and 4% of the population. Somnambulism (sleep walking) is a state of altered consciousness in which there are some features of wakefulness and some of sleep. The individual usually arises from bed (during the first third of nocturnal sleep) and begins walking but with reduced awareness, reactivity and motor skill. Upon awakening, there is usually no recollection of the event. It is more common in children. Management is by reassurance, simple safety measures and gentle encouragement by the family to return to bed.

Sleep apnoea is a physical condition in which the upper respiratory tract becomes partially occluded during sleep. This can cause transient cessation in breathing, which causes the patient to wake repeatedly during the night, reducing the quality of sleep. Sleep apnoea results in daytime tiredness. It is more common in overweight males who snore. Treatment is by continuous positive airway pressure (via face mask) during sleep.

22. MOVEMENT DISORDERS

E – Stupor

Stupor describes the state of being unresponsive, akinetic and mute but fully conscious. Stupor can occur in mania (this case), depression, catatonia, epilepsy and hysteria. Obsessional slowness is a reduced rate of activity due to repeated doubts and compulsive rituals in obsessive–compulsive disorder (OCD).

Hyperkinesis is often seen in children and teenagers. It comprises overactivity, distractibility, impulsivity and excitability. Motor tics are repeated involuntary movements involving a group of muscles. Parkinsonism describes a group of characteristic movements that occur in Parkinson disease and other conditions. These include resting tremor, cogwheel rigidity, festinant gait (an involuntary tendency to making short, accelerated steps when walking) and posture abnormalities.

Movements seen in schizophrenia

Ambitendency involves making tentative incomplete movements, apparent when shaking hands. Echopraxia is the copying of another person's movements, even when asked to stop. Mannerisms are repeated involuntary movements that appear goal directed (e.g. flicking hair). Stereotypies are repeated patterns of movement that are not goal directed (e.g. moving head from side to side). Negativism is the motiveless resistance to commands and attempts to be moved. Posturing is where a bizarre body position is adopted for an inappropriately long time. Waxy flexibility is when the patient remains motionless but allows their limbs to be moved by someone else. The limbs then remain in the new posture.

23. TRANSCULTURAL PSYCHIATRIC DISORDERS (1)

A – Amok

Amok is seen in Southeast Asia, usually in Malaysian men. The features are acquisition of a weapon followed by a series of frenzied attacks, killing or seriously injuring anyone within reach. The attacks can last several hours and are frequently only terminated by the attacker being killed by someone else or killing himself. If he is not killed, amok is followed by a stupor/sleep lasting one day, followed by amnesia of the event. It is thought to be a form of dissociative disorder.

Koro is seen in Asian men, especially of Chinese origin. It is the fear that the penis is retracting into the abdomen. Some have a secondary worry that full retraction will lead to death. Koro is more common in people who have limited access to education.

Dhat occurs in young Indian males. It is associated with anxiety and a belief that semen is being lost in the urine. It often accompanies excessive guilt about masturbation. There may be a belief that semen is 'vital fluid', more so than blood, and the loss of it leads to fatigue.

Latah is a culture-bound condition found in women in North Africa and the Far East. There is an exaggerated startle response, in which women sometimes start repeating the words of another person (echolalia) or obeying their commands. Frequently, there is amnesia after the event.

Susto usually occurs in people living in South America. It is a severe depressive episode usually occurring after a traumatic event. There are often physical symptoms such as diarrhoea and nervous tics. It is thought (within the culture in which it exists) to be caused by separation of the soul from the body. It has some features in common with acute stress reaction.

Amok, from Malay *amuk* = mad with rage; it is the origin of the phrase 'to run amok'. Koro, from Malay *koro* = turtle head – retraction of the turtle's head is seen as similar to koro.

24. BIPOLAR DISORDER (2)

C – Lithium
Bipolar affective disorder is characterized by two or more episodes in which mood and activity levels are significantly disturbed. This should include at least one episode of elevation of mood and increased energy and activity (hypomania or mania) although, on other occasions, there may be a lowering of mood and decreased energy and activity (depression). There is a 1% lifetime risk, with the average age of onset being in the mid-20s. Males and females have an equal risk of developing bipolar disorder, and higher social classes have a higher risk.

Acute episodes of mania are managed with neuroleptic drugs (e.g. olanzapine or haloperidol), with benzodiazepines for agitation. Long-term prophylaxis (mood stabilizer) is most often given in the form of lithium (carbamazepine and sodium valproate may also be effective). Mood stabilizers are prescribed only if there has been more than one episode of mania. Lithium causes sustained remission in 80% of cases. Psychotherapies have a supportive role and can improve concordance with therapy. Electroconvulsive therapy is used for manic stupor and resistant mania but, if used during a depressive episode in a patient with bipolar disorder, it can precipitate mania.

25. NEUROLEPTIC MALIGNANT SYNDROME

B – Hypothermia
Neuroleptic malignant syndrome is a life-threatening neurological condition that can occur with the use of typical and atypical antipsychotics, particularly after an increase in dosage. Symptoms include pyrexia, fluctuating consciousness, muscle rigidity and autonomic dysfunction. Investigations may reveal a raised creatine kinase, raised white cell count and abnormal liver function tests. The first step in the management of this rare but potentially fatal condition includes stopping the precipitating agent and supportive measures such as benzodiazepines, oxygen, maintaining fluid balance and reducing core body temperature. Intravenous sodium bicarbonate can be used in cases of rhabdomyolysis, and dantrolene or lorazepam can be used to reduce rigidity. A dopamine agonist such as bromocriptine may also be required. Symptoms may resolve within a

week of treatment; however, this may take longer if a depot antipsychotic medication is the offending drug.

26. THE MENTAL HEALTH ACT (2)

C – Section 5(2)

Section 5(2) is doctor holding power. It allows the detention of hospital inpatients (under any speciality) by the doctor responsible for their care. It lasts 72 hours (long enough to arrange a review by a senior psychiatrist). Note that, in even more acute situations, patients can be stopped under common law for a short time if there is an immediate threat to their health or if they are an imminent risk to others. Section 5(4) is nurse holding power. This allows detention of informal psychiatry inpatients by nurses if there is no doctor available. It lasts 6 hours, allowing time for a registered medical practitioner to assess the patient.

Section 2 is compulsory detention for assessment when the exact diagnosis and response to treatment is unknown. Its duration is 28 days. Application for detention under this section can be made by the patient's nearest relative or by an approved mental health practitioner (AMHP). It must be agreed upon by two doctors (one of whom must be Section 12 approved). To become approved under Section 12(2), the doctor will have attended a specific Section 12 training course following completion of a relevant period of work experience in psychiatry (usually 3 years of experience or membership in the Royal College of Psychiatrists) and be recommended for approval by two psychiatry consultants.

Section 3 allows compulsory detention for treatment when the diagnosis is already known and treatment is available at the approved mental health unit where the patient will be detained. It lasts for 6 months but may be renewed if necessary. It must be agreed by two doctors (one of whom must be Section 12 approved).

Section 4 allows an emergency admission to hospital when there is not enough time to organize another section of the MHA. Its duration is 72 hours, and there is no right of appeal against it. It can be arranged by one doctor.

Sections 35 to 37 can be requested by a court on advice of a Section 12 approved doctor when a patient has been charged with an offence that may lead to imprisonment. Section 35 is for the purpose of producing a medical report on the psychiatric illness of the offender. The duration is 28 days. Section 36 allows treatment of the patient. It also lasts 28 days but requires two doctors to agree on it. Section 37 is for the detention and treatment of a patient already convicted of an imprisonable offence. This also requires two doctors' agreement and lasts 6 months.

Section 17 allows for set periods of leave from the inpatient unit (with a responsible adult) to be granted by the responsible clinician.

27. SYNDROMES IN PSYCHIATRY (1)

A – Capgras syndrome

Capgras syndrome is a delusional belief that a close acquaintance has been replaced by an identical double. It is most commonly seen in schizophrenia.

Fregoli syndrome is a delusion that a persecutor is able to change into many forms and disguise themselves to look like different people, much like an actor. It is named after Leopold Fregoli, an Italian actor (1867–1936) who was famous for being able to make quick changes of appearance during stage acts. *Folie a deux* is when a delusion in one person becomes shared by someone close to them. A similar effect can occur in three or more people (*folie a trios*, *folie a plusieurs*).

An individual's delusional belief that someone of higher social status is in love with them is known as de Clérambault's syndrome (erotomania). It is more common in women. Couvade syndrome occurs in males around the time of the birth of their child. They experience symptoms similar to those of pregnancy, such as nausea and dyspepsia. They may even suffer abdominal distension and labour-like contraction pains. The cause is not well understood, but symptoms usually resolve soon after birth.

Couvade, from old French *couver* = to hatch.
Folie à deux, from French *folie* = madness.
Joseph Capgras, French psychiatrist (1873–1950).
Gaetan Gatian de Clérambault, French psychiatrist (1872–1934).

28. NEUROTIC DISORDERS (1)

B – Low self-esteem

This man has developed post-traumatic stress disorder (PTSD). PTSD (shell shock) occurs secondary to a traumatic stressor (i.e. one that any 'normal' person would find stressful). Diagnostic features include:

- Experience of a major traumatic event
- Re-experiencing the trauma (nightmares, flashbacks)
- Avoidance behaviour
- Increased arousal (hypervigilance, insomnia, enhanced startle reaction)
- Onset is delayed (but within 6 months) and the features should last ≥1 month

The usual course is recovery, but occasionally symptoms become chronic.

Risk factors for PTSD include:

- Low education
- Lower social class
- Afro-Caribbean/Hispanic ethnicity

- Female sex
- Low self-esteem
- Personal or family history of psychiatric problems
- Prior traumatic events

  Protective factors include:

- High IQ
- Higher social class
- Caucasian
- Male sex
- Chance to view body of the deceased friend/family member

29. PERSONALITY DISORDERS (2)

C – Emotionally unstable, borderline type

The emotionally unstable personality disorder (borderline type) is characterized by emotional instability, disturbed views of self-image, feelings of emptiness and intense but easily broken, relationships. Self-harm is a common feature, often in an attempt to avoid abandonment. The emotionally unstable (impulsive type) personality disorder is similar, but a lack of self-control and violent outbursts are more prominent features. Histrionic individuals crave attention, are preoccupied with appearance and are inappropriately flirtatious. They may display theatrical expressions of emotions, from excessive excitement to unexpected, manipulative tantrums.

30. ELECTROCONVULSIVE THERAPY (2)

E – Treatment-resistant dementia

Electroconvulsive therapy (ECT) may be considered as a treatment option for depression when there are severe biological features, marked psychomotor retardation or when the patient is at high risk of harm to themselves or others. Other indications for ECT include catatonia, prolonged or severe mania and neuroleptic malignant syndrome.

31. CAUSES OF WEIGHT LOSS (2)

E – Malignancy

Malignancy is a common cause of weight loss and should always be considered, particularly in older people who complain of tiredness and a reduced appetite. A full examination and systems review should be carried out to determine a possible site of malignancy.

Thyroid dysfunction is associated with weight change. Hyperthyroidism can lead to weight loss despite a good appetite, and hypothyroidism can cause weight gain without increased intake.

32. PSYCHIATRIC DISORDERS RELATING TO WOMEN'S HEALTH (1)

A – Maternity blues

Maternity blues affects two-thirds of women postpartum. It begins 3 to 5 days after birth and lasts no longer than 10 days. It is characterized by low mood and tearfulness and the patient usually recovers spontaneously. Management is by reassurance. Postnatal depression starts within 3 months of giving birth and usually lasts less than 6 months. It affects 10% of women. Features are similar to those of depressive episodes, but some symptoms of depression (insomnia, tiredness and low libido) are normal postpartum. There may be obsessional thoughts, particularly intrusive thoughts about harming the baby. There may be an excessive concern about the baby's health and the mother's own adequacy as a parent. Treatment may be solely supportive or may include antidepressants.

The puerperium is defined as the first 6 weeks after childbirth. This is a high-risk period for developing psychiatric illness. Puerperal psychosis affects one pregnancy in 500 and has a rapid onset during the first 3 weeks after birth. There may be a prodrome of insomnia and irritability, followed by acute confusion and psychosis. It should be treated as a medical emergency in a specialist centre because there is a suicide risk of 5% and an infanticide risk of 4%. Seventy percent of cases recover fully. The aims of treatment are to keep the mother and child together in a safe environment; electroconvulsive therapy is sometimes required.

Pseudocyesis describes the presence of the signs and symptoms of pregnancy in a non-pregnant woman (e.g. amenorrhoea, breast enlargement and significant abdominal distension).

Pseudocyesis, from Greek *pseudes* = false + *kyesis* = pregnancy.
Puerperium, from Latin *puer* = child + *parere* = to give birth.

33. DIAGNOSIS OF DEMENTIA (2)

D – Pseudodementia

Pseudodementia is recognized in people with severe depression. Their apparent cognitive dysfunction is heavily affected by their lack of motivation. The mood disturbance precedes the cognitive impairment, and patients may not try to answer during formal assessments, often providing 'don't know' responses to questions asked. They are more likely to complain of memory loss, whereas someone with true dementia is more likely to confabulate and try to hide it. Depressive pseudodementia is a diagnosis of exclusion in someone with depression, and management aims to treat the underlying mood disorder.

Creutzfeldt–Jakob disease (CJD) is a rapidly progressive dementia caused by prions (an infectious agent composed only of protein). The prion proteins can be transmitted by neurosurgical instruments and human-derived pituitary hormones. Features of CJD include rapid cognitive impairment, which may be preceded by anxiety and depression. Eventually, physical features become prominent, including muscle disturbance (rigidity, tremor, wasting, spasticity, fasciculations, cyclonic jerks, choreoathetoid movements). Convulsions may also occur. The EEG is characteristic (showing stereotyped sharp wave complexes). Death occurs within 6 to 8 months.

HIV-related dementia (also known as AIDS dementia complex) occurs years after initial infection. It presents with reduced cognitive function, low energy and libido, general apathy and eventually muscle spasticity with hyperreflexia, incontinence and ataxia. It is caused by the virus itself rather than an opportunistic infection. Diagnosis is based on clinical probability.

Hans Gerhard Creutzfeldt, German neuropathologist (1885–1964).
Alfons Maria Jakob, German neurologist (1884–1931).

34. PSYCHIATRIC SIGNS OF PHYSICAL ILLNESS

A – Cushing syndrome

The features of Cushing syndrome are caused by raised levels of glucocorticoids from any source. Causes include steroid use (as in this case), ectopic ACTH secretion and a pituitary tumour (Cushing disease). In addition to the physical features (weight gain, hirsutism, striae, acne, plethora, bruising, thin skin, cataracts), psychological features include depression, insomnia, reduced libido and occasionally psychosis.

35. NEUROTIC DISORDERS (2)

B – Generalized anxiety disorder

Generalized anxiety disorder is defined as generalized, excessive worry for more than 6 months. It is twice as common in females and occurs frequently in early adulthood. Sufferers of generalized anxiety disorder feel anxious or nervous most of the time. There is not one particular trigger, and it can be described as 'free-floating'. There is an underlying worry that 'something bad may happen'. Physical symptoms include trembling, sweating, light-headedness, palpitations, dizziness, abdominal discomfort and muscle tension. Genetic predisposition overlaps with the predisposition to depression. Management options include psychological therapies, selective serotonin reuptake inhibitors, benzodiazepines for rapid anxiolysis and β-blockers for autonomic symptoms. The disease course is usually chronic and fluctuating.

Panic disorder is characterized by sudden-onset, severe panic attacks that are not limited to one particular situation. Panic attacks last a few minutes and are often accompanied by a fear of going mad or dying. Physical symptoms include nausea, hyperventilation, palpitations, chest pain, sweating and light-headedness. Affected people are symptom-free in between attacks. Panic disorder is only diagnosed if there is no underlying disorder such as depression. First-line management is with cognitive behavioural therapy. Panic disorder is most common in young female adults.

Acute stress reaction is a transient phenomenon that occurs secondary to exceptional physical or mental stress in people without a pre-existing psychiatric disorder. It can start after a few minutes after the trigger and may last for a few days. The typical features are an initial 'daze' followed by disorientation and the inability to process external stimuli. There may later be amnesia of the event. If the duration exceeds 3 days, an alternative diagnosis should be considered.

36. FEATURES OF SCHIZOPHRENIA (2)

B – Disorganized speech and behaviour and flat affect

Key symptoms of hebephrenic schizophrenia are disorganized speech and behaviour and flat or inappropriate affect. It has an earlier age of onset and a worse prognosis than the paranoid type.

In paranoid schizophrenia, there are predominantly positive symptoms (delusions and hallucinations) with an increased suicide risk. Paranoid schizophrenia has the best prognosis. Simple schizophrenia is a gradual decline in functioning. There are negative symptoms without positive symptoms. Chronic schizophrenia can be diagnosed if negative symptoms persist one year after positive symptoms. In delusional disorder, it is delusions alone that make up the clinical picture, although very occasional and transient hallucinations do not exclude the diagnosis. It usually starts in middle age. Transient psychotic disorder usually reaches a crescendo of symptoms within 2 weeks with complete resolution within 3 months. It may be precipitated by a stressful life event. Catatonic schizophrenia has a prominence of catatonic symptoms. These are stupor, excitement, posturing, negativism, rigidity, waxy flexibility, perseveration of words and mutism.

37. PERSONALITY DISORDERS (3)

A – Anankastic

People with anankastic personality disorder frequently display an inflexible preoccupation with rules, order and attention to detail (almost like an obsessive–compulsive). They may be very cautious and stubborn, and they may try to enforce their ways on others. Anxious (avoidant) personality disorder is characterized by a tendency to worry, extreme anxiety, feelings of inferiority and by a fear of criticism/disapproval to the point of avoiding people/situations where this might happen. *Dependent personality types* are often passive, relying on others to make decisions. They fear abandonment and find it difficult to cope with daily chores. Such personalities may excessively give priority to the needs and wishes of others, over their own, in an attempt to maintain their close relationships.

Anankastic, from Greek *Ananke*, the goddess of necessity.

38. THOUGHT DISORDERS

B – Flight of ideas

Flight of ideas is accelerated thoughts with abrupt incidental changes of subject and no central direction. The connections among topics are based on chance relationships, such as rhyming words or alliteration.

Schneider's three features of normal thought are constancy, organization and consistency. There are five features of Schneider's formal thought disorder. These are:

- Derailment → a thought derails on to a subsidiary thought
- Drivelling → a disordered intermixture of constituent parts of a thought
- Fusion → heterogeneous thoughts are interwoven with each other
- Omission → part of a thought is omitted
- Substitution → a major thought is substituted with a subsidiary thought

A delusion is a false, fixed belief held with absolute conviction, such that it is not changeable, even by compelling counterargument or proof to the contrary. A primary delusion has no obvious cause considering the patient's circumstances. Secondary delusions are more closely linked with the rest of the clinical picture; for example, grandiose delusions (inflated self-worth) are common in mania, and a persecutory delusion may be seen in paranoid schizophrenia. A bizarre delusion is one which would be seen as totally implausible within the patient's culture.

An overvalued idea is an unreasonable, sustained, intense preoccupation that is maintained with less than delusional intensity (i.e. the patient may accept that it might not be true). An obsession is a repetitive senseless thought that is recognized as irrational but that is unsuccessfully resisted by the person. The motor equivalent of an obsessional thought is a *compulsion* – a repetitive, stereotyped, seemingly purposeful behaviour that is not actually useful and that is recognized as such by the patient. Ideas of reference are thoughts that the events or objects in one's immediate environment have a particular or unusual significance. *Monomania* is the pathological preoccupation with a single subject, and *egomania* is the pathological preoccupation with oneself.

39. PSYCHIATRIC DISORDERS RELATING TO WOMEN'S HEALTH (2)

C – Normal behaviour

Although this behaviour may be seen as eccentric, there is nothing in the history that suggests an underlying psychiatric disorder.

40. FEATURES OF DEPRESSION (2)

B – Delusions of poverty

The three core symptoms of depression are low mood, anhedonia (loss of pleasure) and anergia (low energy). The diagnostic criteria require there to be a history of two out of three core symptoms for at least 2 weeks. In addition, there should be at least two of the following seven symptoms:

- Decreased concentration
- Reduced self-esteem
- Guilt
- Pessimism about the future
- Self-harm ideation
- Disturbed sleep
- Reduced appetite

The severity of depression is classified as mild (four symptoms in total), moderate (five to six symptoms in total) and severe (seven symptoms in total, including all three core symptoms).

Beck's cognitive triad describes types of negative thought that occur in depression. They are a negative view of oneself, a negative view of the world and a negative view of the future.

Aaron Beck, American psychiatrist (1921b).

41. PSYCHIATRY OF SEXUALITY (3)

D – Sadism

Sadism and masochism are forms of paraphilia. Sadism involves pleasure from inflicting pain or humiliating someone. Masochism involves gaining sexual excitement from having pain or humiliation inflicted on oneself. Sadomasochism is a term comprising both sadism and masochism.

Sadism, from the French novelist Marquis de Sade, whose writings describe it.
Masochism, from the Austrian writer Leopold von Sacher-Masoch, whose stories describe it.

42. SIDE EFFECTS OF PSYCHIATRIC MEDICATION (2)

E – Serotonin syndrome

This woman has recently started taking opioids (tramadol). The combination of opioids with selective serotonin reuptake inhibitors (fluoxetine in this case) is associated with the development of serotonin syndrome. Signs include severe hypertension, tachycardia, high pyrexia, myoclonus, sweating and hyperreflexia. Management is initially symptomatic followed by removal of the offending drugs. Other drugs that may contribute to the serotonin syndrome include other antidepressants (monoamine oxidase inhibitors), triptans, herbs (St John's wort, ginseng), stimulants (cocaine, amphetamines), lithium and metoclopramide.

43. SLEEP DISORDERS (2)

A – Night terrors
Night terrors are seen in children, affecting 6% of 4- to 12-year olds; they resolve by adolescence. The child usually awakes suddenly during the first third of the night in a state of panic and fearfulness. There are associated autonomic responses (e.g. tachycardia and dilated pupils). Affected children are not easily comforted, but when they fully awake (usually the next morning), they have no recollection of the event.

Nightmares are frightening dreams in which the individual awakes suddenly and is then fully alert and can remember the dream very well. They usually occur during the second half of the night. Nightmares affect up to 50% of adults occasionally, while 3- to 5-year olds are more likely to experience repeated nightmares.

Non-organic disorder of the sleep–wake cycle is caused by a lack of synchrony with the desired sleep–wake pattern. The problem is often perceived as either insomnia or hypersomnia. Management is by attention to sleep hygiene.

44. SPEECH DISORDERS

E – Perseveration
In perseveration, mental operations are continued beyond when they are relevant. It is highly suggestive of organic brain disease. Examples are palilalia, which is repeating a whole word (e.g. 'knife … knife … knife …') and logoclonia, which is repeating the last syllable of a word (e.g. 'pass the Yorkshire pudding …ding …ding …ding'). Word salad or schizophasia is an incomprehensible mishmash of words and phrases. Dysprosody is loss of the normal melody of speech. Logorrhoea describes fluent, rambling speech – an extreme version of verbal diarrhoea! A neologism is a new word, or an old word, used in a new way.

Expressive aphasia is difficulty verbalizing thoughts, although comprehension is intact. It is seen in patients after a stroke. In receptive aphasia, there is difficulty understanding and, although the patient feels they are speaking fluently, it is not usually possible to make out any words they are vocalizing. In global aphasia, expressive and receptive aphasias are present. Dysarthria is the physical difficulty in controlling movements of the mouth in order to articulate the words.

Mutism is the complete loss of speech. Poverty of speech is reduced/restricted speech (e.g. monosyllabic answers). Pressure of speech is increased quality and rate of speech. Stammering is when the flow of speech is broken by pauses and repetition. Echolalia is the imitation of another person (even if it is in a foreign language). Coprolalia is the explosive exclamation of obscenities, seen in Tourette's syndrome.

The following forms of speech give the examiner insight into the form of the patient's thoughts. Knight's move thinking is demonstrated when speech jumps from one subject to another with no link. Flight of ideas is accelerated thoughts with abrupt incidental changes of subject and no central direction.

The connections among topics are based on chance relationships, such as rhyming words or alliteration. Circumstantiality is the incorporation of unnecessary trivial details into speech, but the eventual goal is reached.

Coprolalia, from Greek *kopros* = dung + *lalein* = talk.

45. SUBSTANCE USE (2)

B – Opiate use

This man is likely to be suffering the effects of opiate use. Examples of opiates include morphine, heroin, methadone and codeine. Effects of opiates (in addition to analgesia) include euphoria, nausea and vomiting, constipation, anorexia, hypotension, respiratory depression, tremor, pinpoint pupils and erectile dysfunction. The treatment of overdose (after ABC) is with the antidote naloxone. This is ideally given intravenously but can be given intramuscularly or by inhalation. An infusion of naloxone may be necessary as the half-life is short. The effects of opiate withdrawal can be very extreme. They include dilated pupils, lacrimation, sweating, diarrhoea, insomnia, tachycardia, abdominal cramp-like pains, nausea and vomiting.

46. PSYCHIATRY OF SEXUALITY (4)

D – Transsexualism

Transsexualism, a gender identity disorder, is the persistent desire to live and be accepted as a member of the opposite sex. There is a feeling that the physical body is inconsistent with the sense of self. There may be a desire to have surgery or hormonal treatment in order to change the body. Dual role transvestism is the intermittent desire to dress as the opposite sex that is not for the purpose of arousal or for any permanent change. The male–female ratio is approximately 3:1. Management is usually by specialists; surgery/hormone treatments can be done, although the long-term outcome is uncertain. There is usually a requirement to live as the opposite sex for a year before starting treatment.

Transvestic fetishism describes sexual arousal from cross-dressing.

47. SYNDROMES IN PSYCHIATRY (2)

A – Cotard syndrome

Cotard syndrome is a nihilistic delusion that one is dead, has lost all one's possessions, does not exist or is decaying and so forth. It can be a feature of severe depression. Ekbom syndrome is a delusional psychosis that one is infected with parasites. It may be accompanied by a physical sensation of parasites crawling around or burrowing into the skin (formication).

Rett syndrome is a neurodevelopmental disorder, similar to autism, where developmental decline occurs after 1 to 2 years of age, following a normal initial development. Typical behaviours include screaming attacks, avoidance of eye contact, poor social interactions, loss of fine motor skills, development of stereotyped hand movements (especially hand-wringing) and ataxia. It almost exclusively occurs in females.

Ganser syndrome is a factitious disorder where people give approximate answers to simple questions that show they understand the underlying theme of the questions asked. Individuals mimic what they believe to be psychotic behaviour (e.g. when asked how many legs a donkey has, they will answer '12' as opposed to 'chicken wing'). (Although '12' is also incorrect, it is a number and – in that respect – a reasonable answer to a 'how many' question.) Ganser syndrome was first described in prison inmates awaiting trial.

Othello syndrome (delusional jealousy) is a feeling of delusional intensity that one's partner is being unfaithful. It is named after Shakespeare's character, Othello, who murdered his wife based on false beliefs of her disloyalty.

Formication, from Latin *formica* = ant.
Jules Cotard, French neurologist (1840–1889).
Sigbert Ganser, German psychiatrist (1853–1931).

48. SELF-HARM

B – 1%

Suicide is important to consider because it is one of the most extreme negative outcomes in psychiatry. It is important to know the risk factors in order to identify and manage those at risk. Discussing suicidal ideation with a patient does not increase their risk of suicide (as is sometimes feared).

Risk factors for suicide include:

- Male sex
- Age >45 years
- Being divorced, single or widowed
- Unemployed
- Social classes I and V
- Psychiatric illness
- Previous episodes of self-harm
- Chronic physical illness
- Recent adverse life events

Protective factors include having children and being religious. The rate of suicide increases in summer months and decreases during times of war.

The annual incidence of suicide is 1 in 10,000 in the UK. After an act of self-harm, the risk of completed suicide within the next year is 1% (i.e. 100 times more than the risk in the general population). The following features of self-harm are indicators of strong suicidal intent: a more violent/dangerous action, careful planning and preparation, making precautions to avoid being discovered, failing to seek help afterwards and final acts (such as making a suicide note or a will). It should be ascertained whether or not the patient intended to die at the time and, if so, what their reaction is to still being alive. (Do they regret being alive and still wish to die?) There is a high rate of recurrence in people who self-harm.

49. THE MENTAL HEALTH ACT (3)

D – 72 hours

Section 4 allows an emergency admission to hospital when there is not enough time to organize a Section 2 or 3. Its duration is 72 hours, and there is no right of appeal against it. It can be arranged by one doctor and the approved mental health practitioner. This allows time for a Section 2 or 3 to be sought. Section 4 orders are not commonly used.

50. TRANSCULTURAL PSYCHIATRIC DISORDERS (2)

C – Piblokto

Piblokto (or Arctic hysteria) is described in Inuit women living within the Arctic Circle. There is sudden-onset hysteria (screaming, crying, etc.) and bizarre behaviour. This may include removal of clothes, coprophagia (ingestion of faeces) and violence. Attacks last a couple of hours, and there is often amnesia after the event. It is thought that piblokto may be related to vitamin A toxicity, as the native Eskimo diet provides large quantities of it through the ingestion of animal liver and kidneys.

Windigo psychosis is recognized in native North American tribes. Affected people believe that their body is possessed with a spirit that craves human flesh. This results in obsessive thoughts and compulsions regarding violence and cannibalism.

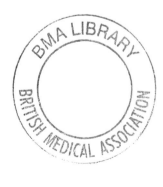